Moving on

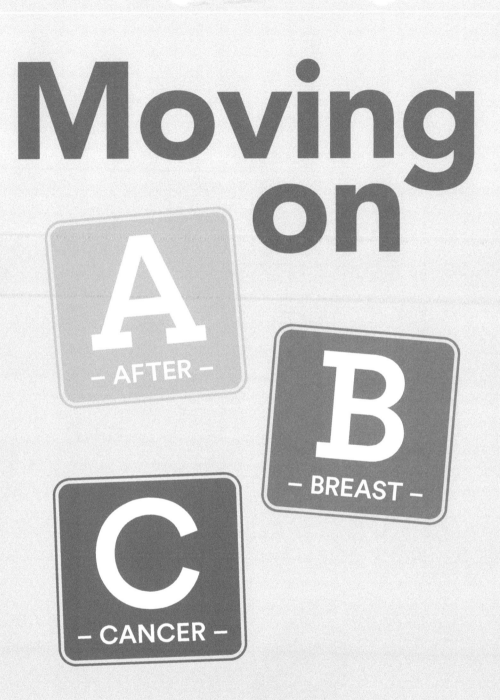

A – AFTER –

B – BREAST –

C – CANCER –

A Complete Approach
Dr Anneela Saleem

MOVING ON AFTER BREAST CANCER

Published in 2016 by
Dr Anneela Saleem
MBChB, Bsc, MRCPCH, DRCOG, MRCGP, FRACGP

A CIP Catalogue of this book is available
from the British Library

ISBN: 978-0-9933707-0-0

Editor Dr Robert Povey

Illustrations by Craig Armstrong

Cover design by Daniel Reed @_DanielReed

Designed and typeset by
www.chandlerbookdesign.co.uk

Printed in Great Britain by
Ingram Sparks

DEDICATION

This book is dedicated to my wonderful
beautiful mother.

She is always by
my side and in my heart.

WITH THANKS

Dr Robert Povey

Craig Armstrong

Daniel Reed

John Chandler

I would also like to recognise the support that I have
received and will be making a donation of proceeds from
this book to a number of breast cancer charities.

Contents

Acknowledgements

It has been a rather thought provoking and consuming process writing this book whilst recovering from treatment. There have been times when I have put it aside but certainly not given up. I wish to thank my family and friends for supporting me along the way; they have all helped me to remain optimistic and enthusiastic. As you will read in My Story I am very close to my family and they have always been there for me. I want to thank my mum for her never ending love and encouragement throughout my life and her strength even when I knew how difficult it must have been for her too. My mum along with my sisters Samia and Naurine looked after my young boys when I was suffering the side effects of chemotherapy and was at my worst. It meant so much to me knowing that my boys were so well cared for; this undoubtedly helped them to come through that period of time unscathed.

My Dad and three brothers, Shahzad, Razwan and Mohsan all gave me a strong shoulder to lean on and plenty of much needed hugs. I gave Shahzad the task of breaking the news that I had breast cancer to my mum, I just couldn't have done it by myself. She had already spoken on a number of occasions about how upsetting it was to see my cousin when she was going through chemotherapy, seeing her with no hair, no eyebrows, unrecognisable. I could only imagine what was going through my mum's mind when he told her. Naturally she was very upset but she soon rallied the family around and reassured me that I didn't have to worry about anything.

It also helped that my mum knew I had met a good man in my husband to be David. We had only been together a few months when I was diagnosed; he was there with me when I was given the news but he has also stood firmly by me and never wavered. Most importantly he also made me laugh through so many upsetting occasions, even on the day that my hair started falling out! It's true what they say; laughter really is the best medicine. David has also been immensely supportive of me writing this book and has read through endless draughts with lots of useful suggestions and has been on hand for plenty of constructive criticism. He has also been the voice of reason and helped me to get support when I needed it and reminded me on many occasions that I needed to slow down.

As well as the support of my family I have also depended on my close friends. Thanks Lisa for getting me into juicing and starting me on the right track. Thanks to Lisa, Michelle and Rina for always being there to support me and make me laugh through the good and bad times. You are all amazing and incredible women.

I also reaped the benefits of the care from Beechwood Cancer Care Centre; they really helped me get through the toughest times. Somewhere I could go to relax and be myself with mutual support and encouragement from other cancer sufferers. They helped me to start embracing the holistic way to my recovery. Anyone reading this should really consider the support of such places. I have also recently been involved in a fundraising charity event for the new Maggie's Centre opposite Christies in Manchester. There are Maggie's Centres across the country and they are there to help people through a cancer diagnosis. I have a new Maggie's family and we are already planning a reunion!

I would also very much like to thank my editor Robert Povey. He very kindly agreed to help me and has been pivotal in shaping the book and steering me in the right direction. Robert has written a number of books himself and so has helped me with the whole process of how to actually go about planning and structuring what to say. He has been extremely patient and encouraging and I am so grateful for all the time and effort he has put into it.

Along the way I have also become more involved in the Asian Breast Cancer Support Group at the Nightingale Centre, UHSM. It has been a real privilege and pleasure to work alongside the founder of the group, Professor Anil Jain. I admire his passion and altruism for helping Asian women to speak more openly about breast cancer. I would like to thank him for writing a foreword for this book and his very kind words.

I have self published this book so have sourced my own design team, Daniel Reed (cover design), Craig Armstrong (illustrations) and John Chandler (book design). They have all been brilliant and have helped make my vision a reality and bring the book to life. I have always wanted the book to be empowering and to be visually positive and user friendly. This has been successfully achieved with their help and enthusiasm.

Thank you again for all having the faith in me and helping me to achieve my goal.

Anneela xx

Foreword

I am delighted to write the foreword for Anneela's book. Anneela joined the Asian Breast Cancer Support Group which I Chair in 2014 and has really become a key member of the Group. Anneela has helped in various initiatives and helped me immensely in achieving various objectives of the Group.

Since joining the Group Anneela has put an immense amount of work in writing her book with special focus on her own experiences as a breast cancer patient. Leading the Asian Breast Cancer Support Group one of the things which I have noticed is that it requires a huge amount of courage for patients to speak about their own experiences of breast cancer. 'Stigma' is not a word just confined to Asian Women but to women from all sections of our society.

As you will note reading the book that Anneela has set out her powerful personal breast cancer journey in a very engaging style. Her poignant story interweaves through personal trials and tribulations, deep support of her family and friends and overwhelming desire to help other patients who may themselves be affected by breast cancer or have family members going through a cancer journey.

Anneela has laced her book with what worked for her and what might work for you. It will widen your knowledge of breast cancer and steps you can take to prevent it or cope with it if it affects you using very simple measures right from healthy diet, exercise to mindfulness or yoga!

Reading Moving on ABC I certainly have come to know more about Anneela and her passion to support other Asian women and I am sure you will imbibe her zeal to help other breast cancer patients.

Professor Anil Jain

Introduction

Breast cancer can take an enormous toll on a woman's physical and emotional well being and will, in most cases, be proportional to the extent of her treatment. What happens next, to a large degree, depends on the individual's approach to the after-effects of cancer. We can try and forget it all, put it behind us, or we can embrace what has happened, accept it and move forward in a more focused and considered way. You may think why bother? But for many women, it is in their own best interest to try and improve their diet, lifestyle and environment. Increasingly, there is more and more evidence to suggest that by making such changes, our risk of a breast cancer recurrence may be reduced. Healthy lifestyle choices can also help us to feel better both physically and emotionally right now.

In this book I explore my own experience of breast cancer, and offer practical advice and support by looking at some of the difficulties and decision making processes I have been through myself. I have struggled with a number of side effects of hormonal treatment, and understand the temptation to stop, but instead of giving up on these proven life-saving treatments, I will suggest ways that may help you to cope with some of the potential side effects.

Fatigue after cancer and its treatment affects just about everyone to some degree.

I anticipated that it would probably take a few months after completing my treatment to make a full recovery. To my dismay even six months later I was not back to full health and I still tired easily. I learned, after much trial and error, that this 'Cancer Related Fatigue' has many similarities to Chronic Fatigue Syndrome and can be managed in a similar way by planning, prioritising and pacing your jobs and activities.

As well as fatigue, symptoms of low mood and anxiety are commonplace in breast cancer survivors. These problems can have secondary effects such as a lack of concentration, poor motivation and sleep problems. A way of managing these difficulties is to learn relaxation techniques and better coping strategies. A helpful technique is a modern-day version of meditation called 'Mindfulness'. I have found that it has helped me enormously to cope with worry and stress and also to keep me more balanced; I will introduce you to some of these techniques. However if you are suffering more severe symptoms that affect your everyday health then it is important to know what to look out for and seek help from your family doctor.

We can also gain many health benefits by avoiding certain foods, not smoking, not consuming too much alcohol and reducing our exposure to environmental toxins. But this book certainly isn't all about what not to do. It is also about the things we can introduce into our diet and about making other positive changes to our lifestyle that arm us with further anti-cancer and immunity boosting properties.

Eating food with optimal nutritional benefits helps to boost our energy levels as well as helping us to maintain a healthy weight. Improving your diet can also help to fight cancer and can be achieved by consuming a diet rich in vitamins, minerals and antioxidants. This can be done whilst still allowing you to eat a variety of tasty and nutritious 'fast' meals. I have always eaten a reasonably healthy diet but now I eat a lot more fresh fruit, vegetables, nuts, seeds, and healthy fats. I also try and cook homemade food most of the time.

'Chemoprevention' is a term used mainly when talking about medications that are used to reduce cancer risk. However it can also be used with regards to our diet and environment. In the future, with a combination of research into prevention and cures, both medical and holistic, it is possible breast cancer survival rates will improve even further. In the meantime, we can try to take better care of ourselves by making some lifestyle changes that can also help us take back some control over our mind, body and soul.

Thanks to ongoing research and a number of treatment breakthroughs in the last 30 years, breast cancer survival rates have improved greatly. However I am sure that there is even more we can do to help ourselves. I have learned a lot by evaluating the current evidence from research studies and from my own experiences. I hope that by sharing this with you I will be able to help you too.

Look after yourself. xx

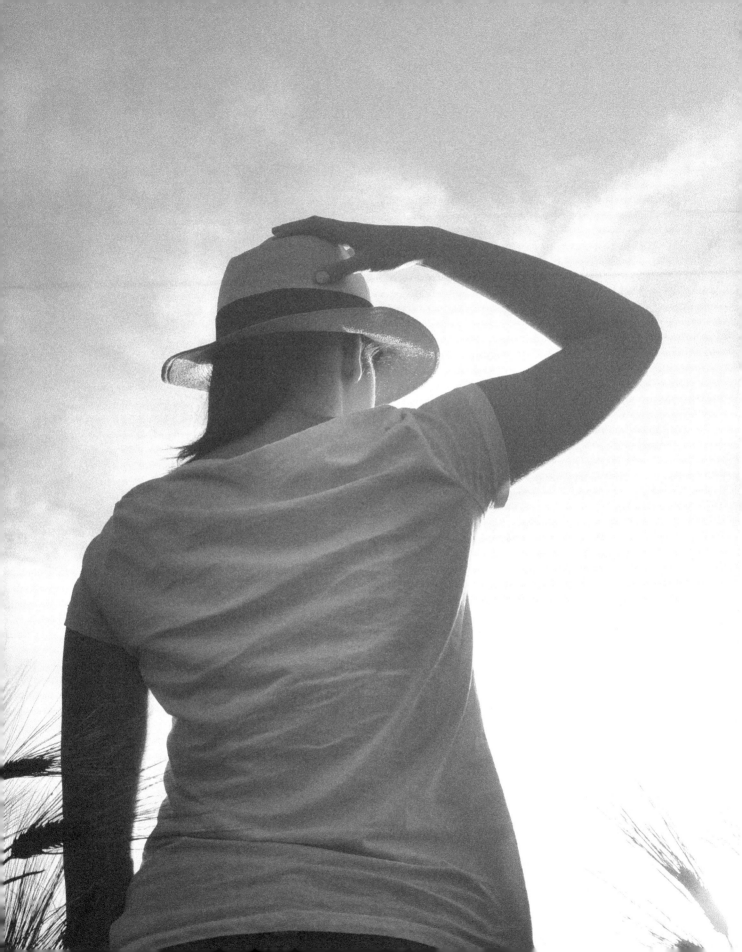

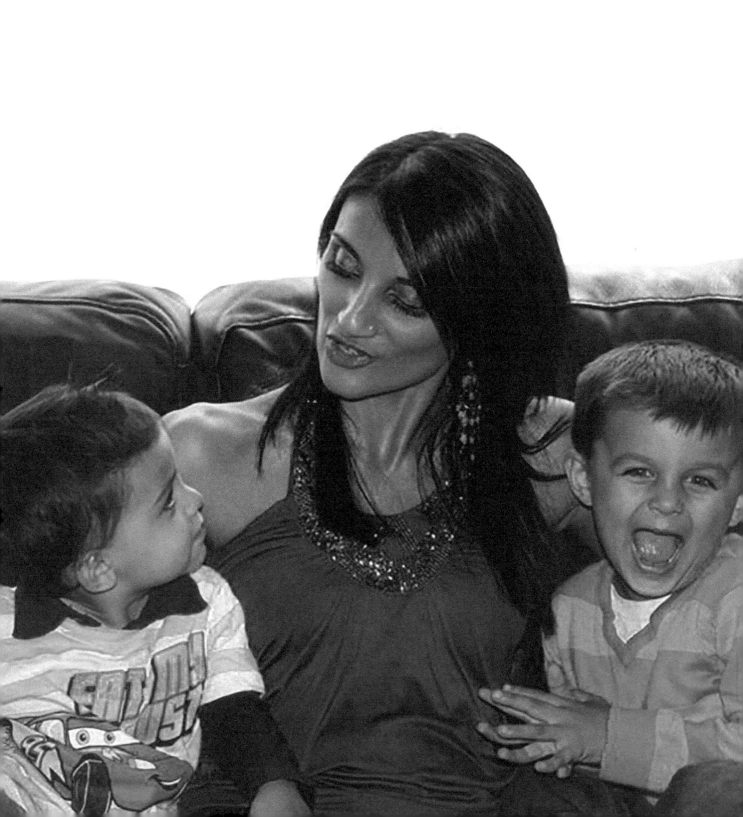

My Story

I was born and raised in Manchester to parents who were first generation immigrants and born in Pakistan. My father came to the UK, leaving his family behind, when he was in his early 20s. My mother arrived with her family when she was thirteen, the daughter of a successful, wealthy Lahore businessman who had travelled widely and decided to experience the opportunities the UK had to offer. Moving to a new country and starting a completely different school life was a rather daunting prospect, and my mother was reluctant to leave behind the family, home and school she loved, to relocate to Manchester. Initially she spoke little English but soon became fluent and fortunately seems to have only fond memories of the transition and subsequent school years.

My mother gave birth to her first child, my older brother, at the age of eighteen. A year later I was born and became the second of six siblings. I have often wondered how my mother coped and have a lot of admiration for the way she bought us up and managed when all of us were very young. When my elder brother was seven and I was six, my mum also had my twin sisters aged one and our new-born baby brother.

My mother was one of thirteen siblings and always taught us to put family first and to work hard. This ethos has contributed to the close bond our family members still have. I did my best to do my bit and learnt at a young age to take responsibility. We didn't have a washing machine or microwave or any of the modern kitchen gadgets that make our lives so much easier these days. I used to go each week with my mother to the laundrette with a pram-full of laundry all bundled up. I also helped at home with cooking and mealtimes and so learnt to cook and appreciate food at a young age. As the eldest daughter I also took a leading role in helping to look after my four younger siblings.

My mother had a challenging life bringing us all up after she herself had just settled in a new country, but she was a very strong and determined woman and just got on with it. She had great pride in us all and always told us that with hard work and study we could achieve whatever we dreamt of. From a young age I grew up with the idea firmly planted in my mind of becoming a 'Lady Doctor'. I was never forced into this career goal but was perhaps given a gentle shove in that direction.

I went to state primary and secondary schools and I studied hard. After being faced with a rather dismissive reaction by the school career's officer to my idea of studying Medicine, I was possibly even more determined to succeed. I went on to pass my 'O' levels with the highest grades on record for the High School and so was well on my way to achieving my goal. I then studied Biology, Chemistry and Maths 'A' levels at College and achieved three A grades and was proud to be the first girl from my high school to go on to do Medicine.

I went to medical school in Leeds. It was daunting when the time came to pack my bags but I soon settled into university campus life. It was a tough slog, but it all went well and over the years I fine-tuned the art of studying and my power of recall in order to pass endless exams. I also took an extra year out half way through my medical degree to gain a Bachelor of Science Degree in Genetics.

Studying was one thing but it really felt like being thrown out of the frying pan into the fire when I started work as a junior doctor. Initially I worked in and around Yorkshire, which as a junior doctor involved relocating and changing jobs every six months. Over the first two years I worked in Hull, Dewsbury, Huddersfield and then Sheffield. Back then we were regularly working 80 to 100 hours each week and were often just walking around like zombies. We would be lucky to get a couple of hours sleep during a typical long weekend shift, which could be for as many as 56 hours long. It felt like some kind of torturous mental and physical endurance test, giving in after having come this far was not an option - and doctors before us had survived it, so now it was our turn.

After two years of being a sleep-deprived doctor I decided to have some well-earned time out and so I took a year out to work and travel abroad. I set off with my backpack, traveller's cheques and around the world ticket. Although very excited I had some reservations since the only way of keeping in touch with my family back then was by post or costly long distance phone calls from special travel booths. I planned to spend a few months working overseas and then to backpack around Australia and New Zealand, with a few weeks in Africa at the end. After just a couple of days to recover from the jet lag I started a three month stint in the Accident and Emergency department at The Royal Perth Hospital. It was an extremely busy hospital as it was also the major trauma centre for Western Australia - a well-run ship where I learned a lot, and enjoyed the work.

After seeing some of the West Coast of Australia I spent about six month's travelling around Australia and New

Zealand and learned to appreciate how few possessions you actually need to get by. It was an inspiring and unforgettable time. I had many wonderful excursions to the islands off the East Coast of Australia including the Whitsundays and Fraser Island. By the time I had made my way up to Northern most tip of the East Coast of Australia my funds had started to run very low, and I had to find more work.

Fortunately, even on a tight timescale I managed to get my medical registration paperwork organised for New Zealand , this meant that when I started this next leg of my travels that I would be able to find work as a doctor. First of all, I met up with a couple of friends from university that were working in New Zealand. We spent six weeks on a road trip taking in the sites around the North and South Island of New Zealand. After seeing the country I then started a six week post as a Locum GP in a small seaside town in the North Island called Mount Manganuii.

It certainly wasn't a hardship to work in such idyllic surroundings on the Bay of Plenty. Whilst I was working I had to consider my plan for my Africa leg of the trip. There was no internet at that time so I couldn't just have a look online and trawl through the reviews. Luckily one day a patient came in to see me, we got talking and he told me that he had just come back from Africa. He highly recommended the group tour he had been on. So I looked into it and the dates for an upcoming tour, my flights and budget all just slotted right into place.

I concluded my travels by going on a six week bush camping trip across Zimbabwe, Botswana and Namibia. I experienced many breath-taking sights such as: the force of the Victorian Falls, wild animals up close on Safari, flying in a rather rickety six-seater Cessna plane into the Okavango Delta, and sand boarding down the vast sand dunes of the Kalahari Desert. I also learnt a lot about myself and other people. I connected with people from all walks of life and in particular learnt not to judge a book by its cover.

Back in the UK, I spent a little time at home in Manchester before taking up a post in the Neonatal Intensive Care Unit in the seaside town of Brighton. For the next seven years I worked and lived in the South of England and London, deciding to specialise in Paediatrics. I worked at St Thomas's and Guys NHS Hospitals, London and also in Dartford, Kent. I proudly passed both parts of my postgraduate membership exams for the Royal College of Paediatrics and Child Health at my first attempts. I worked as a Paediatrician for seven years in all. However, at that time the Paediatric Training Programme had been oversubscribed so there was a bottleneck for higher level training required to become a Consultant. I therefore changed tact and decided to specialise as a General Practitioner instead. It seemed to be the best way forward and I felt in the long run it was more likely to be conducive to family life when the time came. So after some further hospital training posts and a year working as a GP Registrar I qualified fully as a GP in 2004.

After I had just qualified my partner at that time and I decided to have a year working in Australia. I was lucky to land a job in a place called Maleny in Queensland. Maleny is a small township in the hinterland about an hour north of Brisbane, just 40km inland from the Sunshine Coast. The beautiful scenery and it being the home to the majestic Glasshouse Mountains makes it a very popular tourist destination. These Mountains have a strong aboriginal history which makes them even more special and awe-inspiring. I was one of just a handful of GPs in this small rural community and I quickly became a well-recognised figure. I made many good friends some of whom were also my patients. Although the initial plan was to just go for a year, one year rolled into another and altogether I was actually there for five years.

The area was famed for having a permaculture village called Crystal Waters, a place dedicated to protecting the environment and the use of sustainable resources. The people who live there work together in a cooperative and grow a lot of their own food, build their own homes, hold regular markets and they even had their own currency. I had friends who lived there and I was very impressed with their way of life. Many people in Maleny and across the Range also kept 'chucks' (chickens). Most countryside properties seemed to come with a readymade chicken run so it seemed churlish not to give it a go. It was fun having three little chickens scrambling around and feeding veggie scraps to them. Having a ready supply of fresh organic free range eggs was definitely worth the effort. Other delights of rural Australia included waking up to a cacophony of brightly coloured king parrots at five am each day and then pulling back the curtains to spy on wallabies lying on the lawn and soaking up the early morning sun.

My time in Australia also allowed me to experience some alternative and complementary therapies for the first time. Two particularly popular therapies used by many of my patients were Bowen therapy and Reiki. Bowen therapy is a complimentary therapy that uses a very gentle hands-on approach for problems such as back pain and sports' injuries and considering how gentle it is, it is surprisingly successful. Reiki is another complimentary therapy where the practitioner uses very light touch or even holding their hands just over the body. A sequence of movements is used from head to toe to rebalance the body's energy flow and the experience is felt like a heat over the area the hands are placed. It should leave you feeling calm, relaxed and energised. Both are very much mind and body therapies. Although I was interested in a lot of these complementary therapies, because I had been trained in Western medicine with a much more scientific approach I struggled to fully embrace them.

To some extent the different way of life did rub off on me and although I had not practised Yoga in the past, I did during both of my pregnancies. Some of my patients had advocated 'hypno-births' and one of them leant me a book that told me how to prepare for this. The idea was to be able to use only your body's natural endorphins to relieve the pain of childbirth. It seemed implausible after witnessing so many stressful deliveries that I had attended as a Paediatrician. I had always imagined I would go straight for the epidural. However, I decided to give it a go and can honestly say I got in the zone! I actually did succeed in having two completely natural births.

Although I enjoyed my work and time in Australia things didn't work out on a personal front and my relationship deteriorated resulting in a permanent separation during my second pregnancy. It was a terribly stressful time for me but I managed to get through it with the support of my family. I returned to the UK in 2009 with my boys aged almost two and just five weeks old. We moved back into my childhood home in Manchester with my parents and two sisters. I had all the support I could ask for but it was still very hard coming to terms with how things had turned out. After pursuing my education and career successfully it seemed my personal life had taken a nose dive. It felt like I was starting at rock bottom. After a turbulent first year I began to feel more resilient and emotionally strong enough to get back to work and start rebuilding my life.

I began work as a locum GP; initially on a short term basis so that I could become more familiar with some of the GP practices in Manchester. The next two years went well and I settled into juggling work life and being a single parent. I decided to continue working as a locum GP since it gave me a lot more flexibility and more time with the children. Things over the next two years went well; the boys settled into nursery and loved being around their extended family. They had lots of cousins to play with and most weekends we would have a family get together with my mum

at the helm. My dad had no choice but to put his feet up and take a back seat as mum fussed over us all. As the most amazing cook ever she loved to spoil us all rotten. It was great to feel so loved and supported and I felt ready to start looking ahead again.

It was three years after returning to the UK that I met my future husband, David. We both worked in a busy out of hours GP centre and this is where we met. After a little hesitation I agreed to go out for dinner with him but, still being rather cautious, I made sure he knew that it was as 'just friends'. However, the pair of us hit it off straight away and it wasn't long before I introduced my boys and my family to David and his two children.

David and I had both been through some tough times before but we both felt we had met our match and soul mate. It was a wonderful time, falling in love and finding someone I felt I could trust. Things were starting to look up; I seemed to have landed on my feet again. A few months after we met, Dave and I took a romantic short break to New York and started planning our first family holiday. Little did we realise that whilst we were taking in the bright lights, sights and sounds of New York that the strength of our relationship was soon going to be tested.

Six months after we started dating I found two small lumps in my breast quite by chance, while I was applying body cream. The lumps didn't feel particularly worrying and I thought that they were probably just due to cyclical hormonal changes. I was previously fit and healthy. I examined my breasts every so often, but I guess like most people I just didn't think it was going to happen to me so it wasn't paramount on my list of things to do. A few weeks later at work I saw two female patients with breast lumps and, following the guidelines, I immediately referred them to the hospital Breast Clinic for an urgent appointment. It suddenly occurred to me then that I was being rather fool-hardy and that I should really see my own doctor so I could be referred for a check-up too. It was now just a fortnight before we were due to go away on our holiday and I had taken on a lot of work just prior to it. It was a struggle, but I managed to squeeze in an appointment with my GP. She appeared quite concerned and I did start to worry a little bit then.

I saw the Breast Surgeon that same week. He found three breast lumps and said they could all be fibroadenomas (a benign lump) but I needed to have an ultrasound scan (USS) and a mammogram to investigate them a bit further. I wasn't too worried as this was fairly standard protocol, and it was what I had expected to happen. The USS images also suggested fibroadenomas but the Radiologist told me that the borders were a bit 'indeterminate' and that I needed to have a biopsy. Surprisingly my mammogram was normal; however this investigation isn't actually the best way to get an image of breast tissue in younger women. Just two days before going on our first family holiday to Menorca I had biopsies taken from two of the lumps. David and I decided we would wait until we got back from the holiday to get the results. Admittedly, it did hang over us while we were away but I had more or less convinced myself that everything would

be OK so I managed to push it to the back of my mind.

When we arrived home two weeks later, we went back to the hospital to get my results. I doubt that anyone forgets the moment they are told that they have cancer. I can still picture the whole scene as if I was a fly on the wall. I think I knew as soon as I saw the consultant's face. Working as a doctor I had unfortunately had to give bad news many times and often in very tragic circumstances. I still remember him saying to me, calmly and deliberately: "I am very sorry but you have a solid tumour." I was totally shocked and couldn't take it in. I immediately thought the worst. Would I die? What about my kids? Everything seemed to be going so well, this wasn't fair. The kids were doing great, I had just met someone after three years on my own and we were getting along brilliantly. I was working hard and saving. It took some time to sink in; that this was actually happening to me, I had breast cancer.

I didn't want to tell my children but I was advised that I must as they would sense something was wrong. The doctors and nurses at the hospital were truly fantastic. I was given a book written for children called, *Mummy's Lump*. A few days later I told my sons that I wasn't well and read the book to them. It outlines the whole process from having tests, hospital stays and treatment and what that meant for mummy and the family. The book was a great tool and it did make it a lot easier for us all to discuss things out in the open. On one page the woman had no hair and was applying her lipstick while her daughter was playing and putting a headscarf on their pet dog. They wondered: "Are you going to have your hair like that? What? Like that?" They seemed to think it was quite cool and were not upset by it; and luckily this is also how my children reacted when it really did happen. They found it hilarious when they saw the picture of the dad washing dishes surrounded by chaos, saying: "Ha ha, that'll be David."

After breaking the news to my family and friends I seemed to be back and forth to the hospital for numerous tests. Before I had time to take on board what was happening I suddenly felt like I was on an emotional rollercoaster and my life was being consumed with endless appointments and plans. I also threw myself into researching the current guidelines and treatment options. As a junior doctor I had worked for a Consultant Breast Surgeon. That was twenty years before and thankfully treatment has now changed a lot, and for the better. Now there are more accurate and precise tests, new surgical procedures, targeted chemotherapy and other medications, and new technologies. Further tests showed that my lymph nodes were not involved but a Magnetic Resonance Imaging (MRI) scan showed I actually had not three but five distinct tumours.

After discussing the pros and cons of different surgical options with my Breast Surgeon and researching a little myself I came to a decision. I chose to have a total mastectomy with an immediate reconstruction using a Latissimus Dorsi Flap Procedure and a breast implant. This surgical technique uses muscle and skin from the back to help reconstruct

the breast. I remember feeling nervous before the operation but at the same time I desperately wanted to get it over and done with and have the cancer removed from my body. The time soon came around for surgery, just three weeks after receiving my initial diagnosis.

I was in some pain when I woke up from the operation and looked down to see that there were four drainage tubes coming from my new right breast; I was spared a closer inspection since it was covered in dressings. I felt very groggy after the five hour operation but I was also so relieved that the cancer had been removed. It was a few days before I had a proper look once some of the dressings and a couple of the drains had been removed. It was strange really, I still had two breasts but the new one was clearly different, it sat up high and had no areola or nipple, just a disc of skin in its place. It also didn't really feel like it was part of me, this was to some extent because it didn't move when I did but also I couldn't really feel it. I could feel pressure on my breast if I pressed down but the skin over my right breast and across my back was completely numb. I also shortly discovered what I can only describe as a 'phantom itch'. I knew I had an itch but couldn't locate where it was and when I did scratch in the suspect spot I couldn't get any relief.

A few days after my mastectomy the pathology confirmed I had right sided multifocal breast cancer with five tumours and a background of Ductal Carcinoma in Situ (non-invasive stage). It seemed surreal that not only did I have cancer but so much of it. I had little time to take this in since there were other things to consider. David and I spent a lot of time reading about breast cancer and the different treatment options. I knew that chemotherapy and radiotherapy were additional treatments used after surgery to make sure all the cancer cells were removed and to reduce the risk of recurrence. These, and hormonal treatments, are called 'adjuvant' treatments. I looked at the pros and cons of chemotherapy. A computer programme called *Adjuvant Online* is one of the tools oncologists may use to assess if you will benefit from adjuvant chemotherapy.

Another option that came up for discussion was a test that was already being widely used in America called the Oncotype Dx test. (It has been available in the UK since September 2013). It would involve sending some of my cancer tissue over to the USA to be tested privately. However, it would provide more detailed information about how my own individual cancer tissue was actually behaving and provide more precise predictions on whether there was any additional benefit from chemotherapy to my long term prognosis. However when I realised that only one tumour would be sent away, I decided against it. Instead, based on calculations on *Adjuvant Online*, and also because of my relatively young age, it was concluded that I would benefit from having adjuvant chemotherapy.

It seemed that there was no time to waste. Just two months after receiving my diagnosis I started six cycles of chemotherapy treatment which consisted of one of the standard combinations of chemotherapy drugs used to treat breast cancer; 'Fluorouracil, Epirubicin and Cyclophosphamide' otherwise known as FEC. I was to have the six cycles of FEC, once every three weeks from October 2012 through to February 2013. Prior to my diagnosis I had felt really healthy and I enjoyed working out and went to the gym at least 2-3 times a week. It was a scary feeling knowing that I was going to receive treatment that was almost certainly going to make me feel unwell. I had made my decision and felt that really I had to just get on with it.

As anticipated I lost all my hair just two weeks after starting my chemotherapy. Like many I thought that it might not happen, that I might get away with it. No such luck, one evening it just started coming away in handfuls. David came home from work late that evening to find me sitting with quite a substantial pile of hair on the arm of the sofa. He picked it up and had a look of surprise and disbelief; he then decided to try it on. After another two days of my hair falling out and getting everywhere David shaved it all off for me. I won't forget that moment.

Yet this wasn't the worse part by far. I would go to my local hospital on a Monday and spend several hours there having my intravenous treatment. The chemotherapy left me feeling nauseated, bloated, with severe headaches, just wanting to curl up in bed in the dark, my body ached and my veins felt sore and tight in the arm that I received the FEC. I had medications prescribed to ease the sickness but the anti-sickness medication also triggered severe incessant migraines. The steroid tablets made me very snappy and irritable. Thankfully, six to seven days after the chemotherapy drugs were given the major side effects started to ease.

People do respond differently and I really struggled with it all the first week. I couldn't even comfort myself with a nice cup of tea as it tasted just horrid. I also found it incredibly difficult to hold a conversation, my brain couldn't process the incoming information and I struggled to try and give a suitable response. It hurt too much to talk. The second and third week of each cycle I was able to get out a little and do more. However, the third week was always marred by the thought of going through it all again. During this stage of treatment it was very hard looking after my two young children then just three and five years old. Luckily my mum and two sisters helped enormously, I was so grateful for this but it was still difficult for us all.

After the fourth chemotherapy cycle I really felt I could start counting down. There were only two to go so the end was in sight. I had the penultimate one on New Year's Eve 2013; I was in bed by 8 p.m. I believe that when you are fighting cancer a survival instinct seems to kick in giving you an inner strength and resilience to get through it. My mind was rather foggy during the treatment, which was a blessing really as it probably helped me not to over analyse it all. This mind fog, lack of concentration and forgetfulness is often referred to as, 'chemo-brain' or 'chemo-fog'; think 'pregnancy brain' X100. Towards the end I spent a lot of my time just watching daytime TV. I had my whole day mapped out from one show to the next. I certainly

couldn't read a book or do puzzles. The words and figures just stared right back at me. I did small chores around the house, went for short walks when I felt I could and tried to use my exercise bike gently at least 2-3 times a week but often I felt too tired. Thank goodness for *Breaking Bad*, one of the best TV series ever. It is not for the faint hearted but totally gripping. David and I watched the whole five series over the few months that I had my chemotherapy so I always associate the programme with that time.

As a side effect of chemotherapy I also became very anaemic and needed a blood transfusion between my fifth and final cycle. That gave me a welcome boost because at that point my energy levels were so low that I was struggling to get out of bed to even make a cup of tea. The chemotherapy had also had made more of a negative impact on my appearance by this point: my tongue was sore and looked like a geography map; I had been 'chemo-tanned' and my hands and feet had become particularly dark; I had no hair on my head, very patchy eyebrows and I had also lost my pride and joy - my long lashes. Due to all the inactivity I had also gained weight, and my muscles ached and felt weak like jelly. Yet I never for a moment begrudged having the chemotherapy as I wanted the best possible chance of reducing my risk of a future cancer recurrence, especially having two young children. Time passed in a daze but I was getting there, the finish line was almost tangible.

As well as the care I received from my wonderful family I also got through this difficult time with the amazing support of Beechwood Cancer Care Centre. I attended an eight week programme which involved meeting up with the same small group of men and women on a given day each week. When I went there I felt well looked after and I could just be myself, so that even on my worst weeks I would still look forward to going so much that I would literally drag myself out of bed. A lot of the support came from talking to other people who were also dealing with cancer. The mornings involved receiving a course of relaxation treatment; we could choose from one of the following options, Reiki, Reflexology or Massage. This was followed by a one to one counselling session. After this we were served a three course lunch. Then in the afternoon we would get comfortable again in the large lounge area on one of the comfy sofas. We would then be able to completely unwind as a member of staff would take us on a journey somewhere relaxing using a guided visualisation. We would imagine the place while listening to their soothing voice which helped us to imagine all the finer details. This was a new concept to a lot us but over time it became easier to focus the mind and immerse ourselves in it. We learnt to relax and give ourselves the time out that we needed. It opened us up to looking at the holistic way of coming through our treatment and illness.

At last when the chemotherapy was over I had a break from treatment for six whole weeks. It was during this time that I was asked by Beechwood Cancer Care if I would consider taking part in a fashion show for their Ladies Lunch Charity Event. I said yes but admit as it got closer to the date I wasn't so sure if I had perhaps been a bit hasty. After a few weeks reprieve the radiotherapy began and this next stage of treatment involved attending Christies Cancer Hospital every weekday for three weeks. The radiotherapy seemed a breeze compared to the chemotherapy but it was still exhausting travelling to and fro to the hospital each day and sitting around waiting for the next blast of radiotherapy.

From my initial diagnosis it was now a lengthy eight months later before I completed all of my initial stages of treatment. I won't forget the last day of my radiotherapy for more reasons than one as it was also the day I took part in the Beechwood fundraising fashion show and lunch. I had booked the radiotherapy session for 8 a.m. and after it was done I had to dash over to the venue to have my makeup done and practice the catwalk routine with some hunky firemen. It was all very exciting, yet reflective, and some thought provoking speeches were made by relatives of people who had cancer or who had sadly passed away. It did bring it home to me and it could have been an upsetting day but it was actually inspiring and a comfort to see the way people handled themselves and the courage they showed. They had the courage to speak up even though emotions were still clearly very raw but they wanted to share their stories so that others could benefit from the support of Beechwood the way they had. It was such a lovely day, with a lot of warmth and sincerity and it was also a tremendous psychological boost for me.

For months I had been imagining how relieved I would be when the treatment ended. I was on the biggest countdown ever and I was soon going to be free of the drudgery of it all. I was sure I would feel on top of the world when I finally got through it all. The day came and I almost couldn't believe it, such a huge weight had been lifted. I could start to plan ahead and get back to how things were. However, what I hadn't anticipated was how short lived the initial elation would be. Sadly, it didn't take me long to realise that I was utterly exhausted and had little control over how I felt.

Whilst having the treatment there had been a structure, a clear regime to follow, after a while I at least felt I knew what to expect. I could clearly see that I needed to be a lot stronger physically and emotionally before I could go back to work and help other people with their own problems, so I allowed myself six months as a goal to get back to work.

Unfortunately my recovery was also significantly hampered by additional stressful family events that I became preoccupied with. Often I would do too much and can now see that I was actually trying to distract myself from having to think about things. This meant I would often crawl into bed at night exhausted and aching all over. Six months on as planned, but still tired and in turmoil, I returned to work in the Out of Hours

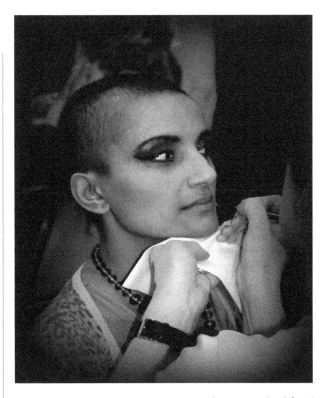

Having my make-up applied for the Beechwood charity event, in March 2013.

GP centre. Everyone was very supportive and I was pleased to return, it seemed on the face of it that my life was finally back on track. What I couldn't foresee was that my immune system hadn't recovered fully from chemotherapy and I just couldn't handle the constant exposure to all sorts of infections. This was impossible to avoid as a GP. I had one virus after another and it just wasn't helping.

At the same time, I was seen by my Geneticist who confirmed that there was an increased risk of me developing breast cancer in my other breast but my results were equivocal so they couldn't be more precise about the extent of the risk. I discussed my options further with my surgeon and we agreed a prophylactic (preventative) mastectomy would be the

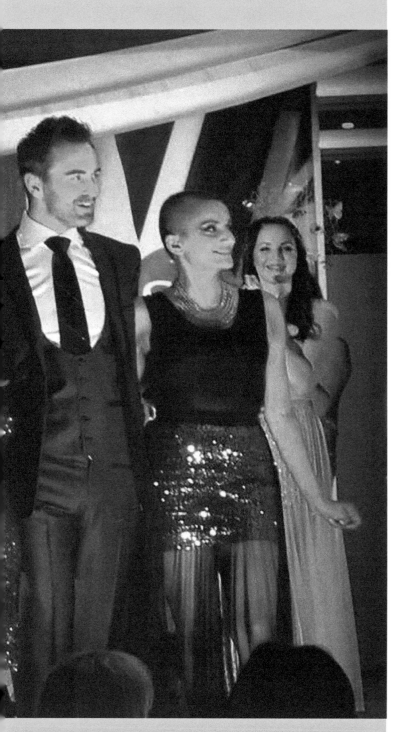

I decided to show off the new hairstyle whilst strutting my stuff on the catwalk.

best way to reduce the odds. Although I had felt this was going to be the likely outcome it was still daunting to have to now think about further surgery; perhaps it wasn't quite all behind me.

At this point, I was also becoming increasingly stressed and irritable, with poor sleep and fatigue. I saw my GP and just burst into tears. I knew I needed help and realised that I certainly wasn't able to continue to work. I was prescribed antidepressants which, after a few weeks, helped me to feel a lot calmer and less tearful. My sleep also improved, which helped reduce how tired I felt all the time. I also went to see a psychologist as I felt I needed to talk to someone who might help me come to terms with it all. I think she thought it was no wonder I was struggling. It was now just before Xmas 2013; my family difficulties had resolved so I was a lot more settled and felt I could now start thinking about me. The psychologist introduced me to the concept of Mindfulness and advised me on some literature and a workshop that I could attend. To begin with I decided to get the book she had recommended but thought the workshop would be overkill. I started to read the book and it made a lot of sense. It showed me that I needed to invest some time in nourishing myself both physically and mentally.

The following week a very good friend of mine came to see me. She herself had had a very difficult year after the breakdown of her long term relationship. It had been a year since I last saw her and she now looked ten years younger. This time she just looked frankly amazing. She had her mojo back, 'How?' I asked. She told me that she had spent time grieving for her broken relationship and that time had indeed been a great healer. She had finally managed to put this period of her life behind her and what was really important for her now was that she had begun to focus on looking after herself. She had been into juicing for over twenty years but had now taken it on board on a much more committed level. She drank freshly made juices three times a day, had healthy snacks and a nourishing evening meal. This had given her a real energy boost and helped her to correct a lot of bad habits. She was avoiding sugar, processed foods, takeaways, caffeine and alcohol. She was also exercising every day. She was looking after herself and most importantly she had her positive attitude back. I happily slotted in with what she was doing, letting her take charge.

I have always considered myself a healthy eater but as a busy doctor and a mum I would often grab things to eat on the go such as low-fat ready meal or a pre-packed sandwich with a coffee or diet cola. Even going to the gym involved speeding from station to station working hard at it, thinking about what jobs I had to do next and never having time to relax in the Jacuzzi or steam room. That first week my friend came to stay everything we had was fresh or home-made. We had smoothies for breakfast; fresh tasty juices 2-3 times a day packed with raw vegetables and super foods. We snacked on roasted nuts and seeds and in the evening we had hearty salads or warming homemade soups. I also allowed myself to rest when I needed to. Even after one week my eyes and skin looked brighter and I had increased energy

levels. I began to feel more recharged and more positive. I came to realise that I had to pay more attention to my recovery to good health and that I could help the process along.

I had already been searching online for information or books to help me try and understand and cope with how I felt after breast cancer treatment had finished, but nothing really grabbed me or answered my questions. So I started asking the questions that I wanted answers to then decided the best way forward was to look at the original research or evidence. I also decided that I should attend the mindfulness workshop to help me explore how I dealt with stress. This was one of the best decisions I made.

Along the way I had maintained friendships with other women going through the same thing as me and as we talked the overriding feeling was that people often didn't know how we felt and that we felt the pressure, 'to get back to normal'. That somehow the cancer was no longer significant, yet we were not coping due to stress and anxiety, worrying about the future and struggling with fatigue. We weren't particularly handling it well, needing medication, sleeping pills, or falling into bad habits with over-eating, drinking too much and possibly distracting ourselves by actually doing too much. None of these things would help in the long run. The other thing that was apparent was the way we could share our concerns openly with each other and gain support and strength from this. We were all bonded by being breast cancer survivors, I don't think that this defines who we are but it meant we could help each other.

It was January 2014, which was nine months after completing my cancer treatment, that I had what I call my Eureka moment, I had the idea to write this book. Although I had been through a process that had led me to this point the idea seemed to come to me in an instant. As I thought about the structure of the book and what I wanted to say it filled me with positive energy and determination. I wasn't sure at first which direction this would take but started with considering the difficulties I had faced so far and what I had struggled with. What could I have done differently if I had thought more about my recovery and how to help myself? I had many questions along the way and knew it was necessary to go to the original research at times to make up my own mind. This in itself is a challenge and can be very time consuming. The outline for my book soon began to take shape. I wanted to provide factual information and answers to questions such as why is the incidence of breast cancer increasing and what we can do to stay healthy and cancer free. Just as importantly I wanted to help women consider the importance of managing stress and their emotions and seeking support when they needed it.

Facts & Figures

Breast Cancer Diagnosis and Treatment

Most people reading this book will know exactly what it is like to be given a breast cancer diagnosis or are likely to know someone who has been affected. The ominous six-letter word 'Cancer' can evoke all sorts of powerful emotions and fears in any person. It is likely that until you or someone close to you has cancer the word and everything that goes with it are usually kept at arm's length, something that happens to other people. We don't consider how we would cope if it was us. To do so would surely be too negative, morbid and unnecessary? However, we may now, be sitting on the wrong side of the fence and asking, "Why me?" We may start to worry about will happen next and what the future holds. In order to help you understand your treatment and what to expect next I believe it helps to have a little more knowledge about the different types and stages of breast cancer and how this can affect your treatment options.

Origins of the 'C' Word

Breast Cancer has been around for many years but thankfully so much has changed in how it is diagnosed and the treatment options available. Nowadays, diagnosis is often at a much earlier and therefore more treatable stage and treatment options have increased considerably which has led to much better long term survival.

Historically, when the word originated, the situation was very different. Physicians have used the word cancer for many centuries with the Greek physician Hippocrates (460-370BC) (also often called; 'The Father of Medicine') being credited for the origin of the word. He originally referred to cancer using the terms 'carcinos' and 'carcinoma' , both of these words came from the Ancient Greek word for 'crab'. Several centuries later a Roman Physician,

Celsus, translated the word into Latin, the Latin word for crab being cancer. It may not be immediately obvious why they used the word crab, but cancerous growths would often become so large and visible that the word was meant to describe the appearance of large tentacle-like growths that spread out from the body of the tumour resembling crabs legs. Fortunately this is extremely rare nowadays and cancer can even be picked up by screening when there are no signs or symptoms of the disease.

What is Cancer?

Today the name cancer is given to a group of diseases in which the cells in an area of the body have changed so that they become abnormal and develop the ability to undergo rapid and uncontrolled growth. Fortunately our body's immune system usually recognises when this happens and suppresses or switches off the mechanism so it doesn't continue to progress and the abnormal cells are removed. Unfortunately, as we get older our bodies become less effective at doing this, so generally the incidence of cancer increases as we age.

When these protective measures are unsuccessful the small cancer cells not only appear, they also manage to survive and form a tiny cluster of abnormal cells. In some cancers these cells can remain dormant and unnoticed for many years, whereas in other cancers the cells start to grow rapidly. Over a period of time the number of cells increase until a definite mass or tumour appears somewhere in the body. The cancer is named after the area of the body or the type of tissue it originates from.

Although breast cancer had been recognised for many centuries it wasn't until the first few decades of the 20th century that surgical removal began to be increasingly used. In the 1950s the surgical treatment offered for breast cancer was more or less the same for everyone. This was a *radical mastectomy* which involved removing all of the breast tissue, its underlying muscle and all the lymph nodes in the adjacent armpit. Fortunately over the last 30-40 years several other surgical techniques have been developed. Instead of every woman having extensive surgery, many can now be offered a simple mastectomy (only the breast tissue is removed) or breast conserving surgery; this involves removing just the breast cancer and a margin of healthy breast tissue around it. As well as this advance there are now also a number of additional treatments that can be used after surgery. This is called adjuvant treatment and is used to reduce the risk of a recurrence. These include radiotherapy, chemotherapy, hormonal and targeted treatments.

If we look at each of these areas separately - the initial diagnosis, the surgery and the adjuvant (added) therapy you will begin to see how different everyone's journey can be.

The Initial Diagnosis

Due to the importance of early detection a lot of effort and focus is understandably placed on increasing breast awareness and breast screening uptake. In all cancers early detection is the key to improved long term survival. However, for many people there is a delay between noticing a change in their breasts and actually going to see a doctor. This may be due to a number of reasons, perhaps fear or anxiety about what it might be and maybe not wanting to think about that, not wishing to trouble anyone, being too busy or just not realising the significance of any changes noticed. It is important that people are aware that the signs of breast cancer are not only a breast lump but that it may present in other ways such as an altered appearance of your breasts or nipples, or a lump found in the armpit. (Please see chapter 7, on breast self examination). For many other women in the breast screening age the breast cancer is picked up on a screening mammogram.

After being seen in the breast clinic if there is any concern about a lump or abnormal appearance of the breast on examination or on a screening mammogram then some initial investigations will need to be carried out. These usually involve the following: a Fine Needle Aspiration (FNA), Ultrasound Scan (USS) and a Diagnostic Mammogram. If there are any abnormalities on these preliminary tests then a biopsy of breast tissue is taken from the abnormal area. The biopsy tissue can then be looked at in more detail under a microscope in the pathology lab to determine if the cells from the area of concern are cancerous or not. If they are cancerous then further information is also gathered from the biopsied tissue including what type of cancer it is, the grade of the cancer cells and their receptor status.

I think most people find that once they have been given a breast cancer diagnosis everything seems to go at full steam ahead and that those first few weeks involve frequent visits to the hospital. The reason for this is that if cancer is confirmed then further investigations and usually lymph node biopsies are necessary to provide additional information. These tests are performed in order to plan treatment and will assess the site, size and number of breast tumours present and whether there is any distant spread. Further investigations may include some of the following: Computerised Tomography (CT) Scan, Bone Scan, Magnetic Resonance Imaging (MRI) scan and a Positron Emission Tomography (PET) Scan. The full diagnosis of breast cancer will depend on a number of factors as listed on the next page.

1. The **size** and **number** of the individual tumours.

2. The **type** of cancer, the type depends on which structure in the breast the abnormal cells originate. This is usually the milk ducts or milk lobules but can also involve other cells in the breast tissue or nipple.

3. The **grade** of the tumour cells (i.e. the appearance of the cells under a microscope.) This is graded from 1-3; with grade 3 cancer cells being the most altered in their appearance from normal breast cells and therefore more aggressive in the way and speed in which they can spread.

4. **Hormone Receptor Status.** 70% of breast cancers are oestrogen and/or progesterone hormone receptor positive. This means they have receptors in their cells that the corresponding female sex hormone i.e. oestrogen or progesterone can attach to. When the hormone attaches to the receptor a signal is sent to the cancer cell – stimulating the cell to grow and divide leading to a larger mass of cancer cells.

5. **HER2 Status** (Human Epidermal Growth Factor Receptor 2). About 20 to 25% of breast cancers are HER2 positive. HER2 is another receptor; this receptor is found on the outer surface of breast cells. The number of HER2 receptors on breast cells is controlled by the HER2 gene. In normal cells HER2 receptors are present and they help to regulate normal cell growth and division; however abnormalities in the HER2 gene can cause an excess amount of HER2 receptors on the cell surface. Too many HER2 receptors results in abnormal cell growth and uncontrolled division.

6. **Localised spread.** If the cancer spreads, then it will initially spread to the lymph nodes in the axilla (armpit) on the same side. These lymph nodes will need to be surgically removed if this happens.

7. **Distant spread** At a more advanced stage, cancer can spread further afield to other areas of the body; these cancerous deposits are called metastases. Breast cancer metastases tend to occur in bones, the lungs, liver and/or brain. If a breast cancer has spread further afield the same chemotherapy, hormonal and targeted therapies used to treat the primary breast cancer can also be used to treat the metastases. Surgical treatment and radiotherapy can also be used to target metastases in different parts of the body.

Looking at the list above you may be able to relate this to your own diagnosis (or of someone you know). A diagnosis of breast cancer can often be more complex than you initially realise.

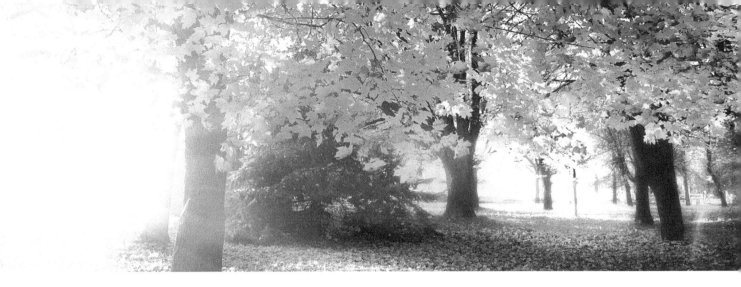

Oncotype Dx Test

This is an additional test that's use is reserved for women with early stage breast cancer; it has only been available in the UK for the last few years and for slightly longer in the USA. The test looks in more depth at the initial biopsy of cancer tissue and helps provide more specific and individual information about the cancer. The Oncotype Dx does this by analysing the activity of a group of genes from the cancer tissue. These genes influence how a cancer is likely to behave and whether the cancer is more likely to grow quickly and/or spread. This knowledge can help to refine treatment in early stage ER + breast cancer by more accurately predicting the risk of breast cancer recurrence into low, intermediate or high risk. If the test identifies you as being in the low risk group then very little or no additional benefit to long term survival will be gained from having chemotherapy and the treatment benefits would not outweigh the risks.

Based on the current evidence for the Oncotype Dx test, in September 2013 NICE approved the test for funding by the NHS. The guidance in the UK is that this test can be used in women who have early stage oestrogen receptor positive (ER+), HER2 negative breast cancer with no involvement of the lymph nodes. The test can identify more accurately the patients in this group that will or won't benefit from chemotherapy. The test is not used in more advanced cases since more extensive treatment such as chemotherapy would be recommended anyway.

In the USA the test is also sometimes used in women with DCIS. Surgery is still required to remove the DCIS but the tissue can then be analysed to work out a low, intermediate or high risk of the DCIS coming back or an invasive cancer developing in that same breast. The dilemma with DCIS still remains that by mammographic appearance alone it is not possible to distinguish DCIS that will develop into an invasive cancer and DCIS that will not. By using the Oncotype Dx test those women found with high risk DCIS will benefit more from further treatment which may include a wider removal of breast tissue or radiotherapy.

Different Types of Breast Cancer

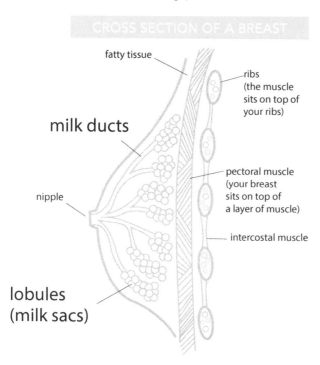

CROSS SECTION OF A BREAST

fatty tissue

ribs
(the muscle
sits on top of
your ribs)

milk ducts

pectoral muscle
(your breast
sits on top of
a layer of muscle)

nipple

intercostal muscle

lobules
(milk sacs)

There are three common types of breast cancer and the abnormal cells in these three types of breast cancers arise either in the milk ducts or the lobules (milk sacs) in breast tissue as seen opposite.

The three most common types of breast cancer are

1 **Ductal Carcinoma In Situ (DCIS)**
Arise in the milk ducts

2 **Invasive Ductal Carcinoma**
Arise in the milk ducts

3 **Invasive Lobular Carcinoma**
Arise in the lobules

The rarer types of breast cancer include Lobular Carcinoma in Situ (LCIS), Mucinous Carcinoma of the Breast, Inflammatory Breast Cancer and Paget's disease of the nipple. These cancers are also usually identified as a lump, a change in appearance of the breast or nipple, or on a screening mammogram. In general most breast cancers are painless; however inflammatory breast cancer results in swelling, redness and tenderness in the area where the cancer is. To simplify things I am just going to give a little more detail about the three most common breast cancers.

Ductal Carcinoma In Situ (DCIS)

Ductal Carcinoma in Situ (DCIS) accounts for about 10% of newly diagnosed cases of breast cancer. In DCIS there are cells inside some of the breast milk ducts (as shown in the diagram opposite) that have become abnormal but have **not** spread into the surrounding breast tissue.

DCIS is sometimes known as a 'pre-cancerous' stage but more correctly should be described as a **non invasive** stage. This is because the DCIS cells have become abnormal in appearance i.e. cancerous, but at this stage these cells **have not** developed the ability to spread outside the breast ducts and in some cases these cells will actually never become invasive. The diagram below shows the difference between normal milk ducts and abnormal cells in DCIS and invasive ductal carcinoma.

DCIS may sometimes be picked up by visible skin or nipple changes overlying the area of DCIS but it is more often detected by a screening mammogram. On a mammogram DCIS looks like an area of small white spots which are caused by tiny deposits of calcium within the area of DCIS , this appearance is called 'microcalcification'. If DCIS is detected a biopsy is taken of the abnormal area to confirm the diagnosis and this helps as the microscopic appearance of the cells can then be examined further to see how aggressive they look.

It is difficult to be certain of the best way to manage DCIS because only about one third will go on to develop the ability to spread outside the breast ducts. At present, however, we cannot say with absolute certainty which cases will become invasive and which cases won't. Therefore the safest action is usually to remove the area of DCIS so that it does not have the opportunity to turn into an invasive cancer. This is particularly important in relatively young women since the likelihood of the abnormal cells becoming invasive over time will be greater.

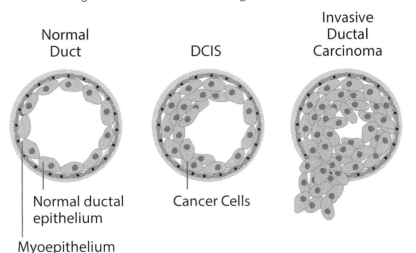

Invasive Ductal Breast Cancer

Invasive ductal breast cancer is the most common type of breast cancer and accounts for 80% of new cases. In invasive ductal breast cancer the cancer cells arise in the breast ducts but have developed the ability to spread outside the ducts into the surrounding breast tissue. This may have been found on screening but it can also be detected by women when they do a 'Breast Self Examination' (BSE) and detect changes in the appearance of their breast or if they find a lump.

Invasive Lobular Breast Cancer

Invasive lobular breast cancer accounts for about 10% of new cases. In this type the cancer cells originate in the cells lining the lobules (as seen on the previous diagram) of the breast and then break through the lobules into the adjacent breast tissue.

Surgical Treatment

Surgery is usually the first step in curative therapy, this is the initial stage of treatment that removes the breast cancer. The following surgical procedures may be required in this process of removing the cancer.

Sentinel Lymph Node Biopsy

This procedure is usually done prior to or during breast surgery. The sentinel nodes are the lymph nodes in the axilla that are closest to breast cancer cells and therefore where the cancer cells may spread to. Involvement of lymph nodes may be suspected if the lymph nodes are enlarged or hard. However, if this is at a very early stage, then it won't always be noticeable on examination or imaging. Before this procedure was discovered and proven to be effective then all of the axillary lymph nodes were removed as a matter of routine. However, an important milestone was reached in the 1990s when sentinel lymph node biopsy was introduced. This procedure involves highlighting the sentinel nodes by injecting a blue dye or a radioactive tracer into the affected breast. These markers then spread through the lymph vessels to the sentinel nodes. This allows the nodes to be found easily by either a blue colour change or by a special machine that picks up the radioactive tracer in them. If these nodes are free of cancer cells then the reliable conclusion is that other more distant nodes will also be clear.

Using this technique the surgeon can identify and surgically remove these sentinel nodes. Usually just 2-4 nodes need to be removed and they can then be examined under a microscope for the presence of

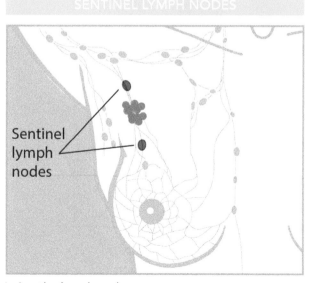

Are the lymph nodes closest to the tumour

any cancer cells. If these nodes are clear then more extensive and unnecessary removal of all the lymph nodes can be avoided.

Axillary Clearance

In total there are about 16-20 lymph nodes in each axilla. Spread to these lymph nodes may be detected by finding an enlarged or firm lymph node on examination, by an ultrasound scan or by sentinel lymph node biopsy. If cancer cells are confirmed to be in these lymph nodes then axillary clearance surgery is performed to remove all or most of the lymph nodes. This is usually done at the same time as or after breast surgery. Since this is a much larger operation than sentinel lymph node biopsy it can be more damaging to the lymphatic system in the axilla and more likely to cause future complications such as lymphoedema.

Local Excision

Local excision is also called a lumpectomy or breast conserving surgery. This technique involves removing just the tumour and a margin of healthy breast tissue around it. Studies show that survival after local excision and radiotherapy for early stage low grade tumours is just as successful as having more extensive surgery so in most suitable cases women will opt for this procedure.

Mastectomy

Complete removal of the breast tissue is called a mastectomy. It may be necessary to remove all of the breast tissue if there is more than one tumour, a large tumour or an aggressive tumour. This can be done with or without a breast reconstruction. Some women will be suitable for an immediate reconstruction which generally involves using a tissue flap from the back or lower abdomen and a breast implant. If radiotherapy is required after the surgery it can damage an implant so an immediate reconstruction would not be ideal in this situation.

> I was diagnosed with a right sided multifocal, grade II, ER +, PR +, HER2 Neg. invasive ductal carcinoma, with no lymph node involvement. I had a mastectomy and immediate reconstruction using my back muscle (latissimus dorsi) to provide a tissue flap. Once the removed breast tissue was fully examined under the microscope it showed that some of the tumours were close to my skin and that there was also a background of DCIS in my breast. The cancer was more extensive than it appeared by imaging alone so I was advised to have radiotherapy as an extra precaution. The radiotherapy did cause my implant to contract and become misshapen but fortunately my breast shape still looks acceptable in clothes so I don't feel the need to try and correct the appearance.

Women may not be suitable for an immediate reconstruction because of uncertainties about the extent of the breast tissue affected and what further treatment they may require. If they are likely to need radiotherapy then it is usually better to wait and have a delayed reconstruction. The other thing to consider is that breast reconstruction is major surgery and usually takes several hours, so some women may not be fit enough to deal with this as well as imminent adjuvant therapy. For them it may be better to remove the cancer in one operation and then consider the reconstruction at a later date. This is called a delayed reconstruction and is usually done a year or so later but can be considered much later too.

Adjuvant Treatment

Adjuvant treatment is the name used for the additional therapy that is used to reduce the risk of recurrence and spread of the breast cancer and includes radiotherapy, chemotherapy, and hormonal therapy. Sometimes the adjuvant therapy can be more demanding than the surgery but this targeted approach has without doubt significantly improved survival rates.

Radiotherapy

Radiotherapy is the use of high energy X-rays to an area of the body to destroy any remaining cancer cells that cannot be seen. It does this by damaging the DNA of cancer cells; it can also affect the DNA of healthy cells, however healthy cells have the ability to repair the damage whereas cancer cells do not. This is why side effects such as tenderness and skin changes often occur in the area treated but this improves over a few days or weeks. Radiotherapy is usually performed several weeks after surgery or chemotherapy (if used) to target the remaining breast tissue and sometimes the chest wall and axillary area on the affected side. This will usually follow a lumpectomy but may not be required after a mastectomy as all the breast tissue has been removed. A course of radiotherapy usually involves daily weekday visits to the hospital over a period of 3-5 weeks. This in itself can be tiring but can also result in fatigue that lasts several weeks or sometimes even longer.

Chemotherapy

Chemotherapy is the use of anticancer drugs to destroy any cancer cells that may have escaped from the breast and are now circulating in the bloodstream or have spread elsewhere in the body. In most cases chemotherapy is used after breast surgery but if a tumour is large it can be used prior to surgery to reduce the size of a tumour. For many this is the treatment that is most feared so any decision to have it is certainly not taken lightly. However the upside is that it has helped hugely to improve long term survival rates.

A course of treatment generally involves attending a chemotherapy suite on an outpatient basis once every three weeks for six to eight cycles and having a combination of drugs given intravenously over several hours. The onset of side effects tends to be after just a few hours and for most people the side effects are worse in the first few days after chemotherapy. This is probably the most difficult part of treatment for most as the drugs make you feel unwell, tired and emotional as well as changing your appearance drastically. It can be hard going back for more, so trying to be as prepared as possible and making sure you have the support you need for the worst days is really important.

Hormonal Therapy

Hormonal therapies are prescribed to men or women with hormone receptor positive breast cancers. They are usually started after surgery; chemotherapy and radiotherapy are all complete and are taken as a once daily tablet for 5 to 10 years. These medications have been pivotal in reducing breast cancer recurrence risk even further. Hormonal therapies include Tamoxifen and Aromatase Inhibitors, such as Letrozole and Anastrozole (as discussed in chapters 8 and 9). Their potential side effects are usually mild but not insignificant and vary from person to person therefore managing side effects is the key to continuing the medication for its full duration.

Herceptin

HER2 positive breast cancers can now be specifically targeted by a drug called Herceptin (brand name for trastuzumab). This is usually given as an intravenous infusion once every three weeks for twelve months. Herceptin works by attaching to and blocking the effects of these HER2 receptors. (This is discussed further in Chapter 9.) Herceptin can sometimes cause severe side effects so careful administration and monitoring of this drug is required especially when it is first commenced.

Improved Survival Rates

Surgery for breast cancer has changed over the years especially with the new techniques that are used for breast reconstruction but the major improvements to long term survival over the past few decades have been due to the use of the adjuvant therapy. Somehow I still have possession of my surgical textbook from my medical school days, 'Essential Surgery' (Burkitt, Quick & Gatt, 1990). So, out of interest I looked up breast cancer and it helps to capture precisely how treatment has progressed. In the 1980s treatment consisted of surgery followed by radiotherapy. Quoting directly from this book, 'the conventional approach is to remove the whole breast (mastectomy) once the diagnosis is confirmed.' It then goes on to say, 'In reality, about 70% of patients presenting with early breast cancer will eventually succumb to the disease.' This meant only 30% long term survival if diagnosed in the 1980s!, which we now know is way off the mark. Thankfully current survival rates are much better and continue to improve.

At that time, concerns were just starting to be raised that some breast cancer cells were not destroyed by localised treatment and they may have already spread locally or elsewhere in the body, but were not yet visible. Trials on chemotherapy in breast cancer were starting in order to try and improve these low survival rates. In the textbook it says, 'Results are so far disappointing but if newer regimes are more effective, this adjuvant treatment may become a routine part of future treatment.' I have now been qualified for over 20 years but reading this was such a stark reminder of how much things have moved on in such a relatively short space of time.

One of the major features signifying progress in the treatment of breast cancer is the ability to specify the type of breast cancer cells and the type of receptors attached to them, and then being able to tailor treatment accordingly. Many women are still managed effectively with just surgery and radiotherapy for early breast cancer. For others, especially those with larger or more aggressive tumours, chemotherapy has greatly improved longer term survival. Targeted hormonal therapy for oestrogen receptor positive tumours and the now routine use of Herceptin for HER2 positive tumours have also had a major impact.

Breast Cancer Survivorship

Everyone who has come through a breast cancer diagnosis and treatment is now a breast cancer survivor. Yet our personal experiences and what effects it has had on us will be quite different. It may have major ongoing implications to our health, both physically and mentally but it can affect us in many other ways too. Along the way we will have learnt a lot from our own situation and no doubt from doing our own bit of research. Each one of us will have some shared experiences but the

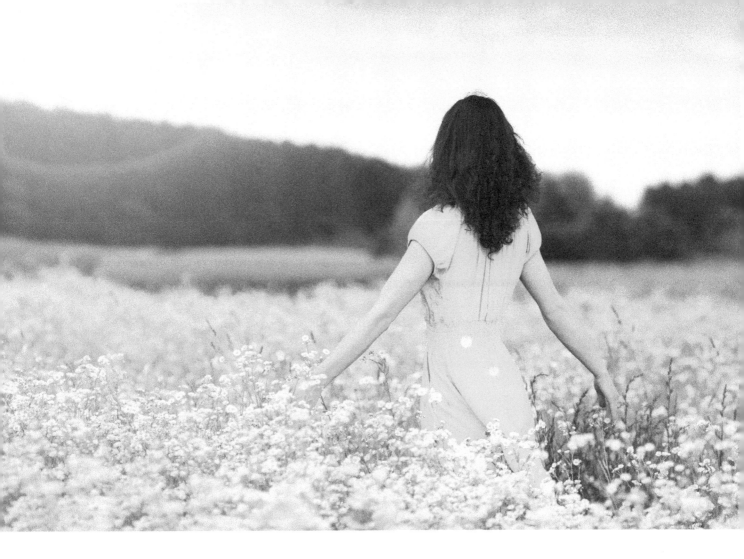

journey we have travelled will be different depending on the type of breast cancer we were diagnosed with and at what stage it was discovered. This will have determined the type of treatment we received and what effects the treatment will have had on us.

The impact of breast cancer treatment also depends on your initial age and fitness levels. Being younger may mean you can bounce back quicker from more gruelling therapy but you may also have to deal with other issues related to having young children, fertility, early menopause and work. On the other hand being older may mean that you have more pre-existing illnesses that make it harder to tolerate some of the more aggressive treatments.

What we can see, is that over the last few decades as treatment has improved the survival rates for breast cancer have also greatly improved. However, we have also seen a large increase in the incidence of breast cancer in developed countries and more women getting breast cancer at a younger age. There may be a number of reasons for this, some of the factors involved are clear to see whereas some are more debatable.

Differences in Breast Cancer Rates

Cancer, alongside other diseases such as heart disease and diabetes, is one of the major health burdens worldwide. Globally, the incidence rates of cancer and these chronic diseases vary greatly. Although breast cancer incidence varies widely around the world, overall it remains the most common cause of female cancer. As you may expect breast cancer rates in the UK, USA and Australasia are much higher than those in less developed parts of the world. One of the reasons is that most breast cancers occur in women over the age of 50 years, so the higher incidence is partly due to a larger elderly population in more affluent countries. However, putting age aside, about 27% of breast cancer cases in the UK each year are said to be linked to lifestyle and other risk factors.

Since age plays such an important role when comparing differences in breast cancer incidence rates across the world, especially between developed and developing countries the incidence rates are usually given as 'Age Standardised Rates' (ASR). To create an ASR the actual incidence figures are adjusted to a population with a standard age structure, this allows direct comparisons to now be made between countries. The ASR reflect what the incidence would be if all countries had the same age distribution. Adjusting for age in this way means that the differences between the countries are not due to one country containing more elderly women than another. If countries in Europe are being compared then European ASR are used and if comparing countries across the world then World ASR are used.

Breast Cancer Rates in the UK

In the UK, USA and Australia breast cancer affects as many as 1 in 8 women in their lifetime; this is based on an estimated life expectancy of 85 years. This means that if all women lived to age 85 years, 1 in 8 would develop breast cancer at some point in their lifetime. It makes up over 30% of all newly diagnosed cancers in women in the UK with lung cancer next at 12% and then bowel cancer at 11%. To put this into perspective these are some recent figures.

In 2013 approximately 53,400 women and 340 men in the UK were newly diagnosed with breast cancer.

Incidence Rates

Cancer incidence and mortality rates are collated from cancer registries. In the UK these are analysed by the Office of National Statistics. The Office of National Statistics (ONS) is an independent government department that is recognised as the national provider of statistics for the UK. The ONS use European age standardised rates so comparisons can be made across Europe. Their latest figures are shown below.

66 new cases per 100,000 women in 1971

125 new cases per 100,000 women in 2011

The original population model for European ASR was created in 1976 and has been updated in 2013 to reflect an aging population across Europe in the last 30-40 years; this makes the new ASR figures higher than previously recorded in 2011. The most recent ASR incidence rates are 163 new cases per 100, 000 women in 2013. (Cancer Research UK, accessed Jan 2016) http://www. cancerresearchuk.org/health-professional/cancer-statistics/statistics-by-cancer-type/breast-cancer/incidence-invasive#heading

Whichever figures we look at it is clear that over the past 40 years, the incidence rates in the UK have increased steadily, and have approximately doubled.

Mortality Rates

The increased incidence of breast cancer has also led to a greater awareness of the disease and this has resulted in more men and women being diagnosed at an earlier stage which then allows for prompt and more successful treatment. Overall better breast cancer awareness and improved treatments have led to fewer deaths. Over the past 40 years in the UK, there has been a 40% reduction in the mortality rates (i.e. the number of deaths from breast cancer).

39 per 100,000 women in 1971
24 per 100,000 women in 2011
(ONS 2013)

Survival Rates

Most people now realise that if breast cancer is detected early there is a very good chance of a full recovery. The survival rates have actually increased by over 50 % in the UK in the last 40 years. This means that now over 85% of women survive more than 5 years after diagnosis and the figure is even higher for those that are diagnosed at an early stage. This compares favourably with a 5 year survival of just 52% in the early 1970s.

Most people facing cancer will look to a five year milestone since a five year cancer-free interval is often seen as a benchmark for longer term survival. For most cancers reaching this milestone is seen as a cure, but it's not quite the same for breast cancer. If it does come back it is most likely to be in the first 2-3 years and usually a recurrence relates to a more advanced stage at the time of the initial diagnosis. The more time that does pass after diagnosis then the less likely it is to come back. However it is important to be breast aware and remain vigilant because it can reoccur after the five year milestone. Overall the odds are much better than for a lot of other cancers and hence we are fortunate to see many more breast cancer survivors. 65% of women now survive for twenty years or more. Some long term survivors you may be aware of are Sheryl Crow (diagnosed 2006), Kylie Minogue (2005), Olivia Newton John (1992) and former USA First Lady Nancy Reagan (1987).

Incidence in Developing Countries

Even after taking age into account we still see a major difference in incidence between countries like the UK, USA and Australia and countries in Africa and Asia. When these countries are compared the statistics are altered to be standardised for the age of a world population. Besides age some of the differences between these countries will no doubt be due to the fact that fewer real cases are actually diagnosed in poorer countries and the quality of recorded data is less reliable. In 2008 the lowest 'World Age-Standardised' incidence rates were a mere 6 per 100,000 women in some parts of East Asia. The rates were also very low at around 20 per 100,000 in Eastern and Middle African women (e.g. Kenya and Tanzania), compared to the much higher world age standardised rates in the UK and USA of around 90 per 100,000 women.

Since breast cancer is hormone related we are able to explain some of these differences. Generally speaking, women in less developed areas of the world have a lower exposure to oestrogen over their lifetime. Pregnancy, breast feeding, later onset of periods and early menopause as well as not using hormonal contraception and/or HRT will all reduce a women's exposure to oestrogen. High oestrogen exposure is a known risk factor for breast cancer.

Having lots of children at a younger age and breast feeding are protective factors. For example in some cultures the use of contraception may be frowned upon or not widely available so that large families will be the norm and partly due to economic reasons these women may also be more likely to breast feed and for longer.

Other major differences are apparent such as lower rates of smoking, drinking alcohol and obesity. So in parts of Eastern Asia the incidence rate is a mere 5% of the UK figure and we could surmise that the type of cancer which affects these women is likely to be largely related to genetic predisposition. Despite the lower incidence in developing countries breast cancer is a huge burden worldwide affecting almost 1.7 million women in 2012. It actually affects about equal numbers of women in developed and developing countries due to the very large population sizes in the latter. In other words although the incidence per 100,000 is much lower in poorer countries there are many more people. The other downfall is that because of poor medical care the number of deaths from breast cancer in poorer countries is higher overall.

Incidence Across Europe (2012 European Age-standardised rates)

We may expect to see major differences across the globe in breast cancer rates but this can also be demonstrated closer to home across Europe. Countries in Europe can also be ranked as to their incidence of breast cancer. The rates in different European countries actually vary quite dramatically and may provide us with further clues. A useful way to learn more about those environmental factors that may be protective or those that increase the risk of breast cancer and other diseases is by collaborating further with other countries.

Highest Rates

Higher rates of breast cancer are seen in Belgium and Denmark at 145 per 100,000 women, whereas the UK incidence is 129 per 100,000. A number of reasons can be hypothesised for these differences and they are likely to be due to a combination of factors. In Belgium and Denmark, for example they have a diet traditionally high in fatty, cured, smoked and processed meats like salami and sausages. These countries also have high rates of smoking and alcohol consumption in women. In addition to this they implemented national breast screening programmes relatively late i.e. after 2000 compared with 1988 in the UK. It is still uncertain whether the later introduction of screening has actually contributed to the higher rates of breast cancer, as areas of Belgium and Denmark that were screened earlier, don't seem to have any lower incidence or improved mortality. Historically these countries may have also had a higher rate of HRT use which may also contribute.

Lowest Rates

At the other end of the spectrum much lower rates of breast cancer are seen across Eastern Europe in countries like Bosnia and Herzegovina, Moldova, Romania and Ukraine. Bosnia and Herzegovina has the lowest incidence in Europe with a mere 49 per 100,000 women affected. Other factors need to be considered here. These countries are amongst the poorest in Europe and may be relatively protected as women have children at an earlier age and they tend to be low users of HRT. They also have low rates of attendance for breast screening which means some of those breast cancers, which never become invasive, are not being detected. However, even though their breast cancer rates are lower, their overall life expectancy is worse.

The four most common cancer types across European countries are breast, lung, bowel and prostate cancers. Eastern Europeans appear to have lower rates of all of these cancers compared with the rest of Europe but are dying from other causes. Instead, they have much higher rates of coronary and inflammatory heart disease, diabetes and strokes. Other European countries like Spain fair much better in both respects with lower rates of the common cancers and lower rates of cardiovascular disease. A lot of this can certainly be attributed to their healthy Mediterranean diet incorporating plenty of fresh fruit and vegetables, fish, olives and olive oil. They are also more likely to cook from scratch with fresh ingredients and not rely on processed foods as much as other countries like the UK.

Migration

A finding of major significance in migration studies is the phenomenon that when people migrate from a developing country to developed countries like the UK and USA they soon take up the cancer incidence rates of their local population. China, Japan and India have about a quarter the incidence of breast cancer compared to the UK, USA and Australia.

In studies that have looked at women who come from Japan it only takes two generations for their risk to increase up to that of the local population. This strongly suggests that the main risk factors are likely to be environmental and lifestyle rather than genetic. Obesity (BMI >30) and being overweight (BMI >25) contribute to an increased risk of some cancers but also other health problems like cardiovascular disease and diabetes which are also much more prevalent in nations with high average BMI figures.

The UK and USA have high adult obesity rates at 25 % and 30% respectively. The numbers that are overweight are also very high at about 60 % and 65% of the population. Japan has the lowest rates of adult obesity in the industrialised world with just 3% of their population affected. This is reflected in their low rates of breast cancer, heart disease and diabetes. Their very low levels of obesity are clearly related to their traditional Japanese diet which essentially contains plenty of fresh vegetables, rice, noodles and fish with low consumption of red meat and processed foods.

Twin Studies

As well as migration studies, studies looking at identical (monozygotic) twins can provide us with further evidence of the importance of lifestyle factors. Identical twins share the same genetic makeup but when they are brought up in different environments, despite showing many similar traits, they sometimes develop different health problems. On the other hand if they have inherited a faulty gene such as BRAC1 gene then they are much more likely to show a similar disease profile linked to that shared gene.

Urbanisation

When a country undergoes urbanisation, unhealthy lifestyles are often adopted such as heavy smoking and a poor diet. In China there has been a dramatic rise in cancer rates over the past ten years; a trend which is seen mainly in the heavily populated cities and not in the rural areas. Increased breast cancer rates can also be explained partly by the aging population and the one child policy (less childbearing years leads to a greater lifetime exposure to oestrogen), but rapid economic growth and subsequent lifestyle changes have played a major role too. Also in China women are likely to have poor breast cancer awareness and there is no national breast screening programme. This leads to other issues such as a delay in diagnosis which inevitably leads to a more advanced stage at the time of diagnosis.

Ethnic Groups

A major issue affecting some ethnic groups in the UK is also the lack of breast cancer awareness. Women in ethnic groups tend not to routinely practise breast self-examinations and there is also a low uptake of screening. In the UK, it is known that South Asian (Indian and Pakistani) women have a lower incidence of breast cancer than Caucasian women but as with other migrating populations the incidence is increasing year by year at a higher rate than the Caucasian population. Also, it was only recently that I was made aware that a much larger proportion of Asian women present with breast cancer at a younger age with a peak age of 45years. A similar scenario exists in the USA with a lower incidence of breast cancer in African-American women compared to the wider population. However, in the USA women getting breast cancer under the age of 45 years are more likely to be African-American and they are also more likely to have a worse prognosis.

For some reason the message is not getting out to these people; awareness needs to be raised in both the health professionals involved and the communities at risk. Professor Anil Jain from the Nightingale Breast Centre, Wythenshawe Hospital, Manchester has created an Asian Breast Cancer Support Group to help tackle some of these issues. From discussions with Professor Jain it is apparent that in some cultures a stigma or taboo is attached to being diagnosed with breast cancer. The reasons for this can be varied and very complex but need to be addressed if we are to help women to recognise signs and symptoms and come forward early.

Lack of education and publicity about breast cancer in ethnic groups and in areas of deprivation may mean some communities may think it is not really a health issue that affects them. Poor awareness and low rates of uptake for screening often leads to a delayed diagnosis with a higher proportion of women not going to see their doctor until there disease is more advanced and this inevitably leads to a far poorer survival rate.

Increased Rates of Breast Cancer Since World War II

In developed countries breast cancer rates have risen steadily since World War II. In many ways the modern world is a much happier, safer and healthier place to live. There is advancing technology, availability of a large variety of good food, more effective medicines and better access to healthcare. Yet in the 1940s the lifetime risk of breast cancer was only about 1 in 22 rather than the 1 in 8 we now see. Even in those families who have a genetic predisposition due to an inherited BRAC I or BRAC II gene, looking back at their family history at the time of WWII only about 40% of women in those generations would have been affected.

REPRODUCTIVE HABITS	LIFESTYLE	FOOD	ENVIRONMENT
Increase in age before having children	Increase in weight	Increase in consumption of refined sugars.	Pesticides. These did not exist commonly until after World War II.
Having fewer children	Increase in alcohol consumption	Increase in consumption of dairy products.	Household toxins from the many cleaning products we now use.
Earlier onset of menarche (periods)	Smoking	Increase in consumption of trans fats found in e.g. solid margarines, biscuits and cakes.	Increase use of personal care products e.g. body creams, bathing products and make up.
Later menopause	Sedentary lifestyle and lack of exercise	Increase in red meat consumption.	
Reduced breast feeding		Increase in use of processed and packaged foods.	
Use of high dose oestrogen pills. Use of HRT		Increased use of artificial sweeteners, preservatives, flavours and colours in food.	

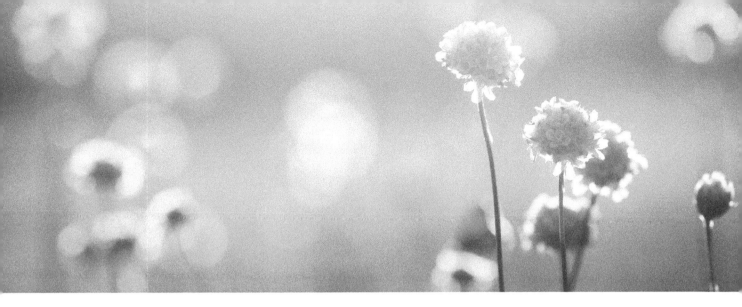

Today if you carry one of these faulty genes it is more likely to be 80%. So it's not all down to your genes. There are many contributing factors even in those that are genetically predisposed.

These factors include women's changing reproductive habits, changes in our environment and the way our diets and lifestyles have changed since World War II as shown in the table opposite.

At a glance you can see that some of these differences could be having an impact on cancer rates. Observing the trends over a period of time doesn't necessarily prove anything but it helps to paint a picture of what may be going on with the incidence figures we are now faced with.

Trends For Other Cancers

Overall, cancer rates in the developed world have increased over the last few decades and have risen from a lifetime risk of 1 in 3 in the 1990s to closer to 1 in 2 more recently. Many of these will be curable cancers so that many more people now survive cancer. In the UK the most common cancer that affects women is breast cancer and in men it is prostate cancer. This is followed by lung and bowel cancer in both men and women. As mentioned previously age is a factor so the rates will generally be higher in the elderly. It is worth looking in more detail at some of these other cancers.

All other cancers 47%

Breast 30%

Lung 12%

Bowel 11%

Female incidence
164,000 cases
UK, 2011

Cancer Research UK 2011 http://www.cancerresearchuk.org/health-professional/cancer-statistics/incidence/common-cancers-compared#heading-Two
ACCESSED JUNE 2015

Lung Cancer

Whereas some cancer rates have steadily increased over the years, thankfully some cancers have actually decreased. Lung cancer used to be the most common cancer overall in the UK up until 1997 but then breast cancer took over. Lung cancer rates are directly related to smoking. In men the incidence of lung cancer has fallen from 108 per 100,000 men to 56 per 100,000 since 1971 (ONS 2011). Greater awareness of the dangers of smoking and public health campaigns to help people quit smoking mean that the rates of lung cancer for men have gone down dramatically over the past two decades. Unfortunately in women the reverse trend is seen as more women have taken up smoking since the 1970s. Smoking is more likely to lead to lung cancer the longer you smoke so we see it diagnosed mainly in elderly men and women that have smoked for many years; almost 9 in 10 occurring in smokers over 60 years old.

Skin Cancer

Skin cancer rates have increased over the past few decades with a change in lifestyle directly related to the greater number of holidays taken abroad and the consequent increase in sun exposure. As well as this, the popularity of looking tanned, leads many to sunbathe and use sun beds too. The sun and sun beds give off Ultraviolet (UV) radiation, which can cause damage to skin cells over time and sometimes a cancerous change. 95% of sunlight is made up of UVA radiation and 5% of UVB radiation, UVB causes skin to burn so is more damaging.

There is a shield of 'Ozone' (O3) gas in the Earth's upper atmosphere that normally absorbs a lot of the harmful UVB radiation emitted from the sun; however over the Southern Hemisphere the protective ozone layer is thin due to damage from environmental pollution, meaning that more UV radiation can penetrate it. (The ozone 'hole' has started to repair and should fully resolve.) This causes the midday sun in Australia to be very intense and potentially more harmful. This and the outdoor lifestyle in Australia have resulted in the age standardised incidence rates for malignant melanoma of the skin almost doubling from about 27 to 49 cases per 100,000 people from 1982 to 2010. Other less aggressive skin cancers such as Squamous Cell and Basal Cell Carcinomas are also very common. Working as a rural GP in Australia I saw many cases of skin cancers and I regularly excised Squamous and Basal Cell skin cancers from patients each week. The dangers of too much sun exposure are now evident, but public health campaigns are starting to get the message across to people. For this reason people in Australia try to avoid sitting out in the sun between 11am and 3pm every day. Generally Australians make the most of the early morning and get up with the birds which can be so loud that you don't really have much choice. Since the sun is too intense later in the day you will find that walkers and joggers are out in force from about 6 am each day.

Hormone Related Cancers

With lung and skin cancers it is quite easy to appreciate the reasons for their incidence rates going down or up respectively. However, with breast cancer it is not as straightforward. Also, the trends seen with breast cancer are seen with other hormonally related cancers such as prostate and testicular cancers. There has been a gradual steady increase in these three cancers over the past 40 years, but a single main causal factor is not responsible. One concern is that these cancers are being stimulated to some extent by a plethora of environmental chemicals that may be disrupting our hormones. This can be highlighted in other ways too, such as the earlier onset of puberty over the last few decades. It is also known that many environmental chemicals inevitably end up in our rivers and waterways and here we can see some further evidence of hormone disruption, with the widespread feminisation of male fish.

'Therapeutic' prescribed hormonal treatments have also been linked to an increased risk of female cancers. A drug called 'diethylstilboestrol' (DES) which is a synthetic oestrogen was used in the 1940s to 1960s in women prone to miscarriage; it stopped being used because it wasn't particularly effective. It was then banned in 1971 because unfortunately what came to light was that there was increased rate of a relatively rare cancer, vaginal cancer, in the daughters that were exposed to it in pregnancy. It has also been associated with an increased risk of infertility and miscarriage in the daughters as well as an increase risk of breast cancer for these women in their 40s. More recently HRT has been thrown into the spotlight with a small increased risk of breast cancer due to its use, this is more so with higher dose combined (oestrogen and progesterone) preparations and in long term use. *(See chapter 10)*

Prostate Cancer

The second most common cancer in the UK after breast cancer is prostate cancer. Prostate cancer carries a 1 in 8 lifetime risk for men. The incidence increases sharply after the age of 54 years with the highest level in men between the ages of 75-79. Overall the incidence has increased greatly since the mid 70s from about 30 per 100,100 to 106 per 100,000 (ONS 2010). In prostate cancer a lot of the increase over the last 40 years is attributed to increased detection.

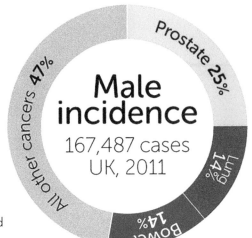

Cancer Research UK http://www.cancerresearchuk.org/health-professional/cancer-statistics/incidence/common-cancers-compared#heading-One

ACCESSED JUNE 2015

A blood test called 'Prostate Specific Antigen' (PSA) can sometimes be a way of detecting prostate cancers early. This test started to be used more widely in the early 1990s and led to an improved diagnosis for many. However, it isn't a particularly sensitive test so it can be negative even if cancer is present and positive when it isn't. Until more effective screening tests are developed, it can still be useful in men who are middle aged or older who have some of the urinary tract symptoms listed below.

Prostate cancer is also often picked up by chance when men are having a 'Transurethral Resection of the Prostate' (TURP) procedure. This is a common procedure used to remove some of the prostate in older men if they have problems due to benign prostate enlargement; these include a poor urine stream and having to get up more often at night to pass urine (overlaps with symptoms below). Some of the cancers diagnosed this way are not aggressive or invasive and may otherwise never have been detected and sometimes never have caused a problem. These accidentally found cancers contribute to the higher rates seen in recent decades. However, the largest group showing an increase has actually been in younger men aged 45-54, with a nine-fold increase in this age group in the last 30 years. This is a huge increase and the reasons for this are not yet known.

Needing to rush to the toilet.

Frequency of passing urine

Nocturia, waking up at night more often to pass urine

Hesitancy , difficulty getting the urine stream going

Straining to pass urine

Weak flow of urine

Dribbling at the end of the stream

Sensation that bladder hasn't fully emptied

Prostate Cancer (C61): 1979-2012

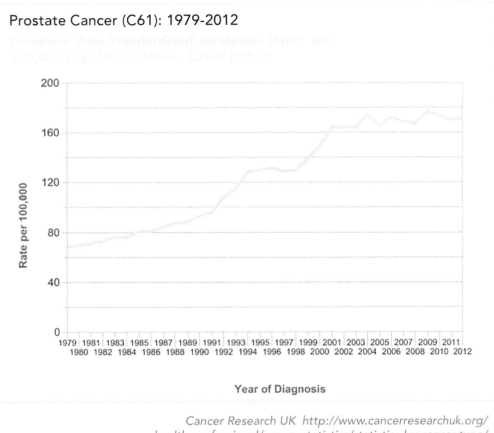

Testicular Cancer

Testicular cancer is another hormone related cancer; it is far less common than prostate cancer with an incidence rate in the UK of only 7 per 100,000 men (2011). Testicular cancer is seen in younger men. Most occur in men aged 15-49 years old and it is actually the most common cancer in men aged 25-49 in the UK. However it shares the same trend as prostate cancer with an increase since the mid-70s when it was only around 3 in every 100,000 men. This time it cannot be attributed to new tests or procedures that are detecting the problem where it may otherwise not have been picked up. Increased awareness of testicular cancer brings about earlier detection but doesn't explain this rise in incidence. It is more likely to be due to environmental and lifestyle changes over the past 40 years.

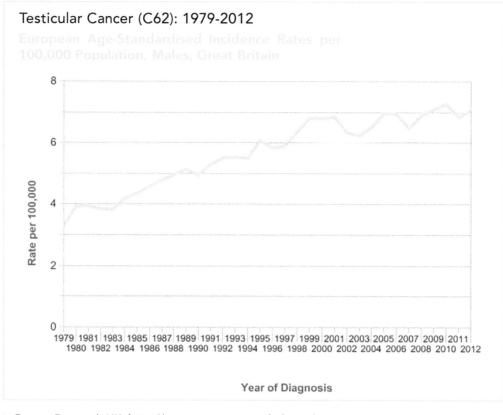

Testicular Cancer (C62): 1979-2012

European Age-Standardised Incidence Rates per 100,000 Population, Males, Great Britain

Rate per 100,000

Year of Diagnosis

Cancer Research UK http://www.cancerresearchuk.org/ health-professional/cancer-statistics/statistics-by-cancer-type/ testicular-cancer/incidence#heading-Two
ACCESSED JAN 2016

I think by looking at these three graphs you can clearly see a similar trend with an increasing incidence of these hormone related cancers over the past 40 years. The actual numbers of people affected per 100,000 for each of the cancers I have shown are different but nevertheless they have the same upward trend. For each of them the overall numbers have more or less doubled. Ideally we want to stop the incidence rates from getting even higher and hopefully actually start to see them come down. In order to do this, we need to address why the rates have increased.

Looking at all these figures will probably get you thinking a bit more; it would seem that everything is not crystal clear. However, if the risk to us becomes greater as a result of lifestyle choices and changes to our environment, then it would seem logical that our risk can be reduced by addressing these issues. Surely we should try and mimic the protective factors found in those countries with the lowest incidence. As well as looking at what goes on in other countries we can look back over time and try to identify historical changes that may also be contributing.

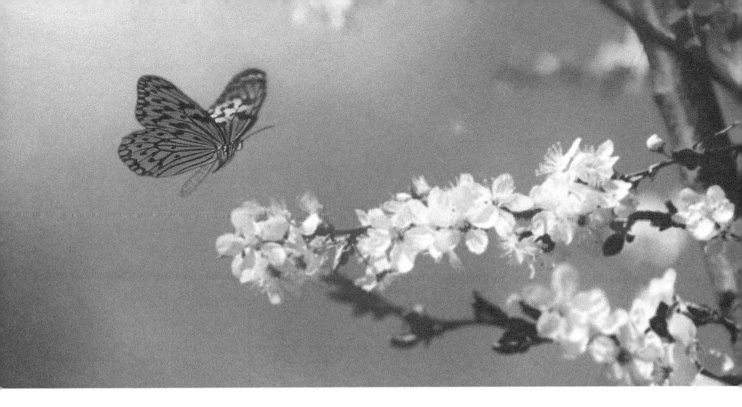

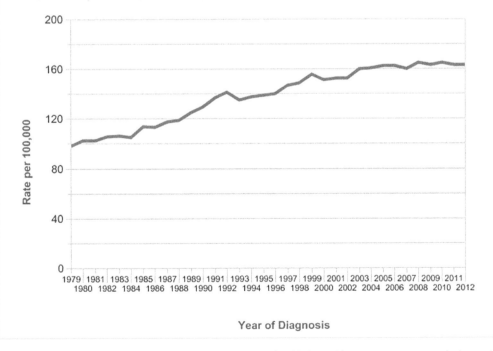

Breast Cancer (C50): 1979-2012

European Age-Standardised Incidence Rates per 100,000 Population, Females, Great Britain

Year of Diagnosis

*Cancer Research UK http://www.cancerresearchuk.org/
content/breast-cancer-incidence-statistics#heading-Two*

ACCESSED JAN 2016

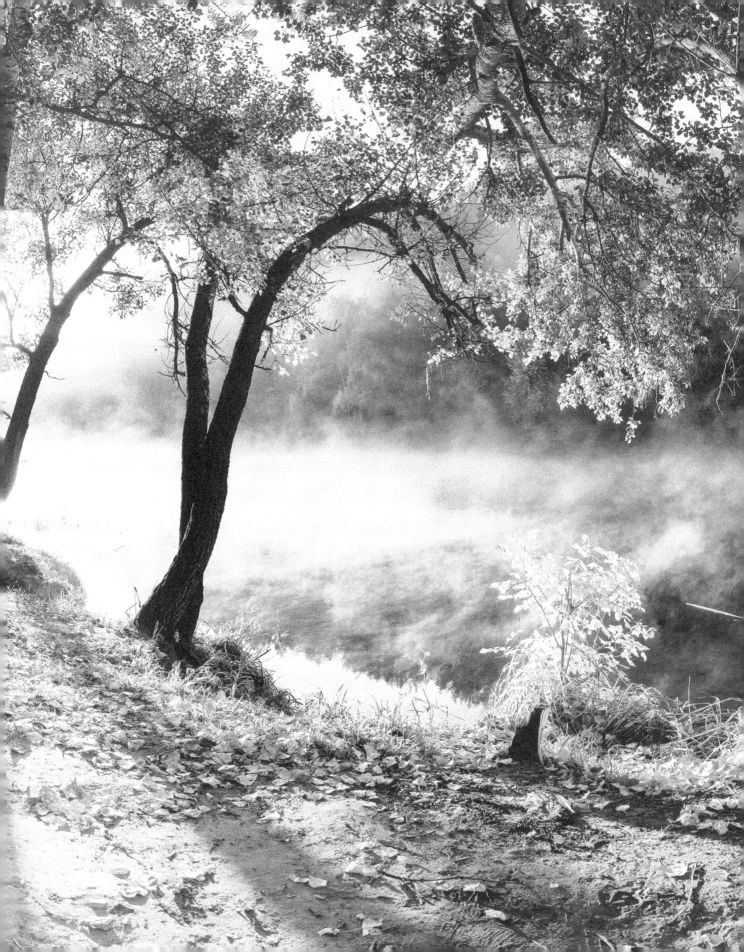

Known Risk Factors

There are often known risk factors that will contribute towards a person's risk of developing a disease; some cancers are clearly linked to particular lifestyle choices. As mentioned in the last chapter I don't think that anyone doubts for a second that smoking is the main risk factor for lung cancer and increased exposure to UV radiation is the main risk factor for skin cancer. Breast cancer rates are increasing but unlike lung or skin cancer we cannot point a finger at one leading causative factor. The two major contributing factors for breast cancer have always been simply being female and getting older. Although being female is the biggest risk factor it is important to remember that men can also develop breast cancer.

About 340 men are also diagnosed with breast cancer each year in the UK. Other risks are related to women's changing reproductive habits over the past few decades and for a small proportion of men and women genetic factors also play a role.

As well as these known risk factors for breast cancer we also know that our diets, lifestyles and environment contribute to the much higher rates of cancer seen in the developed world. Epidemiology is the name given to the study of how often diseases occur in different groups of people and why. These types of study help us to look more closely at the differences between different countries and can help us to identify the other parts of the equation that are leading to the higher incidence of breast cancer seen in more affluent societies.

Male Breast Cancer

Males produce both oestrogen and testosterone sex hormones and when boys reach puberty a small amount of breast tissue develops. This includes a small amount of breast milk ducts similar to those found in female breast tissue. However, during puberty increasing levels of testosterone stops the further development of male breast tissue. Although the major hormonal influences to the developing male occur in puberty, hormonal changes can also occur in men as they age and are more likely to occur if they are overweight.

Men have breasts and can get breast cancer too. Any nipple changes or breast lumps must be checked by a doctor.

Most types of male breast cancers i.e. 8 out of 10 cases are invasive ductal carcinoma. In men the majority of cases occur over the age of 60 and over a third of cases in men over the age of 75 years. Breast cancer in men presents in the same way as in women with changes in the appearance of the breast or nipple or a detectable (usually painless) lump in the breast tissue. Most of the breast tissue in men lies just underneath the nipple and because of this proximity to the nipple; invasive breast cancer in men often causes nipple changes.

Men are also more likely to develop Paget's disease of the nipple. Paget's disease is a rare type of breast cancer which causes nipple changes such as an inverted nipple, dry or inflamed non-healing skin involving the nipple or areola, or a blood stained nipple discharge.

Causes of Increased Oestrogen Production in Males

If men have a hormonal imbalance that causes an increased production of oestrogen then they will be more at risk of breast cancer. This may happen in the following conditions.

Obesity. Like women, men can produce additional oestrogen in fatty tissue so men that are overweight are at an increased risk of male breast cancer.

Chronic Liver Damage A number of disease processes can cause liver damage which may then result in an increased production of oestrogen. The liver damage caused by excessive alcohol consumption is linked most closely to male breast cancer.

Klinefelters The risk of male breast cancer in men who have a chromosomal disorder called Klinefelters contributes to an increased risk by about twenty fold compared to other men. In this rare condition the man carries an extra X (female) chromosome (XXY instead of XY) which results in him producing larger amounts of oestrogen. Although men with this condition are at a much higher risk it only accounts for a small percentage of male breast cancer cases.

Hormone Receptor Status

90% of breast cancers diagnosed in men are hormone receptor positive and these cancers are treated in the same way as hormone receptor positive breast cancers in women. Most men undergo a full mastectomy to remove all of their breast tissue; this may be followed by chemotherapy in the same way as women. Usually men will also require radiotherapy to the chest wall due to the proximity of cancer tissue to the underlying chest wall. Hormonal treatments are also used; most men with breast cancer are treated with Tamoxifen and most trials of the use of hormonal treatments in male breast cancer are with this drug. The side effects are similar to those that affect women including hot sweats, mood disturbance and loss of libido. See Chapter 8 for further ways to deal with these potential side effects. Men may also suffer from erectile dysfunction as a result of Tamoxifen but there are treatment options to help with this. Men or women that are affected by sexual problems should discuss this with their doctor as there are a number of ways that this can be improved.

Other Issues for Men with Breast Cancer

Men generally have less breast tissue then women so changes to the breast may be more visible at an earlier stage however if men ignore these changes either because of lack of awareness or if they are reluctant to go to their doctor or share these changes with anyone then clearly the cancer will progress and unfortunately many cases present at an advanced stage.

The lack of awareness and lower incidence also means that there is a lot less literature or support specifically for men facing a breast cancer diagnosis. Thankfully some support can be received from social media groups and more men are creating more awareness by speaking up about their breast cancer journeys and publicising the issue. Some other difficulties that may affect men are regarding their sexuality or a feeling of being emasculated by being diagnosed with what is perceived as a 'female cancer'. This will be something that can hopefully be managed with further support including Counselling, Cognitive Behavioural therapy or practising Mindfulness Based Cognitive Therapy for Cancer (see Chapter 16).

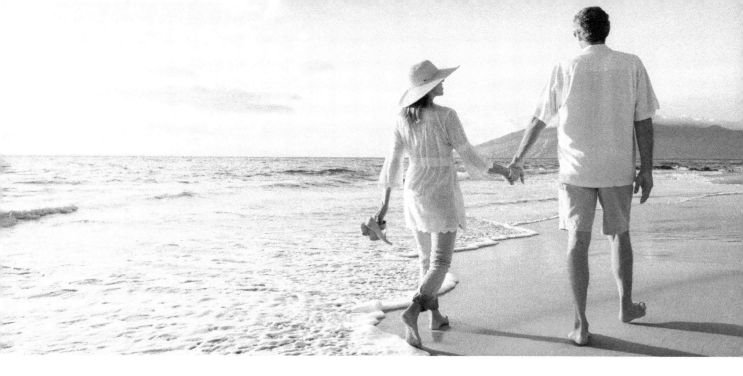

Age is a Major Risk Factor

Just getting older increases the risk of breast cancer, 80% of breast cancers are diagnosed in women over the age of 50 and most commonly in women aged between 60-64 years. One of the reasons that incidence rates have increased in the UK is that we have an aging population. Over the last 3-4 decades the average life expectancy for women has increased from 75 years in the 1970s to nearer 85 years in 2015.

However there is some disparity since 1 in 3 women diagnosed with breast cancer are over the age of seventy yet NHS screening mammograms stop at the age of 70 years (soon to be extended to 73 years). Although women over the age of 70 are no longer automatically sent a reminder they can still request a screening mammogram every three years. Any woman over 70 years old can get details of her local breast screening unit from her GP practice and then arrange an appointment directly. It is also important for older women to be aware that there is this risk and to practise regular breast self-examination (see chapter 7).

Women's Changing Reproductive Habits

Women's reproductive patterns have also changed in a number of ways in the last few decades. These changes include: the earlier onset of menstruation, increased oral contraceptive use, having children at an older age, having fewer children, reduced breast feeding and later menopause. These changes result in an increased exposure to oestrogen over our fertile years. Since many breast cancers are stimulated by oestrogen this increased exposure also plays an important role in the increased incidence of breast cancer.

Familial Breast Cancer

Men or women with a first degree relative with breast cancer are at an increased risk of developing breast cancer. A first degree relative is either one of your parents, a sibling or a child. This risk increases further if there is more than one first degree relative affected. The risk is also higher if their diagnosis is at a younger age, especially under the age of 40 years. However it is also important to know that the majority of men or women who do have such a family history will not go on to develop breast cancer.

A genetic predisposition is only seen in 5-10% of female cases. In these women there is usually a family history of breast cancer and/or ovarian cancer. The most well known mutations are in BRCA1, BRCA2, TP53, CDH1 and STK11 genes but there are now at least 41 other mutations that have also been identified. With these inherited mutations the genes come from one of the parents even if they have not been affected themselves. If you have a positive gene it can greatly increase your risk of developing breast cancer but it does not mean that you definitely will. Preventative surgery greatly reduces the risks associated with a positive gene but it is still important to consider the whole picture including your diet and lifestyle.

You may be wondering whether it is worthwhile having genetic testing if there are other members in your family that have had breast cancer or other types of cancer. If you are unsure then it is worthwhile discussing this with your GP or hospital doctor on an individual basis as every situation is different. The 'National Institute of Clinical Excellence' (NICE) drew up guidelines in 2013 for referral to a geneticist for patients with a concern about their risk of Familial Breast Cancer.

To begin with it is important to establish who your first and second degree relatives are on both your maternal and paternal side and note if any of them have suffered with breast or ovarian cancer and if possible at what age. The table below from NICE Clinical Guidance 164 (CG164) makes it clear which family members are classed as first or second degree relatives.

If you have no personal history of breast cancer and believe you fulfil the criteria for further testing as shown on the next page then discuss this with your GP. This is not an exhaustive list and you can still ask about genetic testing if you have other family history of cancer, especially rarer cancers (eg sarcomas, gliomas) and if these occur at a young age.

FIRST DEGREE RELATIVES	Mother, Father, Brother, Sister, Son, Daughter
SECOND DEGREE RELATIVES	Grandparent, Aunt, Uncle, Niece, Nephew, Grandchild, Half-Sibling
THIRD DEGREE RELATIVES	Great-grandparent, Great Aunt/Uncles, First Cousin, Great Niece, Great Nephew

Is there are history of breast or ovarian cancer in your family? If so, which of these 4 groups matches your family history?	IF SO, do you or your family member meet the criteria in the opposite row/rows?
1 Female Breast Cancers	ONE 1st Degree Relative Diagnosed with Breast Cancer < 40 years old
	OR
	TWO 1st OR One 1st and One 2nd Degree Relative at ANY Age
	OR
	Three 2nd Degree Relatives at ANY Age
2	Having One 1st Degree Male Relative Diagnosed with Breast Cancer at ANY Age
3 Bilateral Breast Cancers	One 1st Degree Relative with Bilateral Breast Cancer where 1st Cancer diagnosed < 50years
4	One 1st or 2nd Degree Relative Diagnosed with Breast Cancer AND One 1st or 2nd Degree relative with ovarian cancer diagnosed at any age.

Looking at the above table, for example, if you have a first degree relative with breast cancer who is male (i.e. your father, brother or son) you would meet the criteria for genetic testing even if you are not affected yourself.

Genetics in Male Breast Cancer

Genetic abnormalities also contribute to an increased risk of breast cancer in men and the above criteria for genetic testing apply to men too. BRCA or other inherited mutations may be present in about 15-20% of male breast cancer cases compared to just 5-10% of women. BRCA2 in particular is linked to male breast cancer and if present results in an increased lifetime risk from 0.12% to 5-10%, it also confers a 20-25% lifetime risk of prostate cancer.

Single Nucleotide Polymorphisms (SNPs)

As well as the mutations seen in Familial Breast Cancer, it is also now known that there are many other lower-risk genetic variations that can increase a person's predisposition to breast cancer. These are acquired in one's own lifetime and do not get passed down from our parents. They are called 'Single Nucleotide Polymorphisms' (SNPs) and these appear to cause an increased risk when combined with lifestyle factors. They are a lot more complex to interpret and not widely available for testing since they may just confuse the issue in many women and there is just not enough data at present to interpret them fully.

I had genetic testing along with my first cousin. She was diagnosed with breast cancer when she was 38 years old and I also had some possible (but difficult to confirm) family history on my father's side of the family. I was faced with the dilemma of what to make of my results when I was told that I had two SNPS. My cousin had just one SNP and we were told that we both shared that one. The geneticist was able to tell us that she was 99% sure that this shared SNP was not disease related. With that particular SNP they had enough data from a library of past gene analysis and computer algorithms to say that it was safe. The geneticist was unsure about my other SNP because there was not enough data available but she agreed that it seemed likely that it had contributed to my risk. She established that I had a 40% risk of getting breast cancer in my other breast. This information led me to my very considered but unwavering decision to have a preventative mastectomy and reconstruction of my healthy breast.

Epidemiological Risk Factors

Other lifestyle and environmental factors such as poor diet, obesity, lack of exercise and drinking alcohol over the recommended limits are associated with at least 30% of female breast cancers in the UK. Several studies have looked at the diet and lifestyle in long term breast cancer survivors to try and ascertain what may be the most beneficial factors to long term survivorship. Learning what is beneficial will give us a better understanding of the protective factors and so should empower and encourage us to make healthier lifestyle choices.

As you can see from the table above some of the risk factors for breast cancer such as age, sex and genetics cannot be

Table of Risk Factors

CANNOT BE ALTERED	CAN BE ALTERED
Age	Smoking
Female	Being Overweight, Diet
Genetics	Excess Alcohol
	Lack of Exercise
	HRT Use

easily changed. At present we cannot alter genes that predispose us to certain diseases but of course there is the possibility that genetic factors could be manipulated in the future.

Modifiable Risk Factors

Some of the risk factors that are known to be associated with breast cancer can be altered. Modifying some of these lifestyle choices can be difficult; especially if they have represented your status quo for many years. The reality is that we can no longer think it might never happen to us. It has happened and so our approach has to change. If necessary this is the time to stop smoking, reduce alcohol to at least within recommended safe limits and lose weight to achieve an ideal Body Mass Index.

Stopping Smoking

If you are a smoker it is very important to try and find a way to 'kick the habit'. It can be useful to start with writing down the pros and cons of smoking and what you like about smoking against why you want to stop. Contemplating stopping smoking is actually the first step to achieving this goal; it is like preparing your mind and paving the way rather than just waiting for that day to come when you may just decide to give it up. Then think about what approach may work best for you, a few lucky people can just decide to stop but for most smokers the cravings are just too strong and the behaviour patterns around smoking just too ingrained.

Recognising where habits and behaviours can be changed and getting help will stand you in good stead in taking that first step forward. Get as much help as you can from your GP and support network. Your local GP practice can offer you lots of help and advice with smoking cessation. UK organisations such as 'Quit' also provide lots of useful and free information to support you in stopping smoking. It's about making that all important decision to just do it. Another useful resource is Allen Carr's (not the comic!) book, Easy Way to Stop Smoking. It is a no nonsense book that says it as it is and it is very motivating and has been very successful in helping many smokers to quit. The objective is to prepare your mind (and indeed he advises you to continue smoking until you finish the book). He puts it to you that rather than thinking of it as giving up something focus more on all the ways you will be rewarded and what you will gain by quitting.

Using nicotine replacement to stop smoking can ease the process hugely by reducing cravings and this means you are much more likely to be successful. Nicotine replacement comes in lots of different preparations including patches to give a steady background dose of nicotine and lozenges, gum and sprays to give you a 'quick fix' if you have a craving. Using patches and one of these other more instant release forms together can be more effective than using one type by itself.

There are also medications called Champix and Zyban that can be prescribed by your GP; they don't contain nicotine but work on receptors in the brain to reduce cravings for nicotine. They are not suitable for everyone due to possible side effects or interactions but they can be very effective.

Champix generally works better than Zyban and with less potential side effects.

The other new arena for smoking cessation is electronic cigarettes otherwise known as E-Cigs. These devices have helped a lot of people to stop smoking however there is wider controversy about whether they normalise the appearance of smoking, especially to the younger generation. There are also concerns regarding possible unknown long term side effects. Besides these concerns they serve a very useful purpose if they are used successfully to stop smoking and then to wean down the amount of nicotine. The danger is that many people may just be swapping over to these E-cigs long term and then we don't really know whether it is safe to do so but they are still arguably much safer than smoking cigarettes. There are certainly a number of options so try to find something that works for you and then plan your stop date.

Maintaining a Healthy Weight

Many people may have an ongoing battle with their weight. Recent studies have confirmed that being overweight does increase the risk of breast cancer and this is partly due to the increased oestrogen that is produced in adipose (fatty) tissue. This seems to be particularly important for post-menopausal women as their ovaries are no longer working so there main oestrogen production is in adipose tissue. This means that having a higher body fat percentage after menopause will increase your oestrogen levels. Therefore losing weight or maintaining a healthy weight is crucial.

Losing weight may not be the most important thing on your agenda immediately after treatment but eating a healthy diet and learning good eating habits should help most women lose weight naturally rather than resorting to extreme weight loss methods or fads. There is little point in trying to live off just cabbage soup or meal replacement shakes. These sorts of diets aren't sustainable and often lead to yo-yo dieting and additional weight gain after the diet ends. This is because the body stores fat more effectively with extreme dieting since it thinks it may be faced with another period of starvation. Subsequently when you do increase your food intake you are likely to pile the weight back on more easily. In order to lose weight in the long term it is important to re-educate how your mind and body respond to food, break negative habits and aim to eat food with optimal nutritional benefits. The approach is to simply cut out refined sugars, processed foods and unhealthy fats and replace them with fruit and vegetables, nuts, seeds, good quality lean protein, healthy fats and whole grains. (See chapters 17-19). By making these changes and maintaining a healthy weight you can reduce the risk of many diseases as well as cancer.

It is worthwhile finding out what support is available; try your local library or community centres. Often there are schemes or clubs you can get involved in that will provide advice and that can support you with weight loss and exercise.

Making your goals small and achievable and recognising that putting in that time and effort for yourself is important. You can start with measuring your Body Mass Index (BMI) and then aim to achieve or maintain a BMI in the healthy range. A BMI target is more useful than just a weight goal as it takes your height into consideration, however it does not take your body frame or bone mass into account. You can calculate your BMI with the following equation but there are many free online BMI calculators where you enter your weight and height and it works out your BMI and what your target weight range is to achieve a healthy BMI.

BMI = WEIGHT (kg) ÷ HEIGHT (Metres)^2

So for a 64kg women measuring 1.6m we would calculate
BMI= 64 ÷ (1.6)² i.e BMI = 64 ÷ (1.6 X1.6)
BMI = 64 ÷ 2.56 = 25

IDEAL BMI	
Less than 18.50	Underweight
18.50 to 24.99	HEALTHY WEIGHT
25.00 to 29.99	Overweight
≥ 30	Obese

Keeping to Safe Drink Limits

Excess alcohol is also a known risk factor for breast cancer and the amounts women consume has risen considerably over the last few decades. It is debatable whether alcohol needs to be stopped completely as it is often a part of socialising and special occasions but we should certainly aim to stay within safe limits. The Department of Health recommended limits per week are 14 units for women and 21 units for men (this is at time of writing). This amount should be spread out over the week to no more than one to two units per day, but you should also aim to have at least two days each week that are alcohol-free. It is worth knowing what makes up a unit of alcohol to avoid under estimating how many units you are actually having. It can be very easy to go over the recommended limits especially with home measures. The number of units in a drink will depend on the volume of the drink and its 'Alcohol by Volume' content otherwise known as the 'ABV'. The ABV is the percentage of the volume of drink that is alcohol. For example, a standard strength bottle of red wine with an ABV of 13% contains about 10 units of alcohol so even a small glass of wine (125ml) contains well over a unit.

How to Work Out Units of Alcohol

There is a calculation that you can do to work out the number of units in any alcoholic drink.

No. Of Units = ABV X VOLUME (ml) / 1000

Some Examples of Units in an Average Drink

DRINK	ABV	VOLUME	UNITS of ALCOHOL
Glass of Red Wine	12 %	175 ml	2.1
Large Glass of Red wine	14%	250ml	3.5
Bottle of beer	5 %	330ml	1.7
Pint of Beer	5.2%	548ml	2.9
Small shot of Spirit	40%	25 ml	1

Having at least two alcohol-free days each week will help you to keep within safe limits and also stops drinking alcohol become a habit or an emotional crutch. Try going for lower strength drinks and swapping to a smaller glass or drink size to cut back. Remember that alcohol has empty calories too so cutting down on alcohol will also help you to lose or maintain your weight.

Other Things to Consider

At present it seems to me that we still lack a clear definitive explanation for the huge rise in breast cancer over the last few decades in the developed world, it has not just gone up a bit; it has doubled. There are many women who are diagnosed with breast cancer who don't have obvious risk factors, so the known risk factors cannot fully explain these trends. Some of these other factors can be highlighted by comparing differences in incidence, environment and lifestyles across the globe and also looking back in time to how our lifestyles and environment have changed over the past few decades. I believe (and there is mounting evidence for this) that other environmental and lifestyle factors are also linked to the steady rise in breast cancer rates. I will explore some of these briefly here, but will then discuss them in more detail in later chapters. The three I will touch on at this point are Nutrition, Personal Care Products and Stress.

As well as trying to alter any known risk factors, I believe that nutrition is the key to helping us stave off cancer. In our busy lives convenience is often desired and nowadays many different food choices are available but often they are pre-packaged or pre-prepared and contain high levels of salt, sugars and unhealthy fats, with additives, preservatives, artificial colours and flavourings. These types of pre-prepared foods may also not be particularly fresh. Eating this way can also lead to a cycle of reduced energy, food cravings, and weight gain but still not provide your body with the healthy nutrients it needs. There is plenty of talk of, 'Sugar being the new tobacco' and there is good reason to be concerned. Sugar is addictive and can make us feel that we are unable to control our desire for it, leading to weight gain and an increase in health problems.

On the other hand leading a healthy lifestyle can offer us some protection against diseases and cancer. We can achieve this by reducing our exposure to avoidable toxins and in particular increasing our intake of nutrient packed foods full of natural : anti cancer fighting, immune boosting and anti-inflammatory properties. A better diet means giving our bodies plenty of vitamins and phyto-nutrients (mainly found in fruit, vegetables, seeds and whole grains). This will not only make us feel better right now with improved mood, energy and immunity, but it can also help us reduce our chances of a recurrence or even the onset of a new cancer.

Whilst we should consider what we put into our mouth, I think we should also consider carefully what we put onto our skin. Just think, our skin is our body's largest organ and has a very large area over which chemicals can be absorbed and potentially enter our bodies. Some medications are designed to use the skin as a site of administration and can be absorbed via this route into our body. Exposure to other chemicals must also be considered and especially women's exposure to them via beauty products, body creams and make up.

It remains a very controversial area but some of the synthetic chemicals used in these products are now known to be hormone disruptors and mimic oestrogen in cell and animal studies. It is very difficult to prove a direct effect in humans but if we are at least aware of this potential risk then we can make a choice about whether to avoid them or not. I recently stayed in a hotel that is part of a new hotel chain and noticed that all their shower gels, shampoos and body creams were reassuringly labelled as being 'PARABEN-FREE'. Paraben-free products can also be found at budget supermarkets, so it does not need to be a costly exercise. Once you start looking out for them on lists of ingredients, you can switch to products without them that suit your skin and budget.

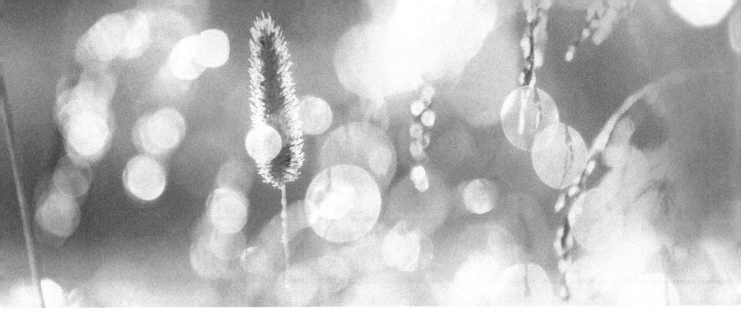

Stress

Stress and anxiety also play a major role in lowering our body's defences. Often our pace of life is fast and furious with little time for proper relaxation. Multi-tasking seems to be a particular skill of women these days and often involves putting everyone else's needs first. We all need time to relax in order to be healthy. When we are stressed our bodies go into a 'fight or flight' response where large amounts of adrenaline are released. This stress response doesn't end there; it sets off physiological and hormonally driven changes which in turn can lower our immunity.

If we can recognize what causes us to be stressed and learn how to deal with stress in a better way, then this will have a positive impact on our health too. There have been a number of studies looking at whether stress can cause cancer, but no definite link has been found so far. This may be partly because it's a difficult area to research. Stress is a very subjective area and what may stress one person may have no impact on someone else. People in the developing world may feel stressed due to lack of food and water; whereas those in more developed countries may feel under stress due to trying to juggle work and family, and so on. People also manifest and deal with stress in different ways so it's pretty impossible to generalise, but one can see how it may have an adverse effect. Learning greater mind and body awareness using techniques such as mindfulness and visualisation can help to lower stress levels.

Exercise is also beneficial for mind and body. It alleviates stress, helps to lift our mood, as well as improving our physical health and fitness levels. Exercise also helps with weight loss or maintaining a healthy weight and independently of this does lower our risk of cancer too. It can also help by giving us some time out and a focus away from all our thoughts. I suggest looking at activities you enjoy and also activities that keep you in the moment, not thinking where you need to be next, not rushing to get it out of the way. Examples are Yoga, Tai Chi and Pilates, but of course any exercise is good.

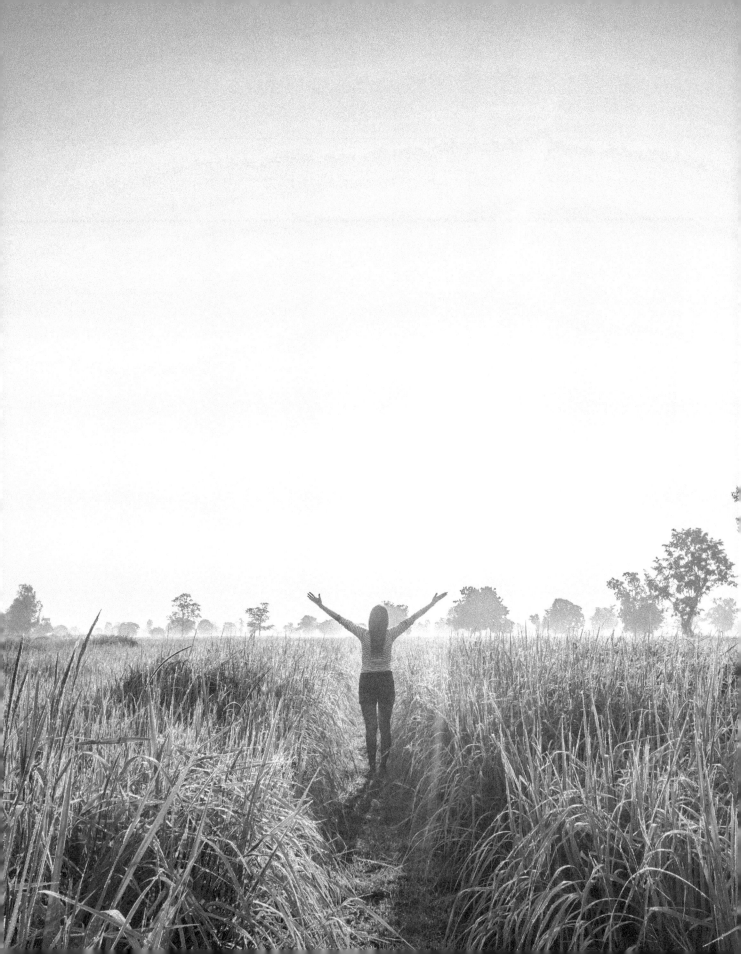

What is the Evidence?

Things have changed unrecognisably over the past couple of decades with regard to the ways we go about sourcing information. When we have a question about something, our first port of call is the internet. In goes the question and out comes the answer. The internet has revolutionised the whole process and it is difficult to imagine how we managed without it. However, with matters of health using Dr Google can often be a confusing and futile exercise that takes you round in circles. We all need to be careful about searching the internet for information on health since it can often give you a distorted picture of the situation and at worst can be frankly dangerous.

Knowing specifically what you are looking for, or what question you want answered, will help. However, not all sites will offer the same advice and the information offered can be contradictory, and this can make it very difficult to know which viewpoint is right. When you search for an answer the quality and reliability of the information provided usually depends on how reputable the source is. Websites like Cancer Research UK and the American Cancer Society are very useful for clinical information but may not provide the answers to more specific questions on healthy lifestyle and diet.

Others like Macmillan Cancer Support, NHS Choices and Patient Info also provide sound and reliable information.

Online forums are another place where people may search for answers and can be a good way of sharing information and providing mutual support. Having access to an online group can also be of immense emotional benefit. However, any advice given is usually based upon individual experiences and people seem more likely to write about things that haven't gone particularly well. Other people who share the same negative experience are also more likely to comment. Although forums present real life situations they don't provide an unbiased overview of the subject. So the content of a forum could also be misleading or even harmful. This doesn't mean that the opinions of small groups of people that have had the same or similar experience is not valid - the opinions can often be very enlightening - but with smaller numbers it is more difficult to be sure how far these experiences have wider relevance.

Even as a doctor I sometimes find the online arena frankly mind boggling and sometimes very deceptive. During the course of my medical training I have been taught how to look at available evidence and apply it appropriately. For physical health problems and treatments there are often clear clinical guidelines based on well researched ideas with replicable results. Yet even here, there are treatment options with different pros and cons that need to be weighed up on an individual basis. There is a huge range of scientific research that helps clinicians to aid decision making, but not all scientific evidence is the same, so it is helpful to understand this in a little more detail.

Evidence Based Medicine (EBM)

Medicine and research have come such a long way over the last few decades, with ever emerging new drugs and treatments. This is fantastic, but the slight drawback is that it can be difficult to keep pace with it all. For a lot of the more clinical aspects of your diagnosis you should be able to rely on your health care team to provide the information you need. However people often feel the need to research things for themselves and if you do start looking online, remember that you do need to be savvy about what you are reading and try to remain objective. This is when you need to consider, 'What is the Evidence?' In Evidence Based Medicine, the evidence from research studies is used to help doctors make decisions about your health. I am not expecting you to become an expert, but urge you to become more aware that the way studies are designed can affect their reliability and the way they are reported can sometimes be misleading; whereas well designed studies are likely to be a lot more reliable and valid.

Which Evidence is Best?

There are different types of study designs used for research purposes. The aim of studies is to ask a question, then come up with a method that attempts to provide accurate answers with statistically significant results and reliable conclusions. A single research study will often not produce conclusive results but it may give rise to further research questions and prepare the way for valuable follow on studies that do lead to more definitive answers.

In general the greater the number of participants in a study and the longer the period of time over which they are followed up, it will be more likely that the results will be accurate. For example, a study of 2,000

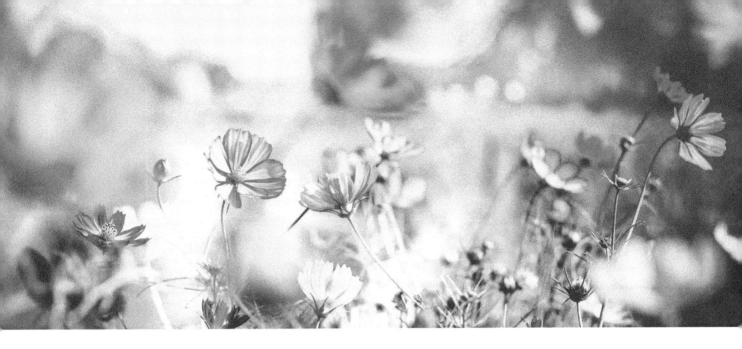

people is likely to be a lot more conclusive than the same study design involving just 20 people. Similarly, when people are followed up for a longer period of time, say 10 years as opposed to just a few months, more reliable results are obtained. When small numbers of participants or short periods of time are involved the outcomes may have occurred purely by chance. Larger numbers and longer durations help to achieve statistically significant results and means you can be more certain that the findings do actually represent a real difference in a real population.

In the same way that size and scale are a major factor, some of the different ways that scientific research is carried out contributes to how meaningful the results are. The basic hierarchy of the best types of study are as follows

Systematic Reviews of Randomised Controlled trials.

Randomised Controlled Trials (RCTs).

Controlled longitudinal studies.

Observational studies

Expert Opinion

Systematic Reviews

Systematic Reviews are collective reviews of all the trials carried out on the same subject over a period of time. This allows the results of all those trials to be pooled and the numbers of participants are added together to help make the findings more statistically significant. For example 20 studies, each with a smallish number of around 50 people would give a total of 1000 people. If similar findings occur in this group as a whole it becomes a lot less likely that they occurred by chance. Systematic reviews can be done on any type of study but a systematic review of Randomised Controlled Trials will have a lot more relevance.

Randomised Controlled Trials (RCTs)

Randomised controlled trials are seen as the gold standard of research studies. In this type of study the participants are randomly assigned to a treatment group or control group with roughly equal numbers in each. These types of research studies are often used to compare two different treatment options to try and deduce which one is better. Evidence obtained from RCTs is even more reliable and valid if the RCT is double blinded and placebo controlled. Using blinding and placebos is important as it helps to remove bias.

Double Blinding

With double blinding both the researcher and patient don't know who is receiving the treatment and who is just getting a placebo, which means that neither of them can subconsciously or consciously influence outcomes in favour of the drug or treatment.

Placebo

A placebo is a drug or treatment option that has no therapeutic benefit and will be given to the control group in a study. Interestingly patients who take a placebo may actually experience a placebo-effect where they show some psychological or physical benefits.

Several such RCTS were instrumental in establishing the benefits of Tamoxifen because they recruited large numbers of women with breast cancer and then followed them up for a number of years. The treatment groups were given Tamoxifen, whilst the control groups just had a placebo. It soon became very apparent that the women on Tamoxifen had significantly better long term survival and lower recurrence rates than those taking the placebo. Once this was clearly demonstrated Tamoxifen went on to be used more extensively.

New drugs fit into this model easily and are usually tested in this way to see if they improve health outcomes such as survival rates. This is not so easy to do for some physical therapies such as reflexology or reiki since both the person receiving and giving the therapy clearly know who is being treated, this can lead to bias in the results. As well as this, the results may be difficult to interpret because it is more difficult to express the outcome in a measurable way.

Longitudinal Studies (looking backwards or forward in time)

Longitudinal studies may be more helpful for looking at physical therapies or the effects of nutrition and our environment on health outcomes. Studies that look forward in time are called prospective studies and involve following up people that have had a drug or intervention against a control group that haven't and seeing what the outcomes are for each.

Retrospective studies look back over a previous period of time. These studies are more open to bias as people may recall only the more extreme things (whether good or bad) or remember only the things that have happened more recently. They are still useful research tools and are often used as they don't involve the same costs as setting up a prospective study.

Observational Studies

Observational studies can be case studies, studies involving smaller groups of people or simply observing trends in a population. These are sometimes used when there are difficulties with the feasibility of designing other types of study. When trends are ob- served then this can often raise questions. Looking at the differences in patterns of disease or behaviour between different groups of people can help research- ers to postulate as to the reasons for these differences.

Expert Opinion

Expert Opinion can also be an important source of information since specialists will have a breadth of knowledge on many different aspects of a particular condition. They will usually have taken part in research and will have their own experience to draw upon. The main things to consider are the credentials of the expert giving their opinion. Anyone can make claims about health and what is good and bad for us. In order to know whether the advice is valid we need to look at the person's training, qualifications and what evidence they are using to back up their claims.

Specific Medical Research Resources

In addition to these different research studies in medicine there are also three major contributors of quality evidence that are widely used in the practice of Medicine. These are the **Cochrane Database,** the **National Institute of Clinical Excellence (NICE) used in the UK** and the **EPIC Studies.**

Cochrane Database

This is a database of high quality and up to date evidence on health research. It is brought together by a global collaboration of doctors, health practitioners, researchers and patient advocates. This database helps health providers to use quality evidence to make decisions about health care. The people involved in Cochrane tend to affiliate with a group depending on their area of interest and knowledge. It is an independent non-profit organisation which is crucial to how it is run since it is not in the pursuit of financial gain. Instead its aim is to improve health care and international collaboration. I mention it since it is a well sited resource that is used in many areas of healthcare.

National Institute of Clinical Excellence (NICE)

Most people in the UK will have heard of the organisation called NICE. This organisation was established in 1999 in order to provide the National Health Service with good quality national standards and guidelines for evidence based healthcare. Each guideline is carefully drawn up by combining the expertise of health professionals and the first hand experiences of lay people and patient advocates. Usually the people involved in making the decisions that form the basis of these guidelines will have an interest or knowledge in the subject being reviewed or updated. This is very important since the public and the very people that are being directly affected get to voice their opinion and preferences too.

The team come together to review new drugs or other treatments by analysing the available research and evidence in that area. They use this information to make decisions on who may benefit from the treatment, what the health benefits are and the cost effectiveness. The representatives involved are asked to consider costs as some new drugs or treatments are very expensive. This will sometimes mean that their use has to be restricted because of the increased demands placed on the NHS and the limited resources available.

One such NICE guideline bought about the national approval of the drug Herceptin. It used to be a postcode lottery whether women with HER2 positive breast cancer would be offered this expensive targeted treatment. This situation was highlighted by breast cancer patients campaigning for the drug and I can certainly recall the campaign since it received considerable media coverage. In 2006, this led to NICE approving Herceptin for use for anyone with early stage HER2 positive breast cancer. Since then this targeted therapy has been widely used in both early and late stage HER2 patients and has dramatically improved the average life expectancy for people that have HER2 positive breast cancer.

Sometimes health care professionals from different specialities and countries work together so that they can gather and compare a larger volume of data. This can be particularly helpful in epidemiological studies. Epidemiology is a field of science that looks at how often diseases occur in different groups of people. Looking at the differences in their disease patterns helps to identify risk factors for a disease. This is important as this information can then be used to try and plan preventative health measures.

One of the largest epidemiological collaborations is EPIC. EPIC stands for European Prospective Investigation into Cancer and Nutrition. There are over half a million participants in the EPIC studies from ten European Countries including the UK. In these studies researchers have followed up the participants for around 15 years. They collect information about their diet, lifestyle and environment to see how these factors may influence the incidence of cancer and other chronic diseases. Studies trying to understand these factors can be difficult to set up so the data from the EPIC studies has been crucial to exploring these issues in more depth. There is no doubt that with such a large number of people followed up for a considerable duration that a lot has been learnt. I will refer to some of these studies in later chapters in the book.

Whatever type of study you are looking at there are pitfalls to be avoided in interpreting the data. How results are presented can sometimes be misleading and this can be illustrated by examining the concept of risk. Generally we want to know if something increases or decreases risk and by how much. Statistics about risks can be presented in two different ways that can mean very different things. They are absolute risk and relative risk. Absolute risk reduction tells you by what amount in numbers or by what percent a risk is actually reduced. On the other hand relative risk is a comparison of risk. The risk or benefits of something can very easily be misinterpreted.

Usually the absolute risk of something will give you a more realistic idea of the actual amount of benefit or harm involved. This is easier to demonstrate by showing you an example, so if we say drug A reduces the relative risk of getting cancer by 50%; this could apply to any of the statistics shown in the left column of the table below.

THE STATISTIC	RELATIVE RISK REDUCTION	ABSOLUTE RISK REDUCTION
Cancer risk reduced from 60% to 30%	50%	30%
Cancer risk reduced from 20% to 10%	50%	10%
Cancer risk reduced from 2% to 1%	50%	1%

As you can see, the relative risk reduction depends on the initial figures. A risk of something being reduced by 50% always sounds impressive. It may not be so impressive if we are talking about a relative risk reduction of 50% but the absolute risk reduction is just 1% (as shown in the bottom row).

A Final Word of Advice

Specific difficulties and questions should be addressed with your doctors and nurses. Do not suffer in silence if you are struggling with some aspect of your treatment. Ask for help to see what options are available to you. Further support can come from groups or forums but it does pay to get reliable advice backed by evidence. A person's individual experience shouldn't have the same influence on you. By nature we are curious and want to find out what we can, so when you are looking for answers

Whilst both sets of results are completely true the way risk is presented may not mean what you think it does. As you can see the relative risk can makes things look much better than they really are. So not only do you have to decide whether the study is a good study you also need to have a little idea of how results can be presented.

try and think a bit about how reliable the information you are reading or being told is. I have read numerous articles, web pages and research papers in the process of writing this book and know just how difficult and confusing it can be trying to make sense of everything you read or hear. I hope that by looking for the answers to the questions I have had and then sharing this with you, that I am able to answer some of your questions too.

PART

2

What Happens Next?

Follow-up ABC and Breast Screening

The time has arrived when you have finally completed your active hospital treatment. But as you might expect it does not all just suddenly stop there. You will now enter a period of follow-up where you will continue to receive ongoing outpatient care and monitoring. During your diagnosis and initial treatment you will usually have had frequent attendances at the hospital so life tends to revolve around these appointments. For most of us we cannot wait for this stage of intensive treatment to finish. However, there is also sometimes a sense of loss or worry as you may have become reassured by the routine of it all. To some extent, being seen regularly may have inadvertently provided you with a sort of emotional security blanket. This period of follow up allows you time to readjust. The breast cancer team can begin to loosen their reigns a little as you begin to get back to some sort of normality.

So What Happens Next?

You will continue to be seen and reviewed by your treating hospital, usually for a period of five years. Hospital protocols will vary but follow-up is usually at six monthly intervals. These appointments may alternate between your Breast Surgeon, Breast Care Nurses and your Oncologist. Ongoing support will also be provided in primary care by your GP. Some medical centres may even provide shared care with the hospital. These appointments can be beneficial to the welfare of breast cancer survivors because it allows the opportunity to ask questions and not to push concerns aside. Follow-up also enables doctors to monitor the side effects of treatment and compliance with medications. The doctor will usually examine you as well.

You will also have an annual screening mammogram of the treated breast (unless you have had a mastectomy) and your other breast. After five years, if everything has remained clear, most women will be discharged from breast clinic follow-up and return to the normal three yearly NHS breast screening programme. Younger women will usually continue to have yearly mammograms until they reach the normal breast screening age of 50 years.

At the start of this five year follow-up period most women will also have a special kind of X-ray called a DEXA scan. This stands for 'Dual Energy X-ray Absorptiometry'. A DEXA scan is sometimes also called a 'Bone Mineral Density' (BMD) scan and is used to determine how strong your bones are. The DEXA scan measures your BMD to see if you have a condition called osteoporosis. In osteoporosis the BMD is low which means that your bones are thinner and more fragile than normal and are therefore more likely to break. This is illustrated below. The DEXA scan is not unpleasant and generally only takes about fifteen minutes. Early menopause (which may be as a result of treatment) or the use of Aromatase Inhibitors for post menopausal women are both risk factors for thinning of the bones. A DEXA scan is done at the beginning of your follow up period to give a measure of your baseline bone density. It will then be repeated after 3-5 years to see if any significant thinning of your bones has occurred. If your bones have become measurably thinner over these few years then bone protecting medications can be prescribed to reduce the speed of bone loss or even halt or reverse the disease. DEXA scans can then be used to monitor your response to the medications.

Normal   Osteoporosis

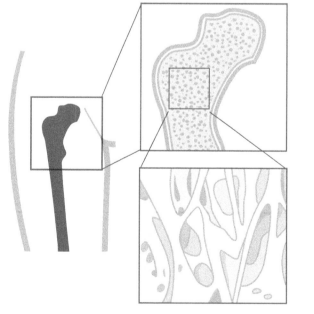
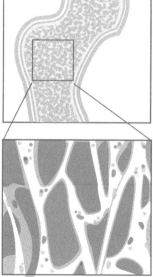

Interestingly, the latest NICE guidelines on breast cancer (2009) suggest that for early or locally advanced breast cancer five year follow-up may offer little benefit in terms of detecting recurrence or mortality. This is a difficult one to weigh up since many women become unduly anxious leading up to a follow-up appointment and so not having to attend the out patient's clinic would avoid this period of anxiety. Also some women may be overly reassured and complacent when given their annual all clear. Although follow-up appointments can be very reassuring it is still very important for you to remain vigilant. You shouldn't rely on an annual screening mammogram and six to twelve monthly breast examinations alone. Abnormal changes could occur in the interval between these appointments so it remains important to routinely practice a monthly breast self examination. Your breasts may have changed a little or more noticeably but if you become familiar with how your new breasts look and feel then you are more likely to pick up any early changes yourself. Women diagnosed with more advanced breast cancer are more likely to benefit from continuing outpatient follow-up.

During follow-up many women may also face the decision about whether or not to have reconstructive surgery. You will need to wait for a period of time to get over your initial treatment but this can also give you some breathing space and plenty of time to consider your options. Generally, there is no time limit to when reconstruction can take place so if you do not feel ready to contemplate further surgery initially you can consider it at a later stage. There are a number of different techniques that are now available so an informed decision can only be made once you have been provided with all of the relevant information. The choices available to you will depend on your particular situation and so these can be discussed with your breast care team.

Regular review and examination may pick up an early recurrence but as more time passes by, the risk of recurrence becomes smaller. In this chapter I would also like to discuss breast screening mammograms as a way of detecting early breast cancer and explain some of the shortfalls that mean you shouldn't rely on this method alone.

What is Screening?

A screening test is used to identify a disease or cancer early by actively looking for it. The reason for doing this is that when it is detected at an early stage it will be a lot more treatable and therefore the chances of long term survival will be much better. Screening programmes therefore exist on the basis that early detection of the disease leads to improvements in long term prognosis. However, National Screening Programmes are a major undertaking requiring huge resources so certain criteria have to be met before a screening programme is approved. For cancer screening programmes some of the criteria are listed on the following page.

The test that is used also has to be good at not only detecting a problem but also not showing a problem when there actually isn't any. In statistical terms this translates to having a low number of false positives and low number of false negatives.

- It has to be reasonably common cancer
- The programme must target the correct population.
- There has to be an early stage that can be identified by a test
- The test has to be reliable
- The test has to be cost effective
- There is effective treatment for the early stage that will prolong survival

The NHS Breast Screening Programme

If you look at the list above you can see that breast cancer fits the bill for being relatively common and having an early stage that is much more treatable. There is a target age range and sex in which most breast cancers occur, targeting younger or older women may not actually be helpful. It can be more difficult to make the decisions about cost but compared to some investigations mammograms are not deemed to be overly expensive. It is not just the monetary cost of the test being measured against the cost of treating the disease but screening programmes also consider the amount of suffering and ill health that can be avoided. However on a national scale, the programme does cost the NHS almost £100 million a year.

Breast cancer screening is available in most affluent countries but there is no consensus on how often and at what age it should be available. In the UK three yearly mammograms to screen for breast cancer are done from age 50-70 years, but the plan is to extend this to women from the ages of 47 to 73 years by 2016. In America the breast screening programme starts at the age of 40 and is recommended annually. At least half of women with private health cover in America do not attend annually. Uninsured (low income) women are able to access USA state screening programmes but generally have a low attendance. In Australia women are offered breast screening every 2 years, from age 50 -74 years.

Breast Screening Mammograms

A mammogram is a special kind of X-ray that was first considered for use as a screening tool for early breast cancer as far back as the early 1960s. Up until then if a woman or her doctor found a breast lump a mammogram would be performed to help locate it. Once it was located a fine needle aspiration or biopsy would be taken from the lump. Ultrasound scans (USS) took over this role in the late 1970s and are very effective

at detecting breast lumps. Mammograms did not become obsolete as they were still useful, especially because it was noted that they could pick up an abnormality called microcalcification which USS could not. This microcalcification usually indicates Ductal Carcinoma in Situ (DCIS) otherwise known as a precancerous or, more correctly, a non-invasive stage of breast cancer. Mammograms can often detect DCIS and other changes or lumps in the breast even before they can be found on examination. The DCIS stage is much more easily treated than invasive breast cancer and if these non-invasive cells are removed they cannot become invasive in the future.

From the first large randomised control trial in New York in the 1960s, many studies have been carried out to look at the ability of mammograms to pick up early breast cancer and so treat it before it has become noticeable. These various studies showed that the women who were selected to have mammograms had a reduced rate of breast cancer deaths ranging between 15-25% compared to those in the control group that did not have mammograms. Breast screening mammograms continue to be a very important way of detecting early breast cancer or early breast cancer recurrence.

These impressive findings prompted the introduction of a UK breast screening programme; this became established in 1988. What puts this into perspective for me is that this was the year I started my medical degree and therefore highlights the advances with cancer detection over the past 30 years. The programme initially led to an increased number of women being diagnosed with breast cancer. However

more were being found at an earlier stage. Many of these women could then be treated with a localised breast excision and radiotherapy, and in many cases this meant the need for a mastectomy and more aggressive treatment could be avoided.

About one third of breast cancers are now found by screening. The Independent UK panel on Breast Cancer Screening estimate that for 10,000 women that are 50 yrs old and then followed up for 20 years, 43 would avoid a death from breast cancer. Despite this, there is concern that about 20-30 % of these early breast cancers would never go on to become invasive. However, it is currently not possible to tell which will or won't go on to develop into a cancer.

Since mammograms have been introduced there has also been a reduction in breast cancer mortality. However, in recent years you will probably have noticed that the pros and cons of having mammograms have been increasingly debated. Many people now believe that a significant proportion of the reduction in deaths from breast cancer are actually related to increased breast awareness along with improved treatments rather than breast screening mammograms alone. The main concerns aired are regarding the potential harm caused from the relatively large number of women who show up as having a suspicious mammogram, who then require a recall and more invasive tests but who actually do not have cancer. It is difficult to weigh up putting these women through unnecessary stress, anxiety and wasted resources against detecting breast cancer early in a few women and improving their chance of long term survival.

This is an important study because it provides much more recent evidence compared to the earlier studies that backed the introduction of screening mammograms. This study aimed to compare the benefits of early detection against the unnecessary anxiety in women who were recalled but subsequently found not to have cancer or who may be over treated. This study was a Nordic Cochrane Analysis (2012) looking at a number of RCTS on screening mammograms (Cochrane Database as discussed in Chapter 5). By reviewing all these trials the specialists concluded that for every 1000 women that have mammograms about 70 (7%) of these women will be recalled. These 70 women will go on to have more investigations to see whether they actually have cancer or not. Clearly this can be a worrying time and can create a lot of anxiety from the point of recall to the time of further investigations and results. For some women the anxiety can continue for longer and may persist to the extent that these women do not return for further screening. If you are recalled further investigations usually consist of an ultrasound scan with or without a fine needle aspiration (FNA). A FNA is minimally invasive although it can still be unpleasant; this procedure allows a small sample of tissue to be removed from the abnormal looking area and this can then be examined further in the pathology lab.

In this Nordic study (as shown opposite) after having an USS with or without a FNA, 60 out of the 70 women recalled could actually be reassured that they did not have cancer. However, the other 10 out of the 1000 women required a biopsy before a definitive diagnosis could be made. Ultimately out of all the 70 women that were recalled for an abnormal mammogram result, only 3 or 4 of them had an actual cancer diagnosis. In conclusion mammogram screening will put a number of women through a worrying time who turn out not to have breast cancer, but it will also pick up a few with breast cancer which is often at an early stage and this is probably a reasonable trade off.

Evidence to support screening comes from a recent follow up study of all Norwegian women aged 50-79; this took place between 1986 and 2009. Within that period Norway's national breast screening programme was implemented. It was started much later and more gradually than in the UK, in the decade from 1995 to 2005. The study findings, 'Modern Mammography Screening and Breast Cancer Mortality' were published in the BMJ, 2014. The researchers compared the deaths from breast cancer in the women invited to screening against those that hadn't been screened. Results showed a 28% lower risk of death from breast cancer in those that were invited for screening. I find this result amongst others a compelling reason for us to continue with the NHS breast screening programme. My perspective is of someone who has had breast cancer so admittedly it will be biased to some degree, but I believe the figures still show a significant benefit.

Also earlier RCTs on mammograms for breast cancer screening may not reflect our

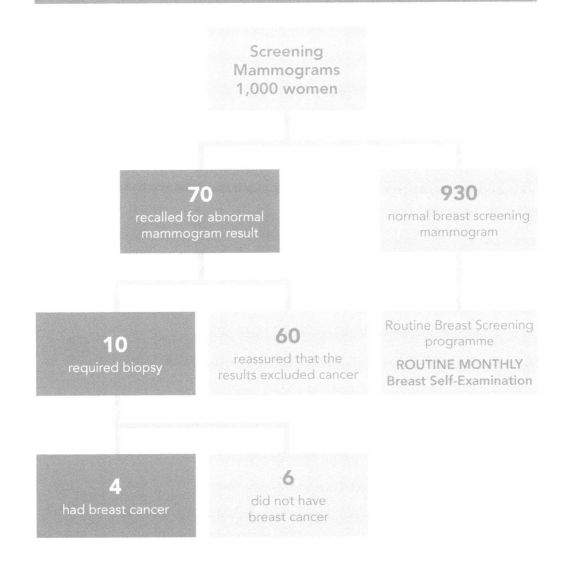

Screening Mammograms 1,000 women

70 recalled for abnormal mammogram result

930 normal breast screening mammogram

10 required biopsy

60 reassured that the results excluded cancer

Routine Breast Screening programme

ROUTINE MONTHLY Breast Self-Examination

4 had breast cancer

6 did not have breast cancer

current knowledge and more up to date treatments. Over the past decade more hospital breast units are starting to use digital mammography. This digital form gives a much better image of breast tissue and is able to detect abnormalities that may be cancerous more easily. This digital view allows the radiologist to zoom in on areas and highlight them in more detail. These mammograms are more accurate and especially so in women under the age of 50 years and women with dense breast tissue. Digital mammography is also less likely to detect artefacts; artefacts are just shadows or abnormalities in the X-ray that aren't a real or actual problem. This can reduce the number of unnecessary recalls and therefore unnecessary further investigations.

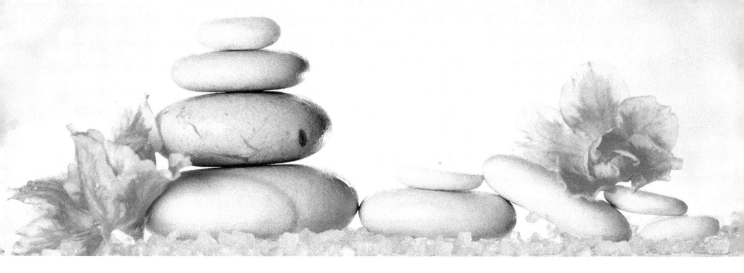

Dense Breast Tissue

Screening can also sometimes provide a false sense of security or reassurance because some cancers may not be detected by mammograms. In this situation getting the all clear can be a little misleading. This is partly due to some women having dense breast tissue (you can't tell by how they feel). Younger women are more likely to have dense breast tissue so traditional film mammograms aren't generally useful in younger age groups.

> In my situation I had found two breast lumps. When I went for tests I was initially examined in the breast clinic and then had an Ultrasound scan, this detected at least three breast lumps. After that I was sent for a mammogram. I felt reassured when my mammogram was actually completely normal. However, a few days later I had a biopsy of two of the lumps and then I had a breast MRI scan. These tests confirmed that I actually had five breast tumours. Then, after I had my mastectomy I was also found to have DCIS in my breast tissue, yet my mammogram didn't show any of these abnormalities. The only explanation for this is that at age 42, my breast tissue was too dense to highlight that anything was untoward.

In the UK target screening group, there may be as many as 10 % of women who have a negative mammogram that actually have a tumour. On this basis it is likely that in the future screening will be done on a more individualized basis taking a person's age, breast tissue density, family history and genetics into account. Studies looking at the benefits of adding in these other factors are currently underway. You just need to be aware that screening mammograms are a very valuable test but not a foolproof test. I get the impression that some women are overly reassured by the screening programme and its benefits and pitfalls need to be raised. This will hopefully help women to adopt a more proactive approach to breast self examination and adopting healthy lifestyles.

Breast Self-Examination

Getting to know your breasts remains very important after breast cancer surgery since it is far better to report any early breast changes in case of an underlying recurrence or new cancer. For many women Breast Self-Examination (BSE) just isn't prioritised or is simply forgotten. However, being a breast cancer survivor means that it is now more important than ever to get into the routine of practising monthly BSE.

When is the best time?

Any time is a good time but you are looking for a change so you need to allow a specified time interval between BSE to be able to do that. Many women's breasts are a bit lumpy and some are more so than others, therefore the important thing is to know if something is different. If you are premenopausal and still having periods, then you may notice that your breasts will tend to be more lumpy and tender just before and during a period. The best time to examine your breasts is five days after your period has finished since your breast tissue will be least affected by fluctuations in hormones at around that time. If you are breast feeding then make sure you also check your breasts at monthly intervals and when each breast is fully expressed or after feeding. If you are no longer having periods then just chose a regular time each month, perhaps at the beginning or end of the month. It can be helpful to set yourself a reminder on your phone or on a calendar.

Post Surgery

If you have had a lumpectomy then you will have some scar tissue in your breast, this may cause some pulling or tethering of the surrounding breast tissue. It is helpful to get to know the appearance of your breasts in a mirror and also how they feel so that you will be able to detect any changes. If you have had a mastectomy it is essential that you check your other breast and your lymph nodes on each side. It is important to check your lymph nodes as this is usually where breast cancer spreads to first. The local lymph nodes are mainly in the armpit (axillary lymph nodes), but there is also a chain of lymph nodes along the upper edge of the collar bone and along the breastbone (sternum). If your axillary lymph nodes have been completely removed, then you should still check the other axilla, along each collar bone and along the breastbone. If you have had a skin-sparing mastectomy and a reconstruction then you should also still look for any skin changes overlying the reconstructed breast or any superficial small lumps.

Know the Signs or Symptoms

A discrete lump

Any new lump in the breast or lymph nodes should be reported to your GP or Breast Consultant.

Skin Changes

Sometimes a superficial lump can result in a visible protrusion. Other visible skin changes that may indicate an underlying breast cancer are as follows

Orange peel appearance to the skin.

Dimpling of the skin

Tethering of the skin

Redness/Rash

Nipple changes

The nipple may become inverted (looking as if it is pulled in) or eczema of the nipple or areola may occur.

Unusual nipple discharge

Any nipple discharge especially if blood-stained or it is a new occurrence.

Pain

Breast pain is not that common with breast cancer but if it is not related to your menstrual cycle or if it is localized it could indicate an underlying infection or a cancer. If it is an infection there will usually be an area of redness with heat and tenderness but this can also occur with Inflammatory Breast Cancer. An infection should completely resolve with antibiotics whereas the latter will not.

Look at Your Breasts

1. Firstly stand up straight in front of a mirror so you can see your breasts clearly.

2. Put your hands firmly on your hips and look at your breasts.

3. Get to know the normal appearance of your breasts. This may well have changed dramatically so start afresh and become comfortable with your new appearance.

4. Look for any skin and nipple changes as shown below

Look For...

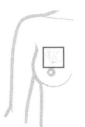 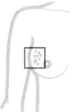 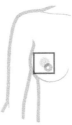 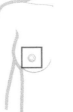 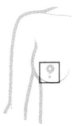 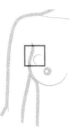

| Skin Change | Dimpling | Redness/Rash | Pulled in Nipple | Nipple Discharge | Lump |

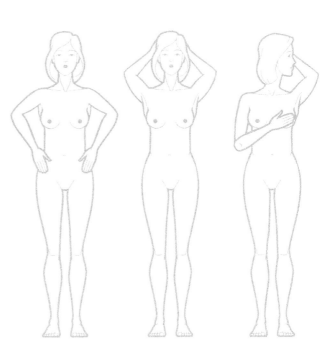

5. Look for any new bulges or visible lumps.

6. Then lift your arms above your head and rest your hands on the back of your head. This will make any skin dimpling, or tethering, or nipple changes more obvious.

Then Feel

7. You can remain standing or lie down to feel your breasts. It is usually easier when lying down supported by a couple of pillows.

8 Put one hand behind the head on the side you wish to examine, this makes it easier to get at all of the breast tissue and the armpit.

9 Then think of the breast as being divided in to 4 quarters (quadrants) by a line going horizontally across the nipple and another line going vertically through the nipple. Then examine each quadrant in turn.

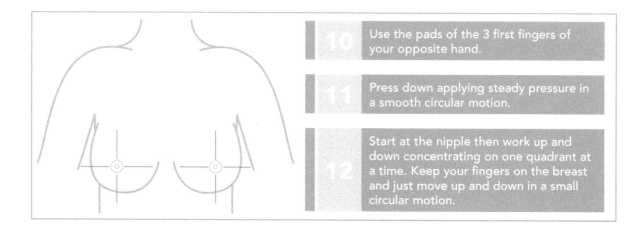

10 Use the pads of the 3 first fingers of your opposite hand.

11 Press down applying steady pressure in a smooth circular motion.

12 Start at the nipple then work up and down concentrating on one quadrant at a time. Keep your fingers on the breast and just move up and down in a small circular motion.

13 First feel superficially then feel deeper before moving on to the next quadrant making sure you include the breast tail that goes up towards the armpit.

14 If you have large breasts then just take your time, you may need to apply a little more pressure when feeling deeper.

15 Gently squeeze the areola around the nipple to look for any nipple discharge.

16 Then relax your arm down and feel deep along the front and back wall of the armpit for any lumps. Make sure you feel all the way deep into the armpit.

17 Then feel along the upper edge of the collar bone and down the breast bone so that you have checked for any enlarged lymph nodes locally as shown in the next diagram.

REPEAT ON THE OTHER SIDE.

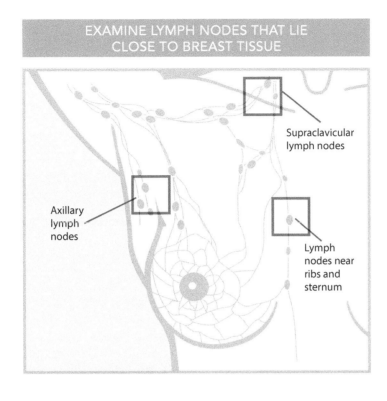

EXAMINE LYMPH NODES THAT LIE CLOSE TO BREAST TISSUE

Supraclavicular lymph nodes

Axillary lymph nodes

Lymph nodes near ribs and sternum

Monitor for Signs of Lymphoedema

Lymphoedema is a build-up of fluid into soft tissues as a result of damage to part of the lymph system. Lymphoedema in the arm can occur when axillary lymph nodes are removed or damaged by surgery or radiotherapy. Therefore, as well as routinely examining your breasts and adjacent lymph nodes it is also worthwhile keeping a look out for signs of lymphoedema. After surgery it is normal to have some swelling present in the breast, chest and armpit areas depending on the extent of the surgery but this should gradually resolve over the initial 1-3 months. However, if you notice swelling in the arm, then you should get this looked at early in case you have developed lymphoedema. Lymphoedema usually appears gradually, and it may even be weeks or months after treatment before it is noticeable and sometimes it starts years later.

The lymphatic system is a network of lymph nodes and lymph vessels and is an important part of our immune system. Normally fluid from our bloodstream enters our tissues from tiny blood vessels called capillaries. This fluid provides our cells with the substances it needs for energy. When the fluid then leaves the cells it takes the cells waste products and debris away. This remaining fluid is drained back in to the bloodstream by the lymphatic system. Whilst the fluid is passing through the lymphatic system it is also filtered by lymph nodes that can remove infective organisms (bacteria, viruses, etc.), toxins and cancer cells. You may have noticed that the lymph nodes close to a site of infection often become a little larger and tender; this resolves a short while after the infection has cleared.

Unlike blood, the flow of lymph fluid is not assisted by the pumping action of your heart instead it relies on the pumping action and movement of your muscles and one way valves that help push the fluid back towards the major branches of the lymphatic system and then back into the bloodstream . As a result of damage to structures of the lymphatic system a build-up of fluid may occur into the surrounding tissues. This is usually permanent but if it is recognised early enough it can be managed a lot more effectively and even controlled. These are the signs to look out for.

Signs of Lymphoedema

Swelling in the arm, hand, breast or chest wall

Changes in the appearance of your skin. Your skin may become indurated, making it feel harder or it may look shiny.

Changes in skin texture, your skin may feel rough or dry.

Heaviness or tingling in the arm.

Stiffness in your shoulder, wrist or hand.

Clothes or jewellery may feel tight on the affected side.

Also bear in mind that there are other things that can cause a swelling in the arm. If a swelling comes on suddenly rather than gradually then it may indicate a blood clot or an infection. A blood clot can be life threatening so needs to be treated as soon as possible with blood thinning medications called anticoagulants. An infection is more likely to cause a red, hot and tender swelling and make you feel feverish and generally unwell. Damage to the lymph vessels can compromise the ability of the immune system to fight off infections so an infection can quickly become worse. The ensuing infection could itself trigger lymphoedema.

Preventing Lymphoedema

The risk of lymphoedema after sentinel lymph node biopsy is in the region of 5-10% and if it does occur it is usually very mild. For women that have had an axillary clearance they have a 20% chance of being affected and their lymphoedema is more likely to be severe. It can be hard to predict who will get lymphoedema but some measures reduce the risk of it happening. If you are at risk of lymphoedema due to the removal or damage of lymph nodes then it is worth taking some simple precautions to try and reduce this risk as discussed below.

Good skincare

Avoid stiffness

Avoid straining

Report signs early

Good Skincare

It is important to keep the skin supple to protect it from getting dry and cracked. If the skin barrier is not kept intact it is much more prone to becoming infected. It is a good idea to get into the habit of moisturising your skin on your arms once or twice a day and using an upward stroke to help with lymph flow in the right direction. Also keep your nails reasonably short and oil around your nail beds to stop the cuticles and nail folds getting dry. Don't push or cut back the cuticles as this may damage them or cause an infection.

In general try to avoid cuts, grazes and sunburn to the arm on the side where lymph nodes have been removed. It is important to wear gloves for cleaning and gardening to minimise the risk of cuts. If you do get a cut then clean it straightaway then apply antiseptic and dress it. If the skin does start to become red around any cuts or grazes, or is oozing pus, or is becoming swollen or itchy then see your doctor as it is likely to have become infected.

Avoid sunburn by covering up, avoiding the hottest part of the day or using a high SPF (30 +) sun cream. The skin in the at risk arm may not be able regulate its temperature as well as it used to so don't expose it to extremes of temperature such as saunas and hot tubs; the heat may cause a surge of blood to the skin that the lymph system may then struggle to deal with. This may then result in a build-up of lymph fluid in the tissues.

Avoid Arm Stiffness

After extensive surgery you will have been given a programme of arm and shoulder exercises to do by a physiotherapist and hopefully will have been shown how to do them. Aim to do the exercises as instructed and make the time to do them regularly. Your arm may feel stiff after surgery but using your arm normally for light everyday tasks, such as washing, dressing and eating will help with lymph drainage.

Avoid Straining

It is important to avoid straining your arm and the chest and axillary area whilst it is healing. So don't lift heavy loads and avoid vigorous repetitive actions such as gardening e.g. pulling up weeds. If you haven't ventured into online shopping yet it is definitely worth giving it a go, otherwise make sure you go shopping with someone. Also have help at home to unpack shopping and to put it away. When you are doing laundry, don't carry a full load of washing, instead empty the washing machine in stages and hang washing up in smaller bundles. The other thing you should do is pace yourself by spreading out tasks so you are not doing them all in one go. It is also important not to have blood tests or blood pressure taken on the treated side as it may cause trauma or an infection that may trigger lymphoedema. To avoid a restriction in the flow of lymph fluid, wear your watch and jewellery on the untreated side.

Report Signs Early

If you notice any signs of lymphoedema report these early to your GP or breast care team. If lymphoedema is addressed swiftly, treatment is more effective and can sometimes be preventative.

Managing Lymphoedema

Lymphoedema won't respond to elevating the arm or to diuretics (water tablets).

But it will respond to these simple measures.

GOOD SKIN CARE
MASSAGE
COMPRESSION
EXERCISE

Good skin care remains important since the skin in the affected area is at an increased risk of becoming infected. Massage, compression and exercise are all practical ways that will aid the flow of fluid from the tissues back towards the major branches of the lymphatic system. If you develop lymphoedema a specialist nurse will be able to show you the technique of massaging your tissues to help with manual drainage. She will also be able to measure you correctly for a compression sleeve. This fitted sleeve applies compression to the arm and therefore helps move lymph fluid out of the tissues back into the body. If you lose or gain weight and the sleeve becomes loose and feels as if it is no longer compressing or it becomes too tight then you will need to be re-measured. Weight gain can also make lymphoedema worse, so this is another reason for healthy eating and exercise to maintain a healthy weight.

It is important to ask your surgeon when you can start exercising since you will need to have recovered sufficiently from surgery first. Exercises that involve your upper body help ease lymphoedema because when these muscles contract they help to pump the lymph fluid out of the tissue. Stretching exercises are important too since they help avoid tightness in the scar tissue and joints. Initial stretches after surgery need to be quite basic to allow scars to heal but then can be gradually progressed.

Beneficial exercises include swimming, light weights and yoga. Swimming is a good all round exercise as you are using the upper body and arms; the resistance and pressure of the water also helps with draining the tissues. Swimming is also a good overall exercise for cardiovascular fitness as well as upper and lower body muscle toning. Light weight-training or resistance exercises will create good tone and strengthen the arm muscles, which again helps to pump the fluid out of the tissues and back into the lymph system. Yoga is a great exercise for toning your muscles and stretching out any scar tissue as well as helping with your posture and relaxation.

You may also wish to get further advice from a support group as it can really help to talk to other women with the same condition. In the UK the Lymphoedema Support Network and British Lymphology Society can help you to find services and support in your local area. In the USA there is the Lymphology Association of North America (LANA) and National Lymphedema Network.

Moving Forward

Regularly looking for signs and symptoms early will continue to stand you in good stead in keeping well and staying healthy. When you practice BSE and you notice something try not to worry, but do let your doctors know as soon as possible. Your doctors may be able to exam you and simply reassure you. Sometimes they may suggest further investigations. Often these additional tests will prove to be normal. However if there is a problem then it is always much better to deal with it promptly. Being seen routinely in hospital clinics or by your GP gives you a number of opportunities to discuss your concerns. However, if you find a change in your breasts by BSE or elsewhere in your body that you are concerned about, don't hesitate to ring your Breast Clinic for an earlier appointment.

Further Treatment

Once your initial and usually more intensive treatment is complete it is then time to begin focusing on the next step. Whilst you continue to be followed up you may still require other treatments which may involve medication or surgery. In the next two chapters I will explain how further hormonal or targeted treatments can significantly reduce your individual risk of a breast cancer recurrence. I will try and show you what a difference these drugs can make and explain why these further treatments are recommended for some of you.

Hormonal Therapies and the Discovery of Tamoxifen

To understand how hormonal therapies work in lowering the risk of a breast cancer recurrence it helps to understand what hormones are. Hormones are chemical substances produced by different glands in our body and act as messengers between one part of the body and another. Hormones are very important as they help to control and regulate different organs and cells in our body. This system of chemical messengers and glands is called the Endocrine System.

Oestrogen is a female sex hormone that is responsible for the development and regulation of breast tissue and the female reproductive system. It is produced mainly by the ovaries in pre-menopausal women and it also has effects on other areas of the body as shown on the following page.

When breast tissue is biopsied it is sent off to the pathology lab .By examining the biopsy tissue pathologists are able to identify whether the cells are cancerous and then they can determine the type and grade of the breast cancer cells. Once this is established they will look for the presence of hormone receptors and HER2 receptors. All this information helps to plan individualized treatment. Hormonal therapies are only effective in patients with hormone receptor positive breast cancer.

It is now known that that approximately 7 in every 10 breast cancers are hormone receptor positive.   Some breast cancer cells have oestrogen receptors on them and are then said to be oestrogen receptor positive (ER+). Some have progesterone receptors on them and are progesterone receptor positive (PR+). Many breast cancer cells have both receptors on them, making them ER+ and PR+. Oestrogen has a much more prominent role than progesterone in the development of the female reproductive system and also a greater influence on breast cancer cells. When oestrogen enters cells that are ER+ it can bind to the oestrogen receptors. Once this happens the receptors become activated and this

Major Components of the Female Endocrine System

Oestrogen Target Tissues

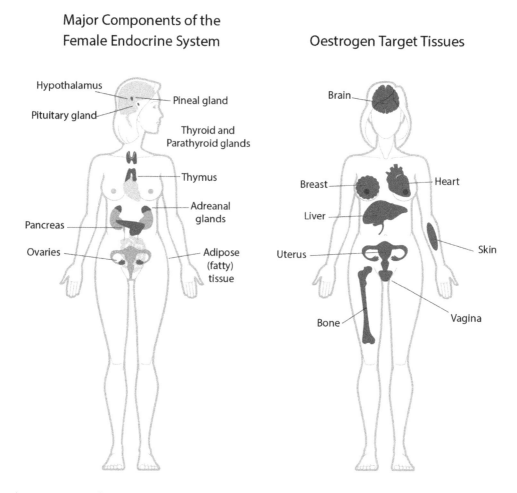

then triggers the increased growth and multiplication of these breast cancer cells.

Hormonal therapies have been developed that can block the effects of oestrogen by either binding to the receptors so that oestrogen cannot or alternatively they suppress the production of oestrogen. These treatments are usually commenced after surgery; adjuvant chemotherapy and radiotherapy have all been completed. The most common types of hormonal therapies come in the form of once daily tablets that are usually prescribed for at least five years. The type of hormonal treatment that is prescribed also depends on whether the woman is premenopausal or menopausal at the time of her breast cancer diagnosis.

Premenopausal women with ER+ breast cancer are generally prescribed Tamoxifen. Sometimes they are also given a monthly injection from a class of drugs called GnRH agonists. Currently, in the UK the GnRH agonist of choice is 'Goserelin' which is more commonly known by its brand name Zoladex. Tamoxifen binds to oestrogen receptors and so stops oestrogen from doing so whereas Zoladex stops the ovaries producing oestrogen in the first place. Postmenopausal women are prescribed Aromatase Inhibitors; these drugs suppress hormones called androgens being converted to oestrogens.

Tamoxifen – A Breakthrough Drug

When Tamoxifen was introduced it was hailed, quite rightly, as a breakthrough drug for the treatment of breast cancer and has helped enormously to improve survival rates over the last three decades. It was the first hormonal treatment for breast cancer and paved the way for the development of another class of hormonal therapy called Aromatase Inhibitors and a targeted therapy called Herceptin (see Chapter 9).

Tamoxifen was first discovered in the early 1960s when it was initially being developed as a morning-after pill. However, it wasn't very effective at stopping unwanted pregnancies and could easily have been forgotten. Fortunately, in the early 1970s further research on Tamoxifen was undertaken by Professor VC Jordan (OBE) who at that time was studying for a Pharmacology PhD at Leeds University, (UK). He started to explore the anti-oestrogen properties of the drug and research its potential benefits in breast cancer patients. The first clinical trial took place in 1971 at the well renowned Cancer Hospital, 'Christies' in nearby Manchester and in 1972 Tamoxifen became a NHS approved drug. However, it was another decade before enough data had been collected from numerous international research trials to show that Tamoxifen definitely improved survival for breast cancer patients. Different health authorities in the UK started to offer it but without a national guideline its use varied between different parts of the country. When it was initially used the course of treatment was only approved for either 1 or 2 years but

it soon became clear that two years of treatment was more effective than just one. More research was necessary in order to establish the optimal duration.

> Five years of continuous treatment with Tamoxifen reduces the risk of recurrence in ER+ breast cancer by 50% and the risk of dying from ER+ breast cancer by at least a third.

Further research funds were made available through the charitable organization Cancer Research UK and gave rise to the Early Breast Cancer Trialists Collaborative Group (EBCTCG) based in Oxford, UK. This well respected group of international researchers published a trial in 1984 showing the conclusive benefits of Tamoxifen. They went on to expand on these studies and published a landmark paper in the Lancet, in 1998 gathering worldwide data from 55 studies and 37,000 women. It soon became clear that Tamoxifen was only effective for women with ER+ Breast Cancer. Also five years of continuous treatment was more beneficial than just two years treatment and there was very little increased risk of adverse side effects.

The Collaborative Group have continued to follow up many of these women with early breast cancer that had originally been selected to receive either Tamoxifen for five years or no hormone therapy. They published their latest review in 2011. By that time they had followed up most of these women for at least thirteen years. Of the 10,645 ER+ women on Tamoxifen the number of recurrences over the first five years was reduced by a half and even after completing the five years of treatment it continued to have a favourable knock on effect. It was found that treatment with Tamoxifen for 5 years substantially reduced breast cancer mortality for at least 15 years after diagnosis.

Further trials such as ATLAS, which explored Adjuvant Tamoxifen: Longer Against Shorter, have looked at the outcomes of ten years treatment against five years. A longer lasting benefit is seen with longer treatment and especially for women who have also got lymph node disease. Their study showed that for every 1000 women that took 10 years of Tamoxifen rather than five years the risk of recurrence was reduced in a further 29 women and there were 19 fewer deaths from breast cancer. This has to be balanced against 16 additional cases of endometrial cancer and two extra deaths from endometrial cancer. However, secondary breast cancer is much more likely to have an impact on long term survival compared to early stage endometrial cancer. Endometrial cancer usually presents early with vaginal bleeding and can therefore be detected early and then promptly treated by having a hysterectomy.

The greater reduction of breast cancer recurrence associated with ten years of treatment may mean this longer course may soon become standard for younger premenopausal women but at the moment this needs to be weighed up on an individual basis. Some women and certainly those that are fifty or above often become menopausal after 2-3 years of taking Tamoxifen. This will often mean that they are more likely to be benefit from having Tamoxifen initially for 2-3 years and then being treated as a menopausal woman and being commenced on an Aromatase Inhibitor for the following five years.

How Does Tamoxifen Work?

Tamoxifen belongs to a class of drug called a 'Selective Estrogen Receptor Modulator' (SERM). It is called a SERM because its actions are selective and change depending on the type of tissue it is acting on. Normally when the ER+ breast cancer cells are exposed to oestrogen their growth and multiplication is stimulated. Tamoxifen works by binding to these receptors without stimulating them and subsequently blocks the ability of oestrogen to do so. Therefore in ER+ breast cancer cells Tamoxifen acts as an anti-oestrogen. Interestingly however in other tissues like the uterus and bones it has oestrogen-like effects, these include stimulating the uterus lining and stimulating bones to protect themselves against becoming thinner and therefore weaker.

Chemotherapy drugs affect normal cells as well as cancer cells. Therefore any cells in the body that are growing rapidly or developing can be affected, this is why hair loss often occurs. The ovaries can also be affected by having chemotherapy and usually stop producing oestrogen which causes periods to stop. This can actually be beneficial in ER+ breast cancer since it reduces the oestrogen stimulus. This may be a temporary or permanent after-effect. If chemotherapy is then followed by Tamoxifen treatment your periods are less likely to return but this will also depend on your age. The closer you are to the age of natural menopause (51 years in UK) the less likely this is.

Tamoxifen alone can cause women's periods to stop but the menstrual cycle usually restarts 6-12 months after the 5 year course, however the closer you are to fifty, again the less likely this is. Younger premenopausal who stop having periods and experience menopausal symptoms are still classed as premenopausal since the ovaries can start working again months or even years after Tamoxifen treatment is finished. Hence it is still important to use barrier contraception to avoid an unplanned pregnancy and falling pregnant whilst on Tamoxifen could cause harm to the unborn child.

Current Uses of Tamoxifen

1. Tamoxifen is used to treat early stage ER+ breast cancer in men and women. It is started after surgery, chemotherapy and, or radiotherapy are completed. When it is taken for five years it reduces the risk of the cancer returning by about a half and it reduces the risk of dying by a third.

2. Tamoxifen can be used after treatment of ER+ Ductal Carcinoma in Situ (DCIS) to reduce the risk of DCIS recurrence and it also lowers the chance of DCIS developing into an invasive cancer.

3. In advanced ER+ breast cancer it can slow the growth of metastatic deposits in other areas of the body.

4. Tamoxifen is also used as a primary preventative measure in women who are at an increased risk of breast cancer because of a genetic predisposition. A number of studies have shown a reduced risk of breast cancer and safe long term use in these women.

5. It can also be used by post-menopausal ER+ women who cannot tolerate an Aromatase Inhibitor.

As with any medication we have to be sure that the benefits of taking Tamoxifen outweigh any potential risks it may have. Most women only experience mild side effects whilst on Tamoxifen and some may not experience any. Yet, sadly it seems that many women struggle to take it for the current recommended five year duration and if women do stop taking it, it is likely to be early on in the course. A charitable organization which is now part of 'Breast Cancer Now' has funded research that highlighted this problem; the findings were published in the British Journal of Cancer in 2013. The research led to headlines in many national papers, for example in The Times, UK, 'Lethal Toll as Women Quit Unbearable Cancer Drug Tamoxifen'.

The study based in Glasgow, Scotland led by Dr Colin McCowan looked at the medical records of 1263 breast cancer patients who had been prescribed Tamoxifen. They were assessed to see how well they adhered to the full five year treatment schedule. They were said to be of low adherence if they completed less than 80 % of the treatment. This was then correlated with the recurrence rates and deaths from breast cancer. They found that as many as 4 in 10 women in the study completed less than 80 % of the full course. From the figures it is estimated that encouraging and supporting women to take the full course could save an extra 400-500 lives in the UK every year.

Possible Side Effects of Tamoxifen

It is worth considering the possible side effects of taking Tamoxifen and then trying to find ways to manage them if they arise. Tamoxifen greatly reduces breast cancer recurrence risk so dealing with any side effects effectively is preferable to stopping this life saving treatment. Remember that the difficulties I discuss do not affect everyone. However, mild side effects are quite common and can still significantly affect your quality of life. Most of the problems are due to Tamoxifen inducing menopausal symptoms. The drug can bring these symptoms on quite abruptly and make them more severe than a natural menopause. As with any medication a careful assessment with your GP or hospital doctor is required to look at the benefits or risks of Tamoxifen and then find the most effective way to manage individual side effects. The following advice should help give you some guidance.

Less Serious but Common Side Effects

If you experience side effects from Tamoxifen they are likely fall into the categories listed opposite.

1. Hot flushes
2. Sexual Intimacy
3. Musculoskeletal
4. Mood changes
5. Eye problems
6. Weight gain

1 Hot Flushes

In general hot flushes are the most common and troublesome side effect of taking Tamoxifen. They can affect up to 80 % of women on hormonal therapies. A hot flush is also the most common symptom of natural menopause and is experienced as a sudden feeling of heat spreading over the body. This can make you look flushed and usually is severe enough to make you want to remove some clothing and start opening windows. Hot flushes also often lead to night sweats that may disturb your sleep. Hot flushes and night sweats tend to be more severe and frequent in the first few months to a year of starting the treatment. After this time they should start to ease, but for some women they do last longer.

Onset of these unwelcome symptoms can be quite difficult to cope with but there are practical ways of minimising them as opposite.

A. Simple measures
B. Diet
C. Exercise
D. Medications

A. Simple Measures

Some simple measures include wearing light cotton clothing since this allows air to circulate more freely around the body and wearing layers allows clothing to be easily removed as and when needed. Sweats are often worse at night and can wake you from your sleep so try and be prepared by using cotton bedding, a low tog duvet and temperature regulating pillows. It is imperative that you try and keep your bedroom cool and airy. Use a fan if needed and keep a refreshing facial spray by your bedside. On warm evenings it can be particularly helpful to put a gel pack in the fridge and then pop it into your bed or in your pillowcase at night to help keep you feeling cool and fresh.

B. Diet

Eating a healthy diet should be part of your plan now and certain dietary changes in particular can help to reduce hot flushes. Everyone is different, so you may see a pattern with particular foods or drinks that make your hot flushes worse. The following are some general recommendations.

Drink plenty of water.

Reduce or eliminate stimulants such as nicotine and caffeine.

If you have caffeine then consume it earlier in the day.

Avoid or reduce alcohol.

Avoid large meals.

Have small regular meals and snacks instead.

Avoid chocolate and spicy foods in the evening if these trigger night sweats.

Eat plenty of fruit and vegetables.

Eat plenty of legumes such as chick peas, kidney beans, lentils and peas.

Eat healthy fats that contain essential fatty acids. These are present in oily fish, avocados, nuts and seeds.

C. Exercise

Maintain a healthy Body Mass Index (BMI) of 20-25 (see chapter 4).

Take regular exercise. Aim for at least 30 minutes of aerobic exercise every day. Brisk walking, swimming and fitness classes are all good examples. Aerobic exercise will not only help with hot flushes but it will also help you to maintain a healthy weight, improve your bone strength and promote a healthy heart.

D. Medications

Some women may consider using over the counter herbal remedies to treat hot flushes and menopausal symptoms. Most contain red clover and black cohosh. Although many menopausal women do find they are of value the regulatory body NICE does NOT recommend their use because of the lack of evidence that they are of any benefit, but also the lack of control over quality and doses. If the dose is not controlled it can be very harmful, for example too much black cohosh can cause liver problems. It is also very important to know that these herbal remedies should be completely avoided by breast cancer patients since they may have some oestrogen like properties. Although Hormone Replacement Therapy (HRT) is very effective for hot flushes it is also contraindicated in women who have had breast cancer.

If flushes are very severe then certain prescribed medications may help. These medications were not necessarily designed for this purpose; they were found incidentally to improve hot flushes in post-menopausal women that were prescribed them for other reasons. The drugs include a number of different antidepressants and a drug called gabapentin. Antidepressants are used more commonly for this purpose so I will discuss them first.

After a period of depression, chronic stress or anxiety, the level of the 'feel good chemical' called serotonin is often depleted. Antidepressants work by boosting the levels of serotonin back to a normal amount. (I discuss this further in Chapter 15). As well as improving mood it seems that serotonin also has a function in the regulation of your body temperature. There are two classes of antidepressants that have been found to help treat both mood problems and also reduce hot flushes.

SSRIs

The first class of antidepressants is called 'Selective Serotonin Reuptake Inhibitors', or SSRIs for short. After the introduction of these drugs it was observed that menopausal women on these antidepressants reported fewer hot flushes. It is not fully clear what the mechanism for this is, but a number of further studies have confirmed this unexpected finding. SSRIs include Paroxetine, Fluoxetine, Sertraline and Citalopram. However, it is very important to note that if you are taking Tamoxifen then you shouldn't take paroxetine or fluoxetine since these particular SSRIs interact with Tamoxifen and make it a lot less effective.

SNRIs

Another class of antidepressant drugs that can help is called Serotonin and Noradrenaline Reuptake Inhibitors. These are known as SNRIs and can also be very helpful in treating hot flushes. The most widely used SNRI for hot flushes is Venlafaxine.

Sometimes even small doses of a SSRI or SNRI can significantly reduce hot flushes. As well as helping with hot flushes, you may notice a reduction in levels of stress and anxiety and a lift in your mood. These drugs can be prescribed purely for hot flushes even if you have no mood or anxiety problems. Your GP will review you regularly when starting any antidepressant medication.

Gabapentin

Gabapentin is another class of medication that can help with hot flushes; it is generally not used first line as it has more potential side effects than SSRI and SNRI antidepressants. This drug is normally used for treating patients with epilepsy or neuropathic pain. Neuropathic pain is a type of pain that is a result of nerve damage and is experienced as a burning, tingling or shooting pain. Chemotherapy or surgical treatment can damage nerves which may result in neuropathic pain. If you are trying to deal with neuropathic pain and hot flushes then Gabapentin may help to control both of these troubling symptoms. In trials on women with breast cancer it has been shown to reduce the intensity and frequency of hot flushes by about 50%.

Gabapentin is always started at a low dose and then gradually increased until it improves the symptoms balanced against any side effects that might occur as the dose is increased. The most commonly seen side effects include unsteadiness, problems controlling movements and lethargy. It is also important to monitor for fever and infections on starting the drug. Less commonly it can cause weight gain. Since it is always started at a low dose any potential side effects are usually minimised and are reversible on stopping the medication.

Sexual Intimacy

A number of issues may arise after a breast cancer diagnosis and treatment that can lead to problems with sexual intimacy. Some of these may be as a result of changes to your body that are affecting you physically or psychologically. It is important to discuss these with your partner and to also ask your doctor for advice. You may find it helpful to talk through your feelings with a counsellor. Counselling may help by allowing you to discuss body image issues or other psychological issues that may be affecting your libido. Meeting other women that have been through breast cancer can also provide you with support as you can often share ideas on how to cope with some of the practical and emotional issues you may face. Your Breast Care team can also advise you of any other useful services that may be available.

Some of the physical problems that can affect your libido can be fairly straightforward to manage. One issue that may arise is vaginal dryness. If this does occur it doesn't usually occur straight after commencing Tamoxifen and can take a few years to be noticeable. If you are nearing the age of natural menopause then Tamoxifen can lead to an early menopause, especially if it is used following chemotherapy. During menopause there is a lack of oestrogen which causes vaginal cells to shrink over time. This makes the lining of the vagina thinner and less elastic, and as a result less moisture is formed.

If vaginal dryness is a problem that is only noticed during intercourse then using a lubricating jelly before penetration will be helpful. The dryness may otherwise cause discomfort with sex and can lead to a vicious circle that reduces desire and libido further. If vaginal dryness becomes noticeable most of the time then a vaginal moisturiser will help. These can be prescribed by your doctor and are also widely available to buy in chemists and supermarkets. They help to actually plump up the vaginal cells and moisturise vaginal skin. They do not need to be applied at the time of sex but are applied once every few days as a maintenance treatment. It is also helpful to do pelvic floor exercises and remain sexually active as this increases the blood flow to the pelvic area and vagina.

If following the above advice for vaginal dryness doesn't help then occasionally your hospital doctor may prescribe a vaginal oestrogen cream to use for a short period of time. Oestrogen creams are generally avoided in order to limit your exposure to oestrogen but in some cases a short course may be deemed necessary and the potential risk of this is thought to be very small.

Musculoskeletal

3

Joint pains and leg cramps may occur whilst taking Tamoxifen. In most cases mild painkillers such as paracetamol or ibuprofen will alleviate these symptoms. If the leg or joint pains are severe then you need to see your doctor to discuss any other possible causes. If one of your legs, especially around the calf area suddenly becomes swollen and painful then you need to seek urgent medical advice in case it is as the result of a blood clot; otherwise known as a 'Deep Vein Thrombosis' (DVT). This can be a rare but more serious potential sided effect of Tamoxifen (see next page).

Mood Changes

4

Mood changes can also be a side effect of any hormonal treatment. It can sometimes be difficult to distinguish whether mood changes are related to medication directly or the toll of cancer and its treatments. If mood changes are affecting your day to day living then it can be helpful to try and learn some new coping mechanisms. As well as individual therapy, it often helps to share your concerns and feelings with others in a group setting. Ask your GP or breast care team if there are any local support groups available. If these measures are not sufficient or you are still struggling with mood changes then medication can help to give you a boost. See chapter 15, 'Dealing with Your Emotions' for further advice.

Eye Problems

5

Occasionally Tamoxifen can cause cataracts or other eye problems. Cataracts usually become more common with age and are caused by the lens of the eye becoming cloudy which results in blurred vision. Although eye problems are an uncommon side effect of Tamoxifen it is worth getting your eyes checked regularly by an optometrist whilst taking the medication.

Weight Gain

Some women notice an increase in their weight within a few months of commencing Tamoxifen. Some of this may be due to fluid retention. There may be a number of factors that can contribute to weight gain such as fatigue or a more sluggish metabolism after cancer treatment and for some women it is due to starting an early menopause. Incorporating a healthy eating plan and regular exercise into your everyday routine will help.

More Serious but Less Frequent Side Effects

The above symptoms, especially hot flushes are relatively common. In a few cases, women may get more serious side effects. The potential risk of these more severe side effects associated with taking Tamoxifen will depend on your own past medical history and your family history. For most previously healthy women the risks of more serious side effects are small and the benefits of Tamoxifen far outweigh any potential serious risks.

Blood Clots

In some women Tamoxifen may make their blood clot more easily and this can give rise to a blood clot in a vein, otherwise known as a 'DVT' (Deep Vein Thrombosis). This is most likely to occur in a deep vein in the calf. Therefore the signs of a DVT are usually a noticeable red and painful swelling in a calf however this can also occur occasionally in the upper arm. It can sometimes be more subtle than this with a less obvious but still localized swelling along with some discolouration, altered texture or firmness of the limb.

In a woman not taking Tamoxifen the chances of a blood clot over a five year period are 4 in 1000 women. For those taking Tamoxifen it is slightly increased to 6 in 1000 women. Usually Tamoxifen would not be prescribed if you have a history of blood clots or a strong family history of blood clots. Keeping fit and active will help to protect you against a DVT. If a blood clot does occur it can be treated by blood thinners known as anticoagulants.

Blood clots can sometimes cause more serious problems so if there are any concerns about a possible DVT seek medical help urgently. If some of the blood clot breaks off and goes to the lungs it can cause a pulmonary embolism (PE). A PE usually causes a sudden onset of sharp chest pains that are worse on taking a deep breath or difficulty breathing. If a blood clot breaks off and goes to the brain, this can cause a stroke. The increase chance of dying from a fatal stroke or a pulmonary embolism due to Tamoxifen is small at less than one in 1000 women.

Tamoxifen acts like an oestrogen in the uterus so can stimulate the uterus and cause changes to its lining; this uterine lining is called endometrium. Tamoxifen can cause an increased thickness of the lining which is called 'endometrial hyperplasia'; if these cells become abnormal then it could develop into endometrial cancer. Fortunately, endometrial hyperplasia or cancer can usually be noticed early because they cause abnormal vaginal bleeding. If you have intermittent (not part of a normal cycle) vaginal bleeding or bleeding after sexual intercourse then you should see your GP or hospital doctor for further tests. Often abnormal bleeding can also be due to a non-cancerous growth such as an endometrial polyp. There is no way of telling this apart from early endometrial cancer without having investigations to look at the uterus. These usually include an ultrasound scan and a hysteroscopy.

A hysteroscopy is the use of a camera passed into the uterus to have a look inside it. A biopsy of any abnormal or thickened areas can also be taken during this procedure and if any polyps are found they can be easily removed at the same time. If biopsies show endometrial cancer then usually it is detected at an early stage and can be cured relatively easily by having a hysterectomy. The total increase risk of endometrial cancer in women taking Tamoxifen that are less than 50 years old is very small or negligible. In older women the additional risk is less than 1%. Your individual risk may be higher if you have a family history of endometrial cancer or if you are overweight or diabetic. Overall, for the vast majority of women the benefits of taking Tamoxifen will outweigh this small risk.

Important Drug Interactions with Tamoxifen

A number of drugs can interact with Tamoxifen because of the way it is metabolized in the body. Usually Tamoxifen is converted by two enzymes to a much more active product called Endoxifen. Endoxifen has the ability to bind to oestrogen receptors on the breast cancer cells by about 100 times more effectively than Tamoxifen. The two enzymes involved in converting Tamoxifen to the active metabolite Endoxifen are enzymes called Cytochrome P2D6 known as 'CYP2D6' and Cytochrome P3A4 known as 'CYP3A4'. There is sufficient evidence to show that if the activity of either of these enzymes is reduced then it can reduce the effectiveness of Tamoxifen. This can happen due to interactions with other medications and some foods.

CYP2D6 Inhibitors

Some drugs inhibit CYP2D6 activity which then reduces the ability of Tamoxifen to be converted to the more active Endoxifen.

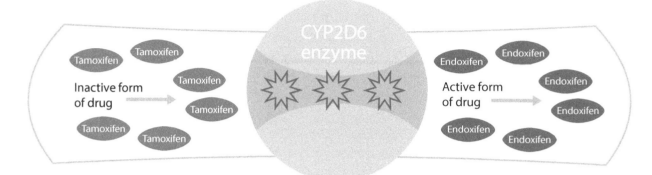

Therefore drugs that are known to be strong inhibitors of this enzyme should be avoided. Some SSRI antidepressants are strong inhibitors and so should not be used with Tamoxifen, they are Paroxetine and Fluoxetine.

The drug information leaflet for Tamoxifen advises against using drugs that that are strong inhibitors as listed in the table below.

CLASS OF DRUG	Strong Inhibitors	Moderate Inhibitors	Mild/ No Inhibition
ANTIDEPRESSANTS	Paroxetine	Sertraline	Venlafaxine
	Fluoxetine (Prozac)	Duloxetine	Mirtazapine
			Citalopram
SMOKING CESSATION	Bupropion (Zyban)		
ANTI ARRHYTHMIAS	Quinidine		
ANTIHISTAMINE	Diphenhydramine (Benadryl)		
ANTACID	Cimetidine		
REDUCING CALCIUM	Cinacalcet		

If you are taking antidepressants and Tamoxifen discuss it with your doctor. Citalopram is a good choice as it is generally well tolerated, can help with hot flushes and only has a mild effect on CYP2D6. Venlafaxine has very minimal or no effect on Tamoxifen, so is another antidepressant that can also be taken with Tamoxifen, it is usually given second line since it can have more potentially troublesome side effects than SSRIs. Another antidepressant called Mirtazapine also has minimal effect on CYP2D6; it is taken at night and can be helpful if you are suffering with sleep problems.

Ultimately it can be a complex and delicate process of asking for help and then finding the combination of medications that are right for you, but this is a process that is well worth embarking on with the support and guidance of your GP and hospital doctor.

CYP3A Inhibition

Cytochrome P 3A4 enzyme known as CYP3A4 is also involved in the metabolism of Tamoxifen and many other drugs. This enzyme is present in the liver and small intestine (first part of the bowel after the stomach). Many drugs are deactivated by CYP3A4 whereas others are activated by it; Tamoxifen is one of the drugs that are activated by CYP3A4. There is a chemical compound found in grapefruit that lowers the amount of CYP3A4 in the small intestine. The most commonly known group of drugs affected by eating grapefruit are statins (cholesterol lowering medications) and statins carry a medical warning not to consume grapefruit with them.

If levels of CYP3A4 are reduced then the full dose of Tamoxifen is not absorbed from the small intestine. In order to avoid this happening you shouldn't have grapefruit or grapefruit juice whilst on Tamoxifen. The effects of grapefruit can last up to 72 hours and will be worse if taken at the same time as Tamoxifen. There is a nutrient called tangeretin which is found in tangerine peel that can also reduce levels of CYP3A4 but since this is in the peel of the fruit rather than the flesh this really shouldn't be a problem.

Summary

Even though Tamoxifen has now been around for over fifty years, further research into its uses and the best duration of treatment continue. One very interesting aspect of this drug is its favourable 'knock on' effect whereby it continues to reduce breast cancer recurrence risk in the five to ten years after it is stopped. More evidence is emerging showing further reductions in risk when given for ten years. It was also approved by NICE in 2013 as a long term preventative treatment for those with an increased genetic predisposition to breast cancer. The tolerability of Tamoxifen varies considerably amongst individuals and I hope that in this chapter I have been able to give you some useful advice that may help. If you are still finding it difficult to cope after trying simple measures then I also hope that you feel more informed about other options that you can discuss with you GP or Breast Care Team. For women that cannot tolerate Tamoxifen an alternative SERM may be more suitable or another hormonal therapy that works by suppressing the ovaries, for example Zoladex could be used. I will talk about this and other therapies in the next chapter.

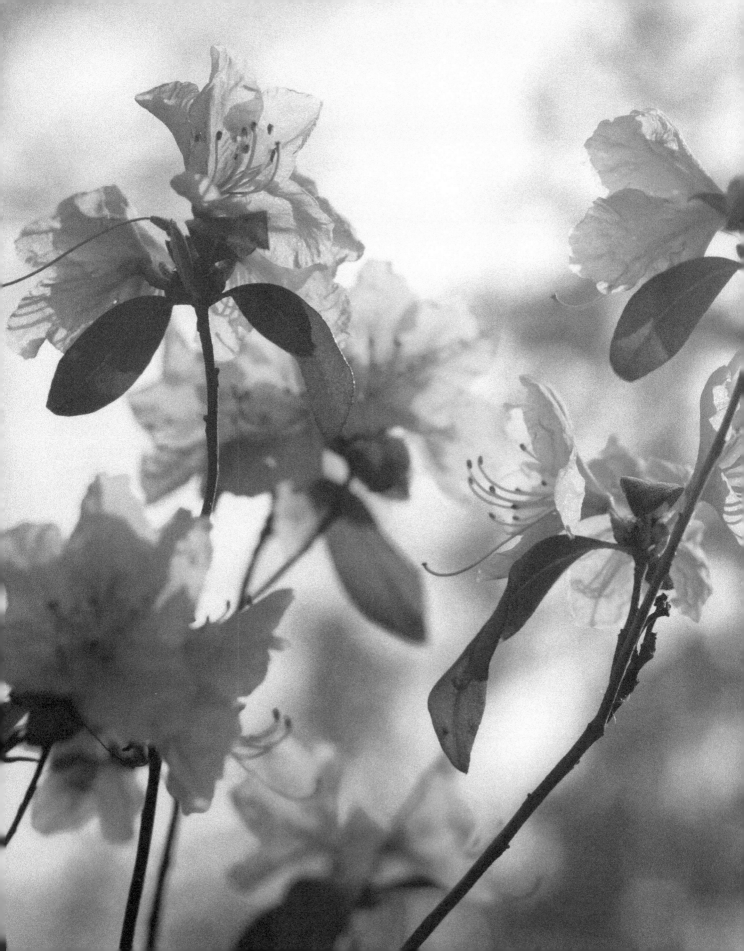

Aromatase Inhibitors

Since its introduction in the late 1980s, the routine use of Tamoxifen for women with ER + breast cancer soon became well established. It was another 15 years before another class of hormonal therapy was introduced. Research showed that these new medications were also very effective at reducing breast cancer recurrence but they were only useful for postmenopausal women with ER+ breast cancer. The reason for this lays in the different ways our body's produce oestrogen before and after the menopause. In premenopausal women the production of oestrogen occurs mainly in the ovaries. Whereas after the menopause women's ovaries stop working, ovulation no longer takes place and the ovaries can no longer produce oestrogen.

However, this does not mean that postmenopausal women do not produce any oestrogen. They can still make small amounts by changing hormones called androgens (male sex hormones) into oestrogen. Both men and women make androgens but in men they are present at much higher levels, these higher levels give men their masculinity. Androgens are made in the adrenal glands (which sit on top of the kidneys) and are then released into the bloodstream. They can then be converted to oestrogen by an enzyme called Aromatase. This enzyme is mainly found in fatty tissue and so this is the main site of oestrogen production in postmenopausal women.

Aromatase is the enzyme that converts circulating androgen hormones into oestrogen.

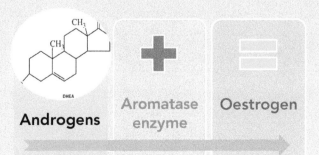

Androgens   Aromatase enzyme   Oestrogen

Aromatase Inhibitors

Medications called Aromatase Inhibitors, as the name suggests, block the actions of the aromatase enzyme and thereby stop the production of oestrogens in peripheral tissues. These inhibitors do not work in premenopausal women because they don't stop the more predominant production of oestrogen by the ovaries. The three main Aromatase Inhibitors (AIs) that are prescribed in the UK are:

Anastrozole   (Arimidex)

Letrozole   (Femara)

Aromasin   (Exemestane)

In the UK, since around 2006, most ER+ post-menopausal breast cancer survivors are now prescribed a daily tablet of Anastrazole or Letrozole. This change came about after the conclusive results of several large trials were published.

One of these, was a trial called ATAC (Anastrozole, Tamoxifen Alone or in Combination). This study began in 1999 and compared the use of Anastrozole instead of Tamoxifen. This involved researchers from around the world recruiting over 9000 postmenopausal women with early stage breast cancer. 84% of them had hormone receptor positive breast cancer. They were then randomly assigned, to take either Tamoxifen or Anastrozole or a combination of both for five years. The combination treatment wasn't any more effective than Tamoxifen alone so that arm of the study was stopped. Initial results were published in The Lancet by Professor Jack Cuzick and his team in 2005.

They were able to show that Anastrazole was actually better than Tamoxifen at reducing disease recurrence in ER+ postmenopausal women. Importantly there were also fewer side effects with the AIs in this group of women. The positive results from this study (as shown below) soon led to the widespread introduction of Aromatase Inhibitors.

In summary, the results showed that for postmenopausal ER+ women taking Anastrazole instead of Tamoxifen over a five year period that there was a

13 % improved disease free survival.

14% reduced relative risk of distant spread (metastases). This reduced the overall incidence of metastases from 12.1 % in the Tamoxifen group to 10.5% in the Anastrazole group over the five year follow up.

40% reduced relative risk of breast cancer occurrence in the other breast. This meant that the incidence of developing breast cancer in the other breast reduced from 1.9% to 1.1 % in the Anastrazole group.

Follow up of the trial participants continued for a further five years after the treatments were stopped and further results were published in 2010. The results also showed that Anastrazole gave a lower breast cancer risk recurrence compared with Tamoxifen but the groups had evened out more over time .

Another influential trial called the ATOLL (Articular Tolerance of Letrozole study) study showed that a person may tolerate one Aromatase Inhibitor better than another. The most common potential side effect that women on AIs find difficult to cope with is musculoskeletal aches and pains. This study confirmed that there could be a lot more flexibility with the choice of medication, since it showed that if a woman couldn't tolerate a particular AI, for example, Letrozole, that she may have fewer side effects with Anastrozole or Exemestane or vice versa.

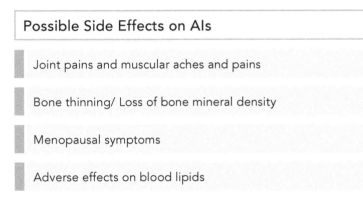

Possible Side Effects on AIs

Joint pains and muscular aches and pains

Bone thinning/ Loss of bone mineral density

Menopausal symptoms

Adverse effects on blood lipids

Joint and Muscle Pains

Joint pains seem to be the most common potential side effect caused by AIs. They can affect as many as 50% of women taking them and they are more likely to arise in women who have had a previous history of joint pains. A review published in the Journal, 'Annals of Oncology' (Jan 2013), states that up to 20% of women on AIs stop taking this medication because of problematic joint pains.

Generally these pains are symmetrical and affect the hands, wrist and knees in particular. Involvement in the hands and wrist may cause other problems such as Carpel Tunnel Syndrome and Trigger Finger. There may also be an increased incidence of muscular aches and pains in the morning leading to stiffness which may mean that it takes a while to get going in the morning. If these side effects occur they don't usually start immediately after starting the medication, instead they usually start several weeks later and tend to peak at around six months.

Interestingly data from the ATAC (as mentioned above) study also showed that those women who 'developed arthralgia within three months of starting endocrine (AI) therapy actually had a lower risk of breast cancer recurrence'. Why this happens is unclear and may be due to some other mechanism that induces both the joint pains and has an anti-tumour effect. Further research is needed since some other studies have reported conflicting results. However, if joint pains are related to a better outcome then it may be of some consolation to those that do get this side effect and may make it a bit easier to live with.

A number of smaller studies also suggest further lifestyle interventions can help. Being overweight has been shown to be a significant risk factor for developing AI induced joint pains. This was more apparent in women with a BMI > 30, and it may be partly due to the extra stress placed on their joints. A small study with just 43 women showed significant reductions in pain with acupuncture. Any form of regular exercise will generally help and some early data suggest that yoga in particular may be of benefit.

Bone Thinning

Postmenopausal women on Aromatase Inhibitors have lower levels of oestrogen as a result. Oestrogen usually helps to maintain bone density and bone strength so reduced levels can lead to an increased risk of bone thinning.

Therefore before being commenced on an Aromatase Inhibitor a baseline Bone Mineral Density (BMD) is measured in order to monitor your bone health. This is done by a special type of X-ray called a DEXA scan and this is repeated at 3-5 yearly intervals or as necessary. When bones are thin they have a low density and are more likely to fracture. Calcium and vitamin D supplements may be prescribed for you since they can both help with bone strength. Other medications called Bisphosphonates can also help to slow down bone thinning. Some studies show that Aromatase Inhibitors may lower vitamin D levels, and since vitamin D is important for healthy bones and joints, it is possible that this could also contribute to bone thinning and Aromatase Inhibitor (AI) induced joint pains.

The additional risk to bone thinning as a result of AIs usually returns back to normal when the AI is stopped. Everyone responds differently so the best drug for you will depend on whether you have any side effects and your previous medical history. For example, if someone already has osteoporosis and then DEXA scans show that this is getting worse whilst on an AI then they may be better switching over to Tamoxifen. However, in most cases Bisphosphonates, calcium and vitamin D can be used effectively to reverse some of the bone thinning. Walking and weight bearing exercises using light weights or resistance are also beneficial for bone strength.

Menopausal Symptoms

General measures to help with symptoms of menopause should be taken in the same way as with Tamoxifen (see Chapter 8). Aromatase Inhibitors are used in women who are already going through the menopause or have been through it. However, they can still increase menopausal symptoms as they will lower oestrogen levels further. However AIs are less likely to cause a problem with hot flushes

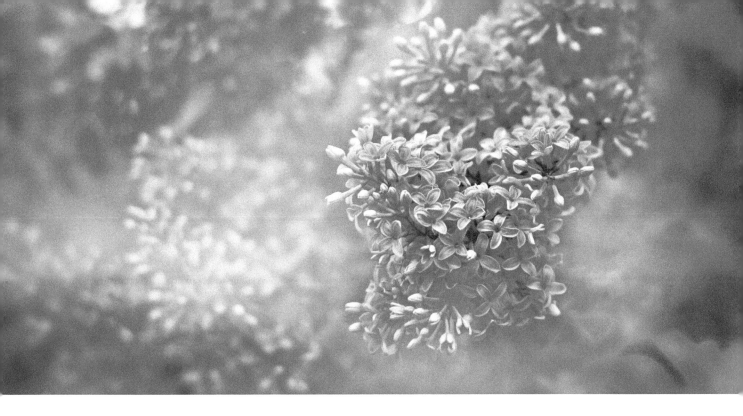

compared with Tamoxifen. The situation may be different for some women that were on hormone replacement therapy (HRT) when they were diagnosed and then had the HRT discontinued immediately. Normally when doctors stop HRT we would advise you to wean off it gradually over about three months to avoid withdrawal symptoms. Stopping HRT abruptly can cause a resurgence of menopausal symptoms. If symptoms are severe and general measures are not really helping then medications can sometimes help. SSRI and SNRI antidepressants can reduce the hot flushes and it is safe to use any of these including Paroxetine or Fluoxetine since they don't interact with AIs.

Lipid Profile

We already know that high cholesterol levels especially of the Low Density Lipid (LDL) variety contribute to an increased risk of coronary heart disease. Some studies show that AIs can increase LDL cholesterol but other studies don't support this finding so it is not entirely clear as yet what effect Aromatase Inhibitors have on cholesterol levels. Concerns about any adverse effect on lipid profiles haven't been sufficient enough to avoid giving AIs to women if they have a history of heart disease. I would encourage all women on AIs to get their cholesterol levels checked regularly at least once a year because of the potential risk. Embracing a healthy diet and regular exercise will also help to keep your cholesterol level within a normal range.

Other Treatments

Tamoxifen is by far the most common hormonal treatment for pre-menopausal women with ER+ breast cancer. It acts to block the effects of oestrogen on breast cancer cells. However, there are other treatment options available that can also be used in pre-menopausal women to suppress or stop the ovaries from working and so stop the production of oestrogen.

Ovarian Oblation

This suppression of the ovaries is given the general term, Ovarian Ablation. The following methods of ovarian ablation can be used.

Gonadotrophin Releasing Hormone (GnRH) Agonists

Surgical removal of the ovaries (i.e. Oophorectomy)

Radiotherapy to the ovaries (uncommon)

GnRH Agonists e.g. Goserelin / Zoladex

GnRH is an abbreviation for Gonadotrophin Releasing Hormone. This is a hormone produced by an area of the brain called the hypothalamus. The pituitary gland is attached to the base of the brain close to the hypothalamus. It is a very important gland as it controls the activity of most other hormone secreting glands.

In women when the pituitary gland releases FSH and LH it stimulates the ovaries to produce oestrogen and progesterone, this normally creates a feedback loop back to the brain that reduces the brains release of GnRH.

The GnRH from the hypothalamus stimulates the pituitary gland to produce two stimulating hormones called Follicle Stimulating Hormone (FSH) and Luteinizing Hormone (LH).

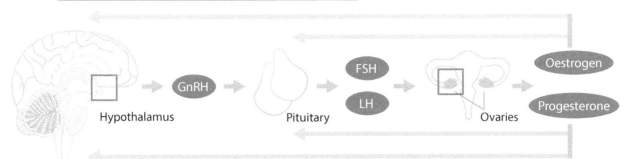

GnRH
Hypothalamus
Pituitary
FSH
LH
Ovaries
Oestrogen
Progesterone

A GnRH agonist causes an initial overstimulation of FH and LSH but then the pituitary gland becomes down regulated and stops releasing FSH and LF all together so effectively blocks oestrogen production

One of the most commonly used GnRH agonists in the UK is called Goserelin often known by its brand name Zoladex. Zoladex is given by a monthly injection just under the skin (subcutaneous) on the lower abdomen. Usually a woman's period stop shortly after the injection is first given. It is common to have some vaginal bleeding in the first few weeks after the initial Zoladex injection but if it doesn't settle then let your doctor know. This injection is usually continued for two years but is sometimes used for longer. When the treatment is finished periods usually recommence but if you are nearing the age of natural menopause when started on Zoladex then your periods may not return.

The side effects seen with Zoladex are due to the reduction of oestrogen and are similar to those of Tamoxifen. Joint pains are more likely to occur whilst on Zoladex compared with Tamoxifen but these are usually effectively treated with simple painkillers. Zoladex like other treatments that reduce oestrogen levels can also cause bone thinning and this will be monitored by periodic DEXA scans and treated if necessary. After the course of treatment is completed any side effects usually disappear. GnRH agonists are also used if ER+ breast cancer has spread to other areas of the body since it can also reduce the growth of these secondary tumours.

Another reminder is that Zoladex should not be considered to be a reliable contraceptive and barrier methods should be used. This is important because if you do become pregnant on Zoladex it can harm the developing baby.

Oophorectomy

Rather than suppressing the ovaries with drugs both ovaries can be surgically removed, this instantly removes the body's main source of oestrogen. Usually this procedure can be done by keyhole surgery otherwise known as laparoscopic surgery. This method is far less invasive than a larger more open incision to remove the ovaries as it involves making just a few much smaller cuts over the lower abdomen. The laparoscope and surgical tools can then be passed through these small incisions and the ovaries can be excised and removed. The recovery time from keyhole surgery is usually much faster and often involves a much shorter post-operative stay in hospital of just a couple of days. Keyhole surgery is not suitable for everyone especially if overweight or if there has been some previous pelvic surgery that has resulted in scar tissue being formed.

This surgical option may be the most appropriate one for women with a positive BRAC1 or BRAC2 gene since they are associated with an increased genetic predisposition to both breast and ovarian cancer. Oophorectomy removes the risk of future ovarian cancer. It may also be an option if the risks of taking Tamoxifen are too high, for example if you have a history of blood clots or endometrial cancer. Removing the ovaries will induce an immediate menopause so methods of managing the symptoms after this surgery are similar to managing the menopausal side effects of Tamoxifen. Oophorectomy may also be used if you are unable to tolerate the different drug therapies that suppress the ovaries.

Radiotherapy to the Ovaries

Radiotherapy to the ovaries can also be used to suppress them and stop them producing oestrogen permanently. This is usually given on an outpatient basis over several days. This method isn't used that often as it may cause localised side effects. These include diarrhoea, bloating and abdominal discomfort which can last a few days or a few weeks. Very rarely there may be damage to localised tissues. The radiotherapy doesn't cause an instant menopause but suppresses ovaries gradually over a few months so it usually takes a few months before periods cease with this method.

HER2 Positive Disease

Human epidermal growth factor (HER2) is a protein receptor that is found on the surface of normal breast cells. If there is too much of this protein it can stimulate the growth of cancer cells. When doctors check the cancer tissue that has been removed as well as looking for oestrogen and progesterone receptors they also look for the amount of HER2 receptors present on cells. If there are high levels of this protein then the cancer is called HER2 positive. About 20-25% of breast cancers are HER2 positive. Often if the cancer cells are HER2 positive the hormonal receptors are negative. However, if the cancer is also oestrogen or progesterone positive,

Normal breast cancer cell

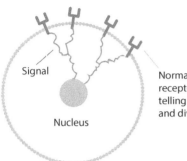

Signal

Nucleus

Normal amount of HER2 receptors send signals telling cells to grow and divide

Abnormal HER2+ breast cancer cell

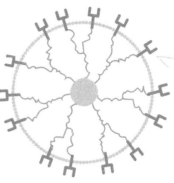

More HER2 receptors send more signals that stimulate the cells to grow and divide too quickly

then hormonal therapies can still be used alongside treatment specifically to treat the HER2 breast cancer.

Until recently HER2 positive cancers carried a worse prognosis as they tend to behave more aggressively. Targeted treatments have now been developed that treat HER2 positive cancers and improve the prognosis so that this is no longer the case. The most commonly used one is called Herceptin (trastuzumab). Herceptin is a drug that can specifically attach onto the HER2 protein on the cell surface. When it does so, it blocks the effect of the HER2 protein on cell growth.

Herceptin was initially trialled in the late 1990s and then used in women with HER2 advanced breast cancer. The financial cost was high at over £20,000 per treatment course with an improvement in life expectancy of just a few months in most cases. This created a lot of controversy and

whether it was offered became a postcode lottery, which in turn created a lot of media attention. Further trials then looked at the benefit to women with early breast cancer. One study was a large international study called HERA (Herceptin Adjuvant) that recruited over 5000 women between 2001 and 2005. The women were given just one year's treatment of Herceptin for early stage HER2 breast cancer. They found that women taking Herceptin had a 24 % reduced rate of recurrence at the end of the four year study period.

Herceptin was established as being cost effective from 2006. Thankfully NICE went on to approve Herceptin in their 2009 guidelines for early stage disease. Review of further studies showed a reduction in relapse of 50% and reduced risk of death by 30%.

Herceptin is usually given after completing other treatments such as surgery, chemotherapy and/or radiotherapy; it is sometimes used alongside chemotherapy. It is administered as an intravenous infusion once every 3 weeks for a year. The initial dose is given more slowly and monitoring for any adverse reactions continues for several hours afterwards. If it is tolerated then subsequent treatments are usually given over 30 minutes with a one to two hour period of observation afterwards.

Mild effects may occur such as headaches, flu-like symptoms, nausea or diarrhoea and are most likely to occur during treatment or immediately after. The potential more serious side effects involve the heart and/or a drop in white blood cell counts which can lead to serious infections. The majority of women will not have a problem. For example, the heart is only affected in about 2-7% of women on Herceptin. At the start of Herceptin treatment and throughout the course of treatment there will be close monitoring for any cardiovascular side effects. Herceptin can potentially cause changes in blood pressure, palpitations or shortness of breath. It can lower the ability of the heart muscle to pump as effectively as usual, thereby reducing its output (the ejection fraction).

To monitor for any heart problems your blood pressure is regularly checked and the heart is monitored by periodic heart tracings (ECG). An ultrasound scan of the heart called an echocardiogram looks at how well the heart is pumping. The echocardiogram is usually done before treatment starts and every 3 months or sooner if indicated. If serious side effects occur then Herceptin is stopped and the abnormality treated. People who already have a history of heart problems or poorly controlled high blood pressure may not be able to receive this treatment due to a higher level of risk. As per usual the benefits and risks have to be weighed up individually.

A fairly new subcutaneous version of the drug was approved by NHS England in September 2013 and is starting to be used more widely. Studies have shown it works just as well as the intravenous form. This is advantageous in terms of ease (a small injection under the skin), avoiding further injury to veins, less time (just takes a few minutes) and the cost savings including reduced staffing, use of hospital facilities and the reduced cost of administering it.

Through further research it has also been found that combining Herceptin with a combination of specific chemotherapy drugs has brought about even greater benefits for patients with HER2 breast cancer. This combination of drugs usually includes Herceptin alongside one from each of the groups below:

Taxane Drugs

Taxol

Taxotere

Anthracycline Drugs

Doxorubicin

Epirubicin

Triple Negative Disease

If breast cancer cells do not have any hormone receptors on them and they are also not HER2 positive then this is called triple negative disease. It has a genetic link and women with BRCA1 mutations are more likely to develop triple negative disease. African-American women are also more likely to develop triple negative disease but it can occur in any ethnic group. As well as these findings it also seems to affect mainly younger women.

In triple negative disease neither hormonal therapies nor Herceptin will offer any benefit. Having said that triple negative disease has been found to be more responsive to chemotherapy than the other receptor positive breast cancers. Breast cancer cells tend to divide and grow relatively quickly in triple negative disease and since chemotherapy works best on cells that are rapidly dividing, when these tumours are found early they are very receptive to certain chemotherapy regimes. If you have been diagnosed with triple negative disease then it might be worth talking to your doctor about genetic testing, especially if you have a close relative who has also had breast or ovarian cancer.

Diet and Exercise for Healthy Bones

Women on hormonal therapies will benefit from adhering to a diet and lifestyle plan that maintains healthy strong bones and keep hot flushes at bay. Any dietary advice given in different chapters in this book will overlap but I think it helps to show how you can target specific issues by adjusting your diet to your needs. Maintaining a healthy weight, having a diet rich in calcium, vitamin D and omega 3 fatty acids will be beneficial for both your bones, joints, skin, hair and nails and for a healthy heart.

Foods Rich in Calcium

Many people think the best source of calcium is from dairy. But there are many non-dairy sources that can provide you with all the calcium you need. When buying dairy produce it is worthwhile buying low-fat diary produce rather than full fat since it has less saturated fat and I would also recommend organic dairy if possible. Aim to consume about 1200mg of dietary calcium a day in your diet. Some good sources of calcium are listed below and following page.

Low fat dairy, 1-2 servings a day. (300-600 mg Calcium)

Alternatively use non-dairy calcium enriched alternatives: soya milk, rice milk, almond or coconut milk.

Fortified soya products such as tofu.

Green leafy vegetables such as: broccoli, green beans, kale and okra. A serving of these can contain up to 100 mg of calcium.

Legumes: chick peas, red kidney beans, pulses.

Nuts especially almonds, Brazil nuts and hazelnuts.

Seeds especially sesame seeds

Oily fish e.g. sardines, salmon, mackerel.

Fruits, e.g. oranges, tangerines, kiwi, rhubarb, prunes and dates.

Foods Rich in Vitamin D

You can get vitamin D from sunshine so exposing your skin to sunshine for twenty minutes every day (if possible!) is good for you. Just try and avoid it around the middle of the day and don't overdo it.

Oily Fish

Egg yolks

Fortified cereals

Good Sources of Calcium	
FOOD	**AMOUNT OF CALCIUM (MG)**
Glass (250ml) of semi- skimmed milk	300mg
Glass of soya milk, fortified almond or other non-dairy milk	300mg
Half a cup of Tofu	200- 400mg
Serving of dark green vegetables	100-200mg
Portion of chick peas (200g)	200mg
Handful of almonds	100mg
Sesame seeds (30g)	250mg
Tin of sardines	350mg

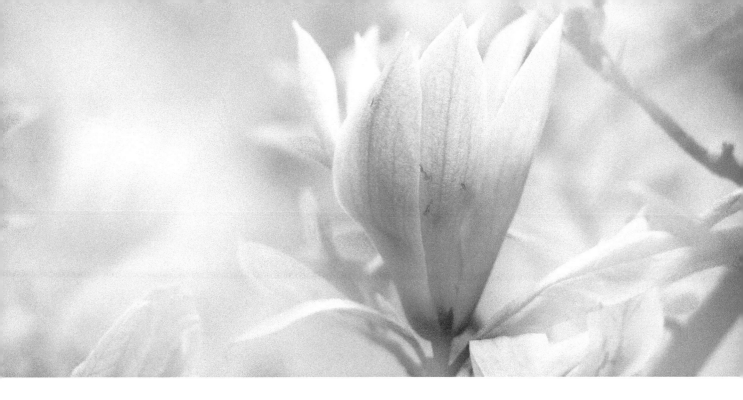

Weight Bearing Exercise

Aim for at least 30 minutes of exercise each day. Any exercise is good for maintaining muscle and bone strength, and cardiovascular health. Weight bearing exercises are particularly beneficial for improving and maintaining your bone density. These include the following:

Walking,

Jogging

Dancing

Sports e.g. tennis, golf.

Weight training using light weights

Summary

As well as remaining vigilant about practicing regular monthly breast self-examination (see chapter 7) I hope you now have a better knowledge of why and when further medical treatment is prescribed .Hopefully I have been able to demonstrate how these tailored treatments have been absolutely paramount to the increased long term survival rates of breast cancer patients.

The next thing I would like you to consider is how changes in our environment may be having an impact on the increased incidence of breast cancer over the last few decades. As well as the oestrogen our bodies make naturally there are external sources of oestrogen that we may be exposed to with or without our knowledge. The ones we know about include the Combined Oestrogen Pill and Hormone Replacement Therapy. However there has been concern in the last few decades that we are also being exposed to increasing amounts of chemicals in our environment that are proven to actually mimic oestrogen in cell and animal studies.

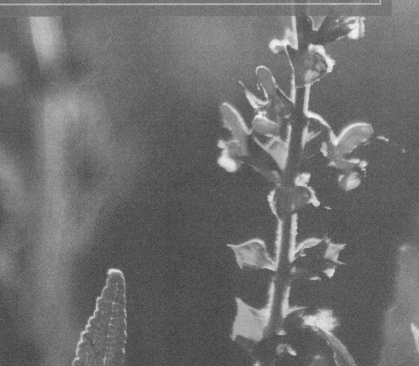

PART

3

Looking After Yourself

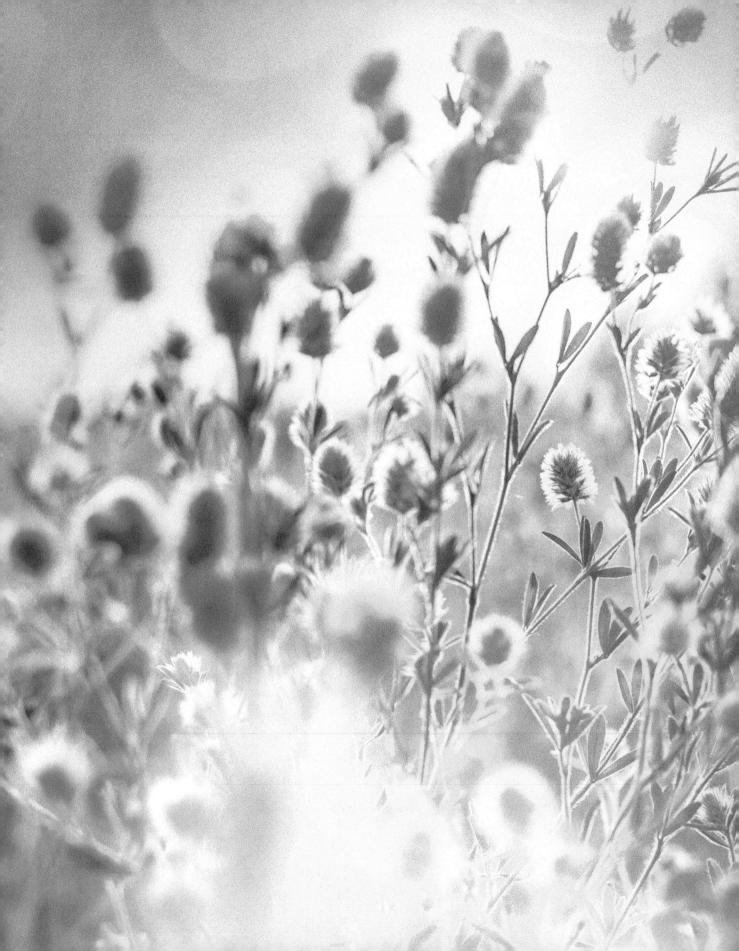

The Role of Hormonal Factors in Breast Cancer

Currently, extensive research is being carried out to explore possible links between certain environmental chemicals and some increasingly prevalent diseases, including cancers and reproductive disorders. This is a difficult subject to unravel since the research is still ongoing, but there are increasing concerns about a number of environmental chemicals that may be interfering with our hormones. Whilst they are being evaluated these chemicals can still be found in many Personal Care Products (PCPs); this term encompasses the many products that we use in our daily grooming. PCPs include all bathing and showering products, antiperspirants, deodorants, skincare and cosmetics.

Your Skin as a Protective Barrier

Not only does your skin affect your appearance but it has many other important roles too - it is your body's largest organ. Your skin acts as a protective physical barrier between your body and the environment, forming the first line of defence against microbes and toxins. Your skin also helps to regulate your body's temperature; when you are hot your skin produces sweat and when this evaporates from the skin's surface it helps to cool you down. When you are cold the hairs on your skin stand on end giving your skin the appearance of goose bumps and this traps a layer of warm air around your body. Your skin is also a highly sensitive organ that allows you to experience pleasurable sensations and receive feedback from your environment through touch. Ultimately when your skin is soft and healthy it makes you look and feel good and its function is optimised.

Sadly however, after chemotherapy or radiotherapy your skin may not be looking its best due to the side effects of these treatments. Chemotherapy tends to cause a number of generalised affects to the skin; these include skin rashes, dry skin, an increased sensitivity to products used on the skin and an increased sensitivity to sunlight which results in the skin becoming darker. Sometimes hands and feet can be particularly affected becoming red, swollen and itchy. Radiotherapy causes similar skin reactions but these are localised to the area being treated. Usually you will have needed one or both of these adjuvant treatments but even if your skin hasn't been exposed to either of these, you should still consider paying a bit more attention to how you look after your skin.

As well as acting as a protective layer between the environment and your body, your skin is also a permeable layer. This means that products rubbed onto the skin can penetrate through the surface of the skin into the deeper layers making the skin a potential entry route into the body for many chemicals. Whilst taking care of your skin it is worth considering what exactly we put onto our skin and whether these products could have any unwanted side effects if they are absorbed into the body.

A number of drugs are actually administered by applying them to the skin, these are called topical medications and include anti-inflammatory gels, analgesic patches, HRT patches and nicotine patches to name a few. If these drugs can be effectively absorbed into the body this way, then surely it is possible that other chemicals can also enter the body via the skin.

Environmental Chemicals

Our biggest risk of exposure to chemicals and potential toxins is through our diet so having a healthy diet is important. However, knowing what we are using in our Personal Care Products is also essential since some chemicals and toxins can be absorbed via the skin too. The presumption is that the chemicals in PCPs are safe, yet many of these substances were introduced decades ago without the rigorous testing and regulations that now exist. Government environmental agencies have explored some of the safety concerns and through the available research and their long history of safety data generally feel able to reassure us of an absence of risk for many of these chemicals.

However, through recent evaluation a number of chemicals that were previously used in PCPs have actually now been classified as being potentially harmful. As a result, in recent years an increasing number of chemicals have become restricted in their use or are in the process of being phased out altogether.

The Role of REACH

In the EU the European Chemical Agency assess the safety of chemicals in the European market and makes decisions about their use. Substances that are identified as being of Very High Concern (SVHC) to our safety are put onto a

REACH Candidate List of substances. REACH is a European Union regulation, which aims to improve and protect human health and the environment. The letters stand for Registration, Evaluation, Authorisation and restriction of Chemicals. Presently, there are over one hundred and fifty chemicals on the Candidate List. To fulfil the criteria for entry onto this list a chemical is either thought to potentially cause cancer, alter DNA or damage reproductive systems. Once a concern is raised about a chemical it is assessed further and if it is found to be harmful then it is put onto an Authorisation List. Once it is on the Authorisation List manufacturers have to abide by the restrictions set by REACH and a realistic period of time is then given to phase out the chemical. Once at this stage, authorisations to use the chemical can only be given to manufacturers in essential and very specific circumstances where no other suitable alternative exists.

The Endocrine System

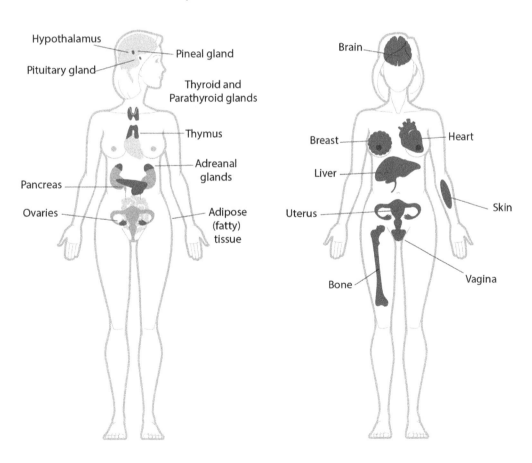

Major Components of the Female Endocrine System

Hypothalamus
Pineal gland
Pituitary gland
Thyroid and Parathyroid glands
Thymus
Adreanal glands
Pancreas
Ovaries
Adipose (fatty) tissue

Oestrogen Target Tissues

Brain
Breast
Heart
Liver
Skin
Uterus
Bone
Vagina

The environmental chemicals that we need to consider in relation to breast cancer risk are those that may interfere with our endocrine (hormonal) system. These are called Endocrine Disrupting Chemicals (EDCs). In women the endocrine system includes the ovaries, pancreas, adrenal glands, thyroid, the pituitary gland and others as shown on previous page. Hormone sensitive tissues include the breast, uterus, ovaries, and bones.

- Oestrogen plays an essential role in female sexual development.

- Along with other female sex hormones, oestrogen is essential for the normal development of female sex organs and breast tissue during puberty.

- A complex feedback mechanism exists between the brain's hypothalamus, the pituitary gland at the base of the brain and the ovaries. This gives rise to a cyclical production of female sex hormones that regulates menstruation and controls reproduction.

Too Much Oestrogen – What Does It Do?

At least 70% of breast cancers carry oestrogen receptors (ER+) and as a consequence oestrogen can stimulate these breast cancer cells. A woman's lifetime exposure to oestrogen is increased if she doesn't have children, has children later in life, and doesn't breast feed or only breast feeds for a relatively short period of time. This increased oestrogen exposure as a result of these changing reproductive habits is now known to increase the risk of breast cancer. I believe that as well as being aware of these factors, we should also be aware that we may be unwittingly exposed to oestrogen-like chemicals from external sources.

Hormone Replacement Therapy

The health concerns related to an increased exposure to oestrogen can be demonstrated by the use of Hormone Replacement Therapy (HRT). When women go through the menopause their ovaries stop working so that ovulation and the ovarian production of oestrogen stops. This leaves only the much smaller amounts of oestrogen that are made in other areas of our body. HRT has been used over the past 50+ years to treat the symptoms of menopause by replacing dwindling female sex hormones.

There are two main types of HRT. Women that have had a hysterectomy use HRT that contains only oestrogen. For women that still have a uterus a combination of oestrogen and progesterone is required; this is called 'Combination HRT'. The progesterone in the combined HRT is necessary as it stops overstimulation of the lining of the uterus; this lining is called the 'endometrium'. If oestrogen is used alone in these women this can cause an unwanted thickening of the endometrium which can increase the risk of endometrial cancer.

The prolific use of HRT waned just over a decade ago when medical opinion about HRT's safety was changed dramatically. This occurred as a result of scientific research that found an association between HRT and an increased risk of breast cancer.

Two of the largest studies on HRT took place in the 1990s. These were the

1. Women's Health Initiative (WHI) in the USA
2. Million Women Study (MWS) in the UK.

The findings of these two revealing studies were published during 2002 and 2003 and had a major detrimental impact on the use of HRT.

1 Women's Health Initiative Study (WHI)

In 1993 the Women's Health Initiative (WHI) study started to recruit postmenopausal women in the USA to take part in a randomised control trial (see Chapter 5) to look at the effects of HRT on a number of health problems including heart disease, strokes and breast cancer. By 1998 they had recruited almost 70,000 participants ranging in age from 50-79; the large number of women involved helped to increase the reliability and accuracy of the findings. At the beginning of the trial these women were asked questions about their previous or current HRT use and then divided into two similarly matched groups. One group were given HRT and the control group were given a placebo. Most women were given combined HRT, but if they had had a hysterectomy then oestrogen-only HRT was used.

The intention was to monitor the women over the following five years to explore whether the HRT led to different health outcomes in the two groups. However, the combined HRT arm was stopped early in 2002 as these women had not only an increased risk of breast cancer but also heart attacks, strokes and blood clots. The findings showed that for one year of HRT treatment an additional 8 women per 10,000 developed breast cancer. However there were some beneficial effects which included the relief of menopausal symptoms, a reduced risk of bowel cancer and a protective effect on bone density

2 Million Women's Study (MWS)

The Million Women's Study (MWS) was an observational study (see Chapter 5) looking at the health of over one million UK women aged between

50 to 64 years. The participants were recruited by sending invitations to women that were already attending for screening mammograms. The major criticism of this study is that the recruitment method could have led to bias because those women that already had concerns due to breast changes, or a suspicious mammogram finding and concerns over their current HRT use may have been more likely to respond and take part in the study. However the results along with other studies do seem to confirm a degree of risk.

The study was designed to investigate the effects of combination HRT and oestrogen-only HRT on the incidence of breast cancer. Questionnaires were used to gather information on the women's past and current HRT use. These women were then followed up for several years to see whether their use of HRT had any effect on the incidence of breast cancer. In the MWS they found that as many as a third of women were taking HRT at the time of the study and almost half of the one million women had used HRT at some point in time.

In current users of HRT they found that the risk of breast cancer was increased. This was seen especially in women using combined HRT and the risks were increased further the longer the HRT was used. Those women using combined HRT preparations for ten years were found to have an increased breast cancer incidence of an additional 19 per 1000 women compared to women that did not use HRT. Whereas, for oestrogen-only HRT used for ten years the women were found to have a smaller increased risk of just 5 per 1000 women. In past users, it was shown that the increased risk of breast cancer returned back to normal within five years of stopping HRT.

The findings of the MWS are shown in the table below.

MILLION WOMEN STUDY	10 years Combined Oestrogen and Progesterone HRT	10 years Oestrogen-Only HRT	PAST HRT Users
NO. OF ADDITIONAL CASES OF BREAST CANCER	19 per 1000 women	5 per 1000 women	Risk returned to normal after 5 years

In the 1990s when these studies were commenced the use of HRT was very widespread as women were keen to control their menopausal symptoms and doctors believed that its benefits far outweighed any risks for most women. However, as a direct result of these two trials, HRT use fell dramatically and a subsequent dip in breast cancer incidence was seen.

When Is HRT Used?

HRT is still prescribed to women struggling with menopausal symptoms including hot flushes, night sweats, poor sleep and mood changes, but now that it has been shown to cause a small increased risk of breast cancer, it is no longer seen as the most ideal treatment for menopausal symptoms. However, it can still be useful for women that are suffering severe menopausal symptoms that are significantly affecting their quality of life. HRT is also beneficial for bone health so may be of use for women that are at an increased risk of osteoporosis (bone thinning). When doctors prescribe HRT they will assess each woman's symptoms and medical history individually to determine whether the benefits to them outweigh the risks.

The findings of the WHI and MWS have resulted in several recommendations. These guidelines include prescribing the lowest possible dose of oestrogen to alleviate symptoms, shorter durations and closer monitoring. For women undergoing menopause at around the average age, hot flushes and night sweats usually settle after 2-3 years so attempts to come off it around this time should be made if not before. Generally it is advisable for women not to use it for longer than five years and with regular yearly review by their doctor. The longer that HRT is used then the higher the increased risk of breast cancer is, but this risk returns to normal within a few years of stopping HRT.

When Shouldn't HRT Be Used?

HRT is contraindicated in women that have a family history of hereditary breast cancer and those that have had a breast cancer diagnosis themselves. Women that have been taking HRT at the time of breast cancer diagnosis are advised to stop it immediately. This is recommended whether the breast cancer is hormone receptor positive or not. Women with breast cancer that have undergone an early menopause due to the side effects of treatment cannot receive HRT.

Endocrine Disrupting Chemicals (EDCs)

The use of HRT is carefully monitored and its potential side effects are known but many people are unaware that we may also be repeatedly exposed to external oestrogen-like chemicals from unexpected environmental sources. Some synthetic chemicals have been shown in cell and animal studies to interfere with the normal production or action of female sex hormones or to mimic oestrogen. They are known as Endocrine Disrupting Chemicals (EDCs) or oestrogen mimickers.

These synthetic chemicals are widely used for a variety of purposes in PCPs including cosmetics and perfumes as well as in household cleaners, plastics and many other products that we regularly come into contact with. There is a theory that our exposure to these chemicals from an early age could partly explain the changing patterns of earlier onset of puberty, problems with fertility and the younger age distribution of women getting breast cancer over the past few decades. 2010 was the first year in the UK in which 10,000 women (out of a total of 50,000) diagnosed with breast cancer, were under the age of 50 years. One in 5 women diagnosed with breast cancer in the UK are now in this younger age group.

These oestrogen-mimicking chemicals have been considered largely harmless in the past, since they are present at much lower levels in manufactured products compared with the levels of oestrogen that are produced naturally by our body. Yet there is increasing concern that these very small amounts may be absorbed into our body and become deposited and stored in fatty tissue allowing them to accumulate over time. Our breasts consist of mainly fatty tissue and so they become a potential target area.

Differences between Oestrogen and Oestrogen Mimickers

Reassuringly oestrogen-mimickers have been shown to be thousands of times less potent than the naturally produced oestrogen made in our bodies. So then, why the concerns about these chemicals that may mimic oestrogen, if these are much weaker oestrogens? The main differences between these chemicals and naturally produced oestrogen are as follows.

1. Our own oestrogen production is regulated by a complex feedback mechanism that maintains a healthy and balanced environment within our body. Hormones are usually released in response to stimuli which bring about a stable and balanced hormonal response. Even small amounts of artificial and hormonally active agents may disrupt this at a cellular level.

2. There are restrictions placed on the amounts of each chemical that can be used in the manufacturing of individual products. However, these 'safe' levels of chemicals have only been looked at in isolation. Therefore we still do not know whether their effect is amplified when they exist in combination with other potential endocrine disruptors or other chemicals found in the products we use each day.

3. In general, these EDCs are present in very tiny amounts within personal care products, but it is unclear at present what concentrations are found within cells.

4. We don't know what components these chemicals are broken down into and what potential dangers these by-products may have.

5. We do not know over what length of time it may take for them to accumulate and what effects this may have.

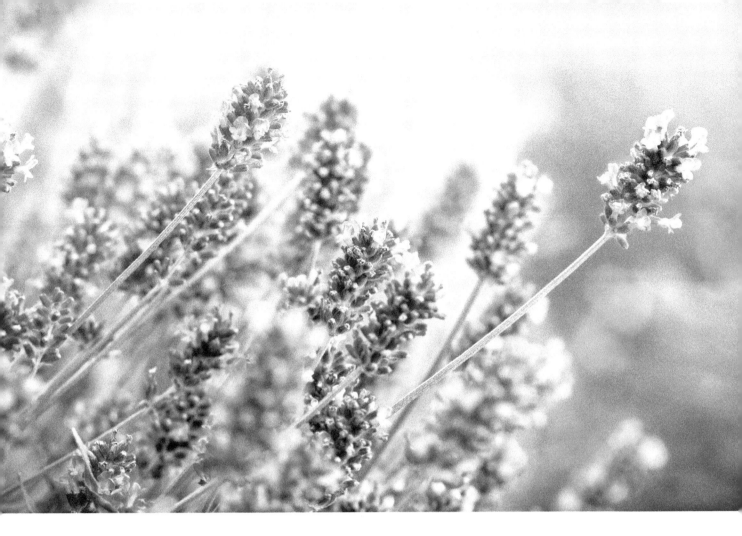

As a result of research on EDCs and possible links to health problems, governments and manufacturers are taking more responsibility for the use of a number of chemicals. Some cosmetic, food and manufacturing companies have already started re-examining their products and have stopped using some chemicals where there appears to be a significant risk. The use of chemicals in PCPs is something I had never considered before being diagnosed with breast cancer. However I am now convinced that we do need to be more thoughtful about what goes into our bodies whether it is from what we eat and drink or from products applied to our skin. Until all the chemicals of very high concern have been fully assessed I suggest that you become more vigilant and aware about chemicals that may act as endocrine disruptors so that you can reduce your exposure to them wherever possible.

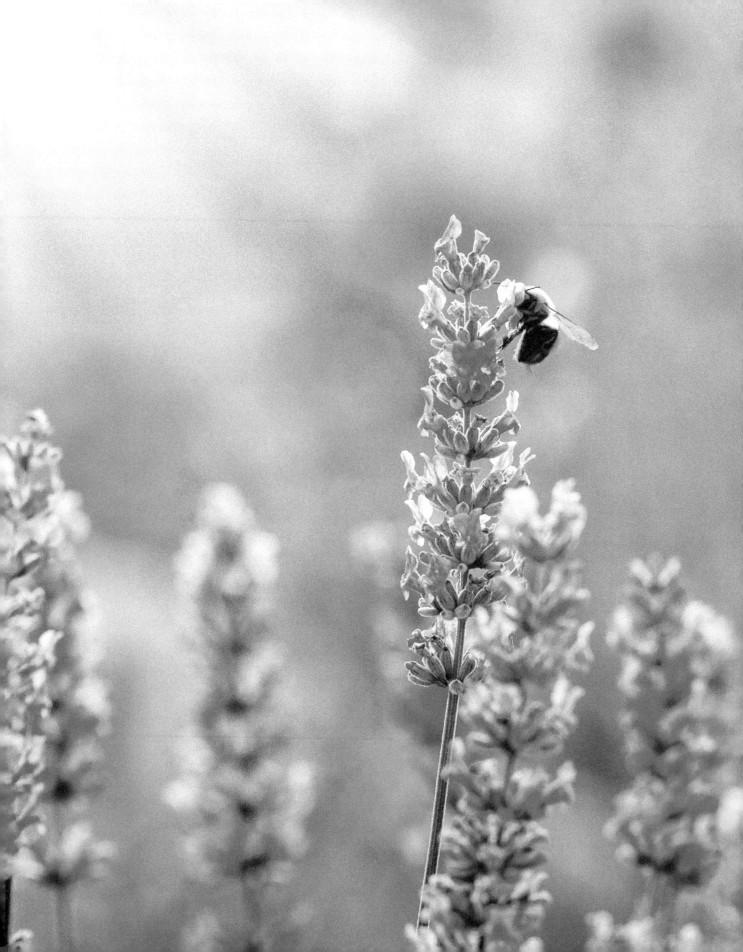

Reducing Your Exposure to EDCs

There are many conflicting reports and opinions on environmental chemicals that may possess endocrine disrupting properties. This difference of opinion is very evident especially amongst Environmental Groups and The Cosmetics Industry. Some breast cancer charities such as Breast Cancer UK and Breast Cancer Care Fund are also raising concerns and campaigning against the use of Endocrine Disrupting Chemicals (EDCs). However, other breast cancer charities remain resolute in their belief that there is no proven link with breast cancer. Breast cancer survivors often try to thrash out the debate on forums but are clearly just as divided and so it remains a huge area of controversy.

Having read a lot of the available research I am now convinced that it is worth considering how you can reduce your exposure to certain environmental chemicals. I have provided you with a summary of the available research to enable you to make your own carefully considered choices. I have also included some tips at the end of this chapter on practical ways to reduce your exposure to these environmental chemicals if you choose to. Opposite is a list of the chemicals that have been suggested as being the main culprits in interfering with our hormones and therefore potentially increasing the risk of breast cancer.

List of Potential Endocrine Disruptors

Parabens

Phthalates

BPA

Triclosan

Perflourinated chemicals

Parabens

Parabens are a group of EDCs which are widely used in Personal Care Products (PCPs) and are also used in some food and pharmaceutical products. This group of synthetic chemicals act as broad-spectrum preservatives and they appeal to manufacturers and consumers alike as they extend the shelf-life of many products by inhibiting the growth of bacteria, yeast and moulds. They are also colourless, odourless and non-irritating and so for these reasons as well as their low cost, they have been widely used in PCPs since the 1950s.

Synthetic parabens are often used in a huge variety of PCPs including hand soap, body wash, face creams, body lotions, hair care products, toothpaste, spray tans, sun creams and makeup. They are generally believed to be safe since the amounts in an individual product are restricted to very low levels. Also in cell studies parabens have been shown to exert a very weak oestrogenic effect by as much as tens of thousands of times less potent than the oestrogen our body makes naturally. Naturally occurring parabens are also present in some plant foods such as blueberries, strawberries, carrots and olives. In these foods they are present at minute levels e.g. <0.003% in blueberries. These natural sources in food exist alongside powerful antioxidants and phytonutrients so their overall effect is certainly beneficial.

Synthetic parabens exist in PCPs in concentrations of less than 1% and often much lower. If parabens are present they are usually listed on the product's label of ingredients and often can be easily identified if you read the label. The most commonly used parabens include methylparaben, propylparaben, butylparaben and ethylparaben. These preservatives share a common chemical structure called para-hydroxybenzoate or are esters of these. Forgive me, but the reason for discussing the complexities of parabens is that sometimes parabens are not immediately recognisable on product labels since they can have other perfectly legitimate names. For example, methylparaben may also be called: methyl p-hydroxybenzoate, methyl 4-hydroxybenzoate and p-hydroxybenzoic acid methyl ester.

However, before you admit defeat and throw in the towel, PCPs that don't contain parabens will usually emphasise the fact that they are 'PARABEN-FREE' which makes them a whole lot easier to identify. The current evidence available on the safety of parabens has been considered by the Cosmetics Industry and although they still proclaim their safety they are starting to produce more paraben-free products allowing for more consumer choice. When parabens are used as a food preservative in processed foods they are given a specific E number, these are methylparaben (E218), propylparaben (E216) and ethylparaben (E214). The easiest way to avoid these is to eat less processed food and instead cook meals using fresh ingredients or use foods where preservatives have not been added.

The potential adverse effects of parabens on our health wasn't really questioned until more recent years and only became widely debated after a small but influential study about parabens was published in 2004. This study was led by a researcher called Dr Darbre from The University of Reading, UK. She is a Molecular Biologist with a PhD in Oncology. It was a small study involving just 20 women with breast cancer who each required a mastectomy. The breast tissue removed at surgery was then analysed for parabens. This research study raised the concern regarding parabens since it indisputably confirmed the presence of up to six different parabens in each woman's breast tissue. Dr Darbre concluded that their presence did not mean they had caused the cancer but she had clearly shown that parabens had managed to get into the breast tissue of these women with breast cancer. She also explained that these parabens had entered the body via the skin since they were intact and were not broken down. If they had been ingested they would have been broken down by the liver into their different by-products.

Dr Darbre and Consultant Surgeon, Mr Lester Barr (Chairman of Manchester, UK, Genesis Breast Cancer Prevention Charity), teamed up to do a further study published in 2012. This was a study of 40 women between 2005 and 2008 who all had a mastectomy for primary breast cancer. Their breast tissue was sampled from the four areas covering the breast and then analysed for parabens. One or more parabens were found in 99% of the 160 samples analysed. The reason it was taken from the four quadrants around the whole breast is that the site of breast cancer is highest in the upper outer quadrant (UOQ) towards the armpit and there are different theories for what the reason for this may be.

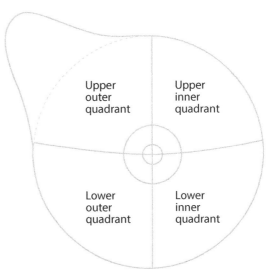

Taking samples from each quadrant allowed comparisons of paraben levels to be made between each area of the breast. This study showed that the concentration of parabens was higher in the UOQ and there have been theories that the predominance of parabens in the UOQ could be related to the use of underarm deodorants. Antiperspirants generally haven't contained parabens for a number of years now but they are still sometimes present in deodorants, however seven of the women in the study group said they never used underarm deodorant. Therefore this study suggests that other areas of our skin are the routes for parabens getting into breast tissue rather than just coming locally from underarm products. This study could not conclude that parabens caused the breast cancer but their presence in breast tissue did fuel the ongoing debate as to whether they play a role.

Studies That Confirm the Widespread Presence of Parabens

Studies involving thousands of people have shown that parabens are present in most men, women and children. One of these is The Nhanes Study on Parabens (2005-2006) involving a diverse group of over 2,500 men and women, and children over the age of six years from the USA. The results showed 99% of the group had methylparaben in their urine. The proportion with other parabens was also very high (42-92%) and reflected their proportionate presence in PCPs. These findings are probably to be expected considering how widely used these chemicals are. On average men and women use at least 5-15 PCPs a day respectively, each possibly containing parabens or other endocrine disruptors. Significantly greater amounts were detected in women compared to men by about 3-5 fold; this reflects women's greater use of cosmetics and body care products.

As a result of their far-reaching uses other studies have shown that parabens are also present at very low levels in our wider environment. They have been detected in the wastewater from treatment plants, in rivers and even drinking water sources. They can also be found at low concentrations in agricultural soil.

Restrictions on the Use of Parabens

Media coverage of the research findings involving breast cancer patients and parabens did create some high impact but rather misleading headlines that caused a stir but were soon forgotten. The previously mentioned study of 40 breast cancer patients led to the following newspaper headline in The Daily Mail, Jan 2012. 'Chemicals found in deodorants, face cream and food products is discovered in tumours of ALL breast cancer patients'. This headline is grabbing but can clearly be misinterpreted.

However, due to sufficient evidence of their endocrine disrupting properties and following years of debate the European Commission is acting to regulate the use of some parabens. Recent European measures to reduce their use include the following. Five (lesser used) parabens have already been banned completely in Denmark since 2011. Also in Denmark, the much more widely used propyl and butyl paraben have been banned in all products for children under three years old. In the rest of the European Union the use of propyl and butyl parabens have only been banned in leave-on products for children under the age of three; these include products such as nappy creams, body oils and lotions. The EU also put regulations in place in 2014 to reduce the allowed maximum concentrations of propyl and butyl parabens in any product from 0.4% to just 0.14%. Although these measures are reassuring, my question is, shouldn't these restrictions be extended? As young children the majority of us will have already have been exposed to parabens in PCPs. I suspect the restrictions will be increased over time but until them we can make a choice to limit our own and our family's exposure to them.

Phthalates

Phthalates are another group of synthetic chemicals that have also been shown to act as endocrine disruptors in cell and animal studies. They are used in PCPs to hold in moisture, act as a lubricant and make products less brittle. They are also more widely used in plastics to make them softer, more flexible and durable. These desirable properties mean that they clearly have a broad range of uses.

Phthalates may be present in many PCPs especially shampoos, conditioners, perfumes, make up, nail polish and hairspray. Their presence in very small quantities in these and many other products often comes under the label 'parfum' or 'fragrance'. In this guise the individual ingredients of parfum don't need to be listed and often there are hundreds of ingredients in a scent, so it just wouldn't be feasible to list them all on the label. Phthalates are widely used in scents to make them evaporate more slowly which makes the smells last longer. Products that contain only natural ingredients to give off a scent usually specify this at the bottom of the list of ingredients.

In terms of structure and safety they are divided into two groups, those with 'high' and those with 'low' molecular weight. The high phthalates are deemed safe, they don't act as endocrine disruptors and account for about 85% of the European market. However, the low phthalates have been shown to act as endocrine disruptors and include dibutyl phthalate (DBP), diethylhexyl phthalate (DEHP) and butyl benzyl phthalate (BBP). These three phthalates are all on the REACH Candidate List of Substances of Very High Concern (SVHC). Low phthalates are commonly used in cosmetics and PCPs so again put women at a potentially higher risk of exposure to them and any adverse effects.

Occupational exposure of phthalates and other environmental chemicals in the plastics industry demonstrates the potential risks of these chemicals in humans. Employees in these industries clearly will have a greater exposure to them and they have been shown to have a higher incidence of certain diseases including hormonally related cancers and reproductive problems. High exposure amongst premenopausal women working in the plastics and rubber industries results in at least a two fold increase risk of breast cancer. These women also have an increased risk of having sons born with hypospadias (a congenital abnormality of boys' genitalia.) Male workers are also affected and have been shown to have reduced sperm counts and fertility.

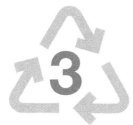

Avoid Recyclable '3' Plastics

Phthalates are found in PVC plastics. If the plastic product contains phthalates it is labelled '3' in the triangle sign (the recycling number) which is usually found on the bottom of containers.

Most throwaway water and drink bottles are number '1' recyclables and these are safe. Otherwise you will see 'PET' or 'PETE' on the bottom of plastic bottles. This stands for polyethylene terephthalate and although it has phthalate in its name it is actually very different from this chemical and is not known to be of concern. However it is important to avoid these plastics becoming heated and not to re-use these plastic bottles. They can leach chemicals if repeatedly re-used, recycle them instead.

Restrictions on the Use of Phthalates

There is sufficient evidence of harm already available to begin the process of reducing the use of phthalates. The three low phthalates that are of very high concern, i.e. DEHP, DBP and BBP have already been banned from plastics involved in the manufacturing of children's toys in the EU. A temporary ban was initially introduced in 1999 and this was made permanent in 2005. The US followed suit shortly afterwards. The good news is that in Europe the low phthalates have also been banned in cosmetics for many years. Cosmetics made in Europe are made under much stricter regulations than those from some other parts of the world.

Despite the ban on low phthalates in cosmetics, two major loopholes still exist. They can still be present in imported products or hidden in the 'parfum'. The USA does not have the same bans at the current point of writing however the majority of American cosmetics manufacturers have already followed Europe's lead.

Most forward thinking companies prefer to keep one step ahead and no doubt look at what is happening elsewhere in the world. This has led to many large global companies making the decision to revise their products and not use phthalates. Looking at the progress in the industry it appears that the publication of scientific research and pressure from consumers does seem to be having a positive impact.

Bisphenol A (BPA)

BPA is one of the most common chemicals we are exposed to and like parabens and phthalates it is also ubiquitous. BPA has been used since the 1960s in the manufacturing of hard plastics which are then used to make items such as food storage containers, drinking bottles, baby bottles and toddler cups. BPA is also used in resins that make the lining of some cans for food and drinks. Recyclable plastics with '7' in the triangle on the bottom contain BPA. BPA is unstable so traces may be released from plastic containers and bottles into the food and drink they carry. This is much more likely to occur when they are heated at high temperatures. So babies who are at a vulnerable stage of development are potentially at risk from milk heated in BPA plastic bottles.

Cell studies show that the presence of BPA increases the growth of breast cancer cells and therefore BPA exposure remains an area of concern. Its effects can also be demonstrated by the results of studies on occupational exposure to BPA. A Canadian case-control study published by JT Brophy and his colleagues in 2012, in the journal Environmental Health, explored whether there were any links between certain occupational environments and breast cancer risk. They found that premenopausal women who had worked in the automotive plastics or food canning industry for ten years or more were at an increased risk. The high occupational levels of phthalate or BPA resulted in a two to five fold increase risk of breast cancer depending on the level of exposure. The risk was more evident in women compared with men and may reflect the higher proportion of women working on the shop floor in these industries.

Restrictions on BPA

You may have noticed that baby bottles are now labelled 'BPA-free' in the UK (Canada, USA and China). This is one of the very first plastic products from which this chemical was banned. The EU banned baby bottles containing BPA in 2011 so they were no longer allowed to be imported and had to be removed from shelves. When there is a concern for the safety of young children then my own view is that this should be extended to protect older children and adults. The effects of BPA could take many years to accumulate. Since the ban on BPA in bottles and cups for young children you will see that there are many more BPA-free water bottles and plastic storage containers available and so it is now possible to change over to these quite easily. Reducing the amounts of processed and packaged foods you consume will also reduce your exposure to BPA that may be present in the packaging.

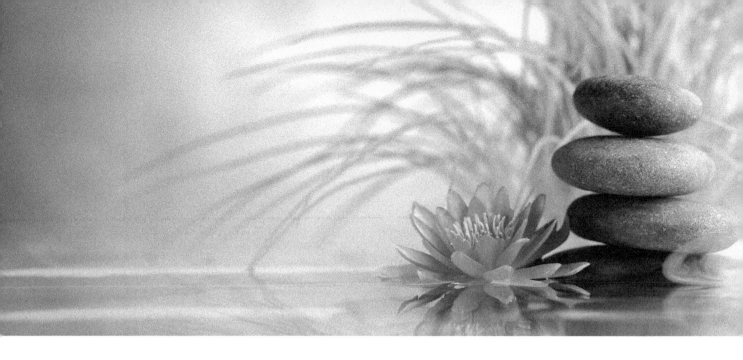

Triclosan

Triclosan is a synthetic antibacterial used in some PCPs but is most commonly found in some antibacterial soap washes. This chemical can mimic oestrogen in cell and animal studies and also disrupt thyroid function. In order to avoid triclosan, look at the label on antibacterial products. Not all antibacterial products contain triclosan, so if you need to use them try and avoid the ones containing triclosan. Many global manufacturers of these products have reformulated their products so they no longer contain triclosan.

There is also a striking argument against the routine use of antibacterial hand wash since this leads to their subsequent entry into wastewater and hence into soil and into the environment. The increased use of sanitizers, antibacterial products and antibiotics in general appears to have contributed to a dampened immune system in humans and is also likely to have played a part in ever increasing levels of antibiotic resistance. 'Public Health England' and 'The USA Centre of Disease Control and Prevention' both recommend that in a normal setting, there is no benefit to washing hands with these products. Although these products remove more bacteria and viruses in the first instance within minutes there is little or no difference.

These public health organisations advise that washing hands thoroughly with just soap and warm water for at least 20 seconds is just as effective. However, sometimes antibacterial products are necessary but preferably you should be more selective about their use. Suitable measures would include reserving the use of these products for dealing with ill or immunocompromised people. This may include those receiving treatment for cancer especially chemotherapy or if someone in your household has a contagious infection such as gastroenteritis. In health care settings antibacterial products remain essential for strict infection control. Whether antibacterial hand wash is used or not a good hand washing technique is also very important.

Perfluorinated Chemicals (PFCs)

Perfluorinated chemicals are a large group of compounds that are designed to repel stains, grease and water, and reduce friction. These useful properties mean that they are vital in many industries such as aviation, car manufacturing, construction and electronics. Their properties are also desirable in many household items. PFCs are used in non-stick cookware, waterproof clothes, some food packaging and to make carpets and sofas stain resistant. They can also be found in moisturisers, eye makeup, nail polish and dental floss.

Issues have been raised about PFCs as some of them have also been shown to act as EDCs in cell and animal studies. Some animal studies show that long term expo-sure can also be harmful to the liver, gastrointestinal tract and thyroid gland. Human studies are less conclusive at present and therefore further research is needed to clarify if there are any potential adverse effects to our health. PFCs are not thought to be absorbed by skin contact with water resistant or stain resistant goods but are absorbed orally. This could occur from the PFCs in products that end up in rubbish dumps and landfill sites, in this way the chemicals may leach into waterways and soil. PFCs are very slow to break down so remain in the environment for a number of years. They also take a long time to be eliminated from the body.

Restrictions on PFCs

Currently two Perfluorinated Chemicals have been found to be sufficiently harmful to human health to warrant a reduction of their use. The first is *PFOS (Perfluorooc-tane sulfonate)*. This was previously used in some fire-fighting foam and to provide a protective waterproof, stain resistant coating to some textiles and leather. In the environment it takes almost nine years for its concentrations to fall by half and this slow breakdown can lead to a build-up of this substance in the environment. By 2002, due to reports about its potential risks to the environment, the main global manufacturer phased out its production. The EU banned the manufacture and use of PFOS in June 2008.

The other PFC of concern is *PFOA (Perfluorooctanoic acid)* and this is on the Candidate List of SVHC for possibly being toxic for reproduction. Similar concerns to PFOS have been highlighted with this PFC but it does not take as long to breakdown, instead it takes about 3 to 4 years. It is less toxic than PFOS but is now being used less due to efforts from the Environmental Protection Agency. PFOA is used in the process of making Teflon but is burned off in the process, so there doesn't appear to be a risk from cooking with Teflon or non-stick cookware of good quality. However, if there are scratches to the surface of non-stick coating, I recommend that you replace the item. Alternative non-stick cookware includes ceramic pots and ceramic- coated cookware.

Pitfalls in the Research on EDCs

1. A major pitfall in research on EDCs is the absence of suitable control groups in many of the research studies. For example in studies of paraben in breast cancer patients, levels were not measured in women that did not have breast cancer. Control groups could have included women with benign breast lesions or women who had mastectomies performed prophylactically .This could have helped to show whether levels of these chemicals are different in healthy breast tissue as opposed to breast tissue with cancer and if there is an increased effect with higher levels of these chemicals.

2. The studies that do show the presence of parabens in breast tissue still cannot provide conclusive evidence to link them with the cause of breast cancer. This is because these chemicals are found in many places so it makes it extremely difficult to isolate them in a real setting. A randomised control study would require one group of women to be directly exposed to an EDC and a control group who are not. The two groups of women would then have to be monitored and followed up for a number of years, looking at the incidence of breast cancer in the two groups. This study has not and probably never will be done since it is just not feasible. Therefore it is quite right to say that there is no conclusive proof that parabens contribute to breast cancer risk in humans.

3. If there is a cancer triggering effect from chemicals it is unlikely to be just one chemical that is having an effect and it is more likely to be due to a 'cocktail' of chemicals . Again this may make it almost impossible to show a cause and effect from isolated chemicals or particular combinations of chemicals.

4. Further research on potential endocrine disruptors would need considerably more funding and it would be difficult to see where that would come from. Due to the issues already mentioned, even with the financial resources needed it may still be impossible to show a direct link with breast cancer and potential EDCs.

Read the Label

If you wish to reduce your exposure to these chemicals it is important to look at the ingredient labels for PCPs and be aware of what is going onto your skin and potentially into your body. Just like food labels, the first ingredient on the list is the one that makes up the largest proportion of the product and so on. The levels of individual potential toxins may be very small and often less than 1%. These levels are heralded as being safe since they are thousands of time less than the levels that are believed to cause harm in humans. The problem that remains, however, is that we do not know what occurs when there is a cocktail of chemicals and whether over time these chemicals accumulate in the body. This is more likely to occur in fatty tissue such as breast tissue, where the chemicals may be stored and hence may cause a problem over time.

Tips to Reduce Exposure to EDCs

1. Look for labelling saying 'Paraben-Free' in your personal care/beauty products.

2. The EU and many global companies do not use low phthalates but if unsure you can ring the manufacturers and ask them.

3. Reduce the use of products if the list of ingredients contains 'parfum' or 'fragrance' unless they certify that these are natural scents.

4. Spray scents onto clothes rather than your skin.

5. Use recyclable plastics with '1, 2, 4 or 5', in the triangle recycling sign;
    - '3' indicates they contain phthalates.
    - '6' stands for polystyrene and these products include Styrofoam cups and plates which may be carcinogenic.
    - '7' plastics contain BPA.

6. Use BPA-free plastics.

7. Do not re-use plastics designed to be throwaway.

8. Microwave foods using glass microwavable containers rather than plastic. Heating plastics can cause chemicals to leach into food and drinks.

9. Wash hands thoroughly with warm soapy water instead of antibacterial products unless in a hospital or dealing with infectious or immunocompromised people.

Summary

You may have noticed a pattern regarding some of these environmental chemicals. The most potentially harmful ones shown from cell, animal or occupational studies are banned in young children initially. These measures are taken since younger children are more rapidly growing and developing than older children, and therefore more vulnerable to any harmful effects from endocrine disruptors. Yet these chemicals have already existed for many decades so as adults we have already been regularly exposed to them throughout our lives. We are also now seeing an ever increasing number of women diagnosed with breast cancer under the age of fifty. Although a number of factors may contribute to this, it is worth being aware of the bans and restrictions placed on certain environmental chemicals and why they are happening.

I believe that we should explore in more detail the concept of cancer prevention through better diet and lifestyle, and also by reducing our toxic burden. This may be leaving your head in a spin but changes can be made gradually. Over time you will find that it really is a very manageable task and is an exercise in being more aware of what you are eating and what you are using on your skin. Just start reading product labels as we do with food and you will soon find other products that you may want to swap over to. This is a rewarding and useful thing to do, especially knowing that it will reduce your own and your family's exposure to potential toxins.

The Debate about Aluminium

We come into daily contact with aluminium in many ways. It is the third most abundant element in the Earth's crust and traces of it are found naturally in food and water. It is also used widely in the manufacturing industry as a strong, durable and lightweight metal. For a number of years there has been a debate about the safety of aluminium in antiperspirants. Aluminium chloride or aluminium chlorohydrate are the active ingredients used in antiperspirants.

These aluminium salts are both extremely effective at blocking skin pores that normally release sweat from the armpit. They do so by forming an insoluble aluminium gel that creates a temporary plug within sweat ducts to prevent sweat reaching the surface of the skin. Sweat glands and ducts are in the superficial layers of the skin. The aluminium component of antiperspirants can comprise as much as 10-25% of the product. Deodorants work by a different mechanism and help to prevent body odour by breaking down bacteria in sweat and masking any odour with a fragrance. Parabens are now generally avoided in both types of underarm products.

It appears that the controversy arose almost two decades ago after a hoax email was widely circulated. The spam email linked aluminium with breast cancer however it did not provide any scientific evidence to back it. The email suggested that the aluminium was blocking pores and therefore not allowing toxins to leave the body. Researchers who argue that antiperspirants may be involved in the development of breast cancer suggest that the use of antiperspirants, especially in combination with underarm shaving, allows aluminium to penetrate into the skin and breast tissue. In cell studies there is some limited evidence of aluminium stimulating the migratory capacity of breast cancer cells. This has not been proven in animal, occupational or human studies but a precautionary method could involve using other methods of hair removal that do not cause a break in the skin.

A number of leading Breast Cancer Charities, the American Cancer Society and the Environmental Working Group, all share the view that these products are safe. I think at present there is negligible evidence of harm from aluminium-based underarm products in humans. However, if you prefer not to use those containing aluminium there is a readily available choice of aluminium-free antiperspirant and deodorant products.

Looking Good, Feeling Good

Being diagnosed with cancer and enduring its treatment is a major life changing event. You may have some long lasting physical and emotional scars but hopefully you can start to look forward and focus on regaining your strength, beauty and confidence in the way you look and feel. Your skin, hair and nails may have taken a bit of a pummelling but should respond well to some nurturing and TLC. This can help to redress some of the toll that treatment has taken out on you and also boost your morale. It is a step in the right direction when you look in the mirror and see that old sparkle coming back.

After reading the previous chapter I would like you to also consider the best way to reduce your exposure to environmental chemicals whilst still taking care of your appearance. I have found that the simplest way to go about this is to go 'au naturelle'. I am not suggesting that you don't wear make-up or don't use skincare products; I love my makeup and love to indulge in a pamper session. In general, I try to avoid personal care products that contain potential EDCs but some other chemicals may also be harmful and possibly damaging to the skin. Personally, I have found that using skin care and cosmetics that are made using natural ingredients is the most straightforward way to achieve this.

Taking this approach certainly makes it a lot easier than trying to read all the small print on the product label and there are many brands that cater for the converted. When I used up most of the paraben-free and phthalate-free skincare and makeup items I already had, I then started replacing them with alternative natural products. In fact it just feels so much better now not to worry about the possible long term effects of putting synthetic chemicals onto my skin, the results are better too. For me, it's a win-win situation.

Other Useful Sources of Information

You can learn a little bit more yourself about some of the products you use by accessing some informative online resources such as the Environmental Working Group and regulators of the Cosmetics Industry. The Cosmetics Industry has to abide by the restrictions on chemicals that are in place. These groups come from quite different standpoints but both provide a lot of useful information.

The Environmental Working Group (EWG)
www.ewg.org.uk

The Environmental Working Group is a charitable organisation that was founded in the USA in 1993. Their advice is to make changes now to protect yourselves, your children and your environment. They have a useful website and also several apps that can be downloaded. One of these is called Skin Deep and it helps to clarify which skin care and beauty products in their opinion are safer to use. The EWG app allows you to enter specific cosmetics and beauty products and then gives them a score, with 0 being the safest and 10 the least safe. The only problem is that they haven't evaluated every product on the market and especially those produced in Europe, however it is still a useful resource. There are also some cosmetic ingredient apps that will tell you what the chemical names on the cosmetics labels are and may give a safety rating on these individual ingredients. If you are using natural skincare and cosmetics then this approach isn't necessary and so it simplifies things.

The Cosmetics Toiletry and Perfumery Association (CTPA)
www.ctpa.org.uk

The CTPA is the official voice of the Cosmetics Industry in the UK. Its members include manufacturers and retailers in the UK. They keep up to date with European Union regulations. In the EU the regulations are certainly stricter than those of the FDA (Foods and Drug Association) in the USA. The EU has banned over a thousand chemicals from cosmetics whereas only a few are banned in the USA. However, the Personal Care Products Council (www.personalcarecouncil. org) in the USA argues that it is unreasonable to have several hundred of these chemicals on the UK banned list because they are not used in cosmetic products anyway. However, even taking this into account the restrictions are reassuringly stricter across Europe.

Research continues on many chemicals used in personal care products. Some of those explored are said to be safe when used in restricted amounts, whilst others continue to be investigated or have been deemed unsafe.

Cosmetics associations share the view that a lot of the research on the possible negative effects on many chemicals is of a dubious standard since most of the studies have been done on animals and therefore cannot be replicated in humans. They take the stance that it is reasonable to consider the chemicals used are safe since there is no conclusive proof of harm in humans. However, they are exploring some of these issues and liaising to try and come up with a general consensus for the global market.

Practical Steps to Reduce Your Exposure to Chemicals in PCPs

If you wish to reduce your exposure to chemical in PCPs then I suggest you start by avoiding products which may contain potential EDCs. This will achieve the most impact and benefits. As you run out of products you can replace them with safer alternatives, this way there is not a major cost burden. Remember that this process is not about being obsessive but you should find that you will be able to reduce your own and your family's exposure to potentially unsafe chemicals and that this aim is definitely attainable.

1. **'All-over' body products.** PCPs that are applied all over the body such as shower gels, body creams, sun creams and fake tan come into contact with a much larger area of skin. This larger surface area allows a greater opportunity for more chemicals to be absorbed into the body. For avid lovers of fake tan then there are paraben-free and phthalate-free fake tans and also an increasing number of natural fake tan and bronzing products.

2. **Bathing.** When we bathe we often soak for at least 20 minutes so bath products should be considered too. Natural bath salts such as 'Epsom Salts' or 'Himalayan Bath Salts' are excellent options for a relaxing and detoxifying bath. To create a preferred aroma and ambience you can also add a few drops of your favourite aromatherapy oils. Natural salts are preferential as they are not only chemical free they also help to draw out impurities and provide your body with trace elements like magnesium. As with any detoxification it is important to drink plenty of water and don't run the bath too hot or you may feel light-headed.

3. **Face cream.** As our skin ages it needs a good moisturiser to help maintain its elasticity, protect it from getting dry and reduce fine lines. Most women apply face cream day and night, massaging it thoroughly into the skin. Personally, I find that natural products do feel a lot better, have good results and are guilt-free. If you want healthy glowing skin your lifestyle will also have a major impact on how your skin looks. Your skin will reap the benefits of not smoking, a healthy diet, a good night's sleep and regular exercise.

4. **Hair products.** When you are massaging shampoo or conditioner into the scalp and hair roots then chemicals could potentially be absorbed. Paraben- free and phthalate free hair products are becoming easier to find and in my opinion seem to last a lot longer than the regular ones. This is likely to be because PCPs that do not contain preservatives tend to contain less water and more of the active ingredients. There is a market for these products and manufacturers are becoming more aware of this and consumers are driving the demand.

5. **Take care of your hands and nails.** Regularly apply natural cuticle oil and use hand cream especially after washing your hands to try and keep your nails and the skin around them in good condition. This will help your nails to become stronger and stop infections arising around your nails. If you are applying nail hardeners or polish try to avoid your nail cuticles and nail folds.

6. **Look for natural cosmetics.** You may find this difficult to begin with especially if you have been using certain products or a favourite colour for a long time but you should be able to find good alternatives. If you can't find something that quite matches up to your most loved products then just stick to those few items you feel you cannot do without. You can use the EWG site or other cosmetic apps to see which cosmetics are safer choices with a low toxic burden.

Botanicals

It is also worthwhile knowing that a lot of the long names you come across on labels may actually be derived from plants. Many beauty products contain botanicals which are ingredients taken from a leaf or plant and have the Latin name. If botanicals are used in a product they are listed with their Latin name usually followed by the common name in brackets next to it. I have given you some examples below, so that when you are looking at your products and now worrying about all those long names, you can decipher which ones you may want to avoid and which ones are indeed natural ingredients.

Examples of Latin Names of Ingredients in PCPs	
LATIN NAME	**COMMON NAME**
Aqua	Water
Tocopherol	Vitamin E
Citrus Nobilis	Mandarin Orange
Urtica Dioca	Nettle
Rubus Fructiosus	Blackberry
Leptospernum Petersonni	Lemon Scented Tea Tree Oil
Actinidia Chinesis	Kiwi

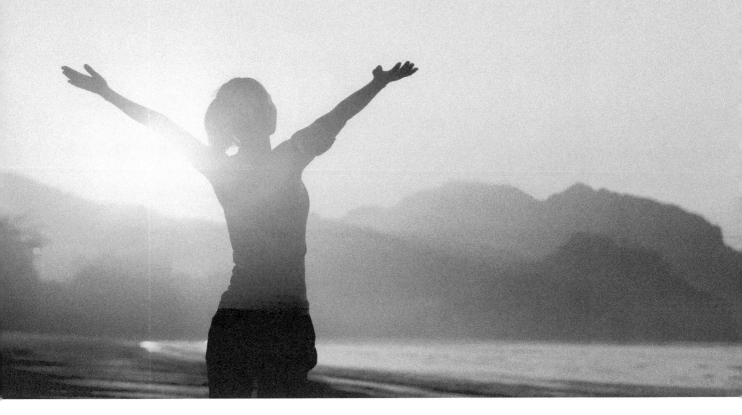

What Does Your Hair Say About You?

Our hair often makes a huge difference to our appearance and gives us our 'look'. Perhaps we shouldn't judge a book by its cover but often how we wear our hair matches our personality and style. We often have enduring relationships with a tried and trusted hairdresser and enjoy the whole experience, after all who doesn't like to get pampered and offload a little. Deciding to go for a different hairstyle is often a well-considered and deliberated event. Previously, I hadn't been very adventurous with my hair (forgetting the perm) and had always had thick medium to long hair. So, like most women, once you get to the point of chemotherapy, one question prevails, 'Will I lose my hair?' Unfortunately with most chemotherapy regimens for breast cancer the answer is predominantly 'Yes.'

There isn't a great deal we can do to stop losing our hair with chemotherapy but sometimes a treatment called a cold cap is offered. This cap contains a gel that is cooled to below minus 15 degrees; this causes the blood vessels supplying blood to the scalp to contract. By reducing the blood flow to the scalp this also reduces the amount of chemotherapy drugs that reach the hair follicles and so reduces the amount of hair loss. The cap is applied for about an hour before chemotherapy and then continued for a further hour after chemotherapy finishes; this amounts to at least four hours in total. Women get variable results from the cold cap and I have certainly seen some successes although some thinning of the hair will still occur.

Just as it can often be shocking and devastating to lose your hair a major part of moving on is when your hair starts growing back. I didn't wear my wig all the time; it was winter so I usually went out with a hat on to cover up instead. At home everyone got used to my baldness pretty quickly and my husband insisted he found it attractive, with favourable comparisons to Sinead O' Connor. If it was a special occasion or I was having a meal out then I would always wear my wig. My four year old son would always look at me rather quizzically, wondering how my hair had grown back so quickly. When I explained it was a wig he insisted on giving it a good tug before he was convinced! I must admit I got somewhat used to being bald and the no-maintenance was a positive aspect. Still the massive change in my appearance with or without a wig made it instantly apparent what a difference a head of hair does make to how you look.

When the chemotherapy finally finished I had been bald for about five months. I wondered how long it would take for my hair to grow back and tried my best to be patient but totally failed. The first wisps of hair started appearing just a few weeks after finishing my chemotherapy and then after a further few weeks I had a very short but even coverage. I spent a considerable amount of time assessing my crop with mirrors positioned so I could inspect my hair growth from various angles, trying to decide when I could bear to show it to the world.

I had agreed to take part in a fundraising fashion event for Beechwood Cancer Care Centre; the event took place just two months after finishing my last chemotherapy session. I wasn't sure whether I was going to wear my wig or not but on the day I decided not to, it just felt right. Whenever I look back at the photos from that day it takes me right back to that day and I am pleased that I didn't wear my wig.

Hair Growth

If you have lost your hair as a result of chemotherapy hopefully you can encourage it to grow back healthy and strong by giving your hair the nutrients it needs and encouraging the blood supply to your scalp. Even if you have not had chemotherapy you hair may have become noticeably thinner or lack-lustre as a result of stress and worry and so will also benefit from some extra care and attention.

The Hair Growth Cycle

Each hair grows from a small pit on the scalp or body surface called a hair follicle. This follicle is supplied with nutrients and oxygen by tiny blood vessels called capillaries as shown opposite. Each hair shaft is made up of a very strong structural protein called keratin. This is the same protein that makes up our nails and the very outer surface of our skin. When a hairs' growth cycle ends the follicle and hair are pushed out of the scalp and then a new follicle forms and the cycle repeats itself.

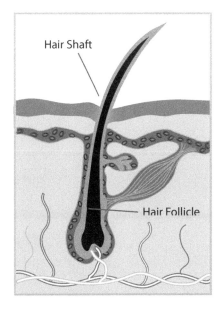

To encourage and stimulate hair growth a good place to start with is applying hair lotion or oil to your scalp combined with some gentle massage. I started using a natural hair lotion on my scalp shortly after my final chemotherapy cycle was complete. It's hard to know whether the hair lotion is what made a difference but it did grow back in good condition. There are many different hair growth and scalp products available but try and look for more natural products. I have given some home-made suggestions below. You may find that your scalp has become more sensitive so natural products are less likely to cause a skin irritation at this stage. As well as being very relaxing just the act of massaging your scalp may also help with re-growth since it increases the blood flow to the scalp.

Coconut Oil

Unrefined coconut oil is an excellent hair treatment which I often used as a teenager and have recently started using again. Studies have shown that coconut oil noticeably reduces protein loss from damaged and undamaged hair. The oil tends to solidify at room temperature so you just need to soften it by standing the glass jar in a bowl of warm water. After a few minutes you should be able to scoop out about 1-2 teaspoons of the oil to gently massage into your scalp. When using it as a hair conditioner scoop out enough to coat the hair fully and massage well into both your scalp and hair, try leaving it on for one to two hours for a deep conditioning treatment. I find that it helps to wrap your oiled hair in (non-PVC) cling film to avoid it dripping onto furniture or clothes. When you have left it on long enough, then shampoo it out twice and rinse you hair well.

Essential Oils

Essential oils are generally used for aromatherapy and relaxation but can also benefit hair growth. DO NOT USE ALONE BUT MIX WITH A CARRIER OIL. Using the oil directly on the skin may cause skin irritation especially if the oils are particularly strong. Store the essential oil in a dark bottle in a cool dark place to keep out sunlight; the sun's ultra-violet light will cause deterioration in the quality of the oil. Good carrier oils are almond oil, jojoba oil or olive oil. Use just a few drops of essential oil at a time and always mix them well into the carrier oil before use.

Peppermint Oil

A few drops of this diluted with 3 teaspoons of water works well. It will stimulate the hair follicles and promote hair growth. It also has a calming relaxing effect.

Rosemary Oil

A few drops of this can be added to olive oil and used as scalp massage oil. It stimulates blood circulation to the scalp and so it also promotes hair growth.

Lavender Oil

This has been used for many years by herbalists to prevent baldness. It has potent natural antibacterial agents that soothe and relax the scalp. It also smells good and can be used to treat dandruff. A few drops will combine well with the rosemary oil in an olive oil base.

Once Your Hair is Growing

When your hair grows back it often grows back differently. It tends to be softer and finer initially but can become wiry or coarser. It can also grow back a different colour and may come back curly rather than straight. Hair generally grows by half an inch every 4 weeks. So after a few months you will hopefully have a satisfactory amount and a good haircut should really make a difference.

If you have never had a short hair do, then at least you have an opportunity to see how it looks. For many women it can give them a more youthful appearance and you may find that you prefer it. Short hair generally needs cutting more often to maintain some style and to also neaten it up around the hairline. If you prefer to grow it longer then why not try out some different styles as it grows back.

It isn't wise to colour your hair very early on when it is first growing back but generally after a few months should be fine. If you cannot wait then you could just start with a semi-permanent colour. If you are dyeing it because it is now a different colour it's probably best to try and bear with it. If it is grey and you want to colour out the grey then try not to do it too often. There are natural henna dyes available in various shades that can also give a good coverage of grey hairs. Henna is also conditioning and coats the hair making it look thicker, regular use will help your hair grow back shiny and strong. Always do a skin-patch test first for hair colouring products, even if it is for a product you have previously used since your scalp may have become more sensitive

Hopefully after a few months or so you will feel confident enough to go out without a wig; not that there is any reason to wait, but I guess most women do. I think part of it, is just wanting to get on with things and being inconspicuous, as opposed to potentially drawing attention to oneself. When my hair was giving me a very short even coverage I didn't mind not wearing a wig or hat at all when I was away on a family break, but I waited several weeks longer before braving it on the school run. I guess I didn't really want the attention from people who didn't know me that well.

Eyebrows

I hadn't really considered that I might lose my eyebrows but they did end up very patchy by the time I had completed my chemotherapy but a good non-smudging eyebrow pencil or powder does wonders. You can also try smearing a small amount of olive oil over your brows to encourage them to grow; a little applied each evening seems to help.

Eyelashes

Losing my lashes was particularly upsetting especially since I was often complimented on their length. When they fell out I decided that like my wig maybe false ones would be a good option for special occasions. Unfortunately, I just didn't have the knack and they pretty much looked disastrous. As your lashes grow back then eyelash conditioning or booster mascaras can encourage them to grow back and help thicken them.

Nails

After chemotherapy your nails may have become short, brittle and uneven. A healthy diet is the key to healthy nails. Since your nails may not be looking their best, aim to avoid further damage. That means always wearing household gloves for cleaning and washing up. This also protects you from the chemicals in household cleaning products. Use hand cream regularly and especially after washing your hands. Almond oil and olive oil are both good for moisturising nail cuticles. Try to apply these oils daily, preferably at night and massage the oil in well. If you don't wish to use natural oils then there are many nail cuticle products available in chemists and supermarkets. This will help to strengthen nails as they grow and soften the cuticles.

It helps if you regularly manicure your nails in order to protect them and encourage growth. File them every 2-3 days to avoid uneven edges and peeling and always try to file in one direction; otherwise the nail can become weakened. If you are using nail polish then apply nail hardener or a base coat to stop the nail polish from staining the nails. Base coats and polish should be applied a little away from the cuticle and nail fold i.e. the skin surrounding the nail. The rest of the nail is made up of keratin so nail polish won't penetrate through; however avoid nail polishes and products that contain formaldehyde. When using nail polish removers try to use acetone free products and wash and cream the hands afterwards to stop them drying out.

Healthy Eating for Skin and Nails

While I had treatment I just wasn't interested in shopping or the preparation of food; it was just too much effort. So, afterwards it was a joy to get my love of cooking back and start trying out new recipes again. The initial phase of moving on is convalescence and recuperating so it doesn't pay to be too hard on yourself or too ambitious at this point. If your diet hasn't been particularly healthy in the past then start now with small adjustments rather than trying to make dramatic changes all at once. However, eating a balanced diet will promote healthy skin, hair, and nails, and will also help you to rebuild your strength and energy levels. To encourage these things then your diet should include adequate amounts of protein, iron and vitamins A, C and E.

Protein and Iron

Keratin is the main structural component of hair and nails and provides them with strength and structure. It is made up of a number of proteins, so protein in your diet is clearly needed to encourage strong hair and nails. Iron is also essential as it ensures a good blood supply to the hair follicle and root. If you are found to be anaemic and low in iron your doctor will usually prescribe iron tablets. Good sources of protein and iron are red meat, chicken, fish, eggs, nuts, lentils and dark green vegetables. The iron in red meat is called heme iron and is more readily absorbed than iron from other sources and is also utilised more readily by the body. Vegetarians can still get enough iron from non-meat sources (non-heme iron) such as lentils, beans, quinoa, broccoli, kale and spinach. Vitamin C aids the absorption of iron so try and combine these plant based iron sources with foods rich in vitamin C.

Omega-3 Fatty Acids

Omega-3 fatty acids are healthy fats; their main health benefits are associated with good cardiovascular health. However, these fats have many salubrious benefits and in particular improve cognitive function, and promote healthy bones, joints, skin and nails. Omega-3s also support scalp health and give hair its shine and lustre. Oily fish are a particularly rich source of omega-3 fatty acids and are also high in protein. Due to its multitude of benefits you should aim to eat oily fish 2-3 times a week. Further information on omega-3 fatty acids is given in Chapter 18.

Vitamin A

Vitamin A is a fat-soluble vitamin. Fat-soluble vitamins include vitamins A, D, E and K. Being fat-soluble gives these vitamins the ability to be stored in fat and then released from fat stores at times when there is low intake. This vitamin is used in making sebum produced from glands in the scalp to provide natural oils for good scalp health and healthy hair. Vitamin A can be found in cow's liver, red meat, poultry and dairy. Orange vegetables, such as carrots, pumpkin and squash and dark green leafy vegetables, such as kale, spinach and Swiss chard contain a precursor to Vitamin A called beta-carotene. Beta-carotene can then be converted to vitamin A in the body. (Further information on the antioxidant Vitamins A, C and E are given in Chapter 20).

Vitamin C

Vitamin C is a water-soluble vitamin so it cannot be stored in the body and therefore a daily supply from our diet is needed. Vitamin C is beneficial to our skin and hair because it helps to produce a protein called collagen which gives structure and strength to your hair and skin. In addition it is also an antioxidant and so boosts our immunity. Vitamin C also helps us to absorb iron when combined with iron-rich foods at meal times. Vitamin C can be found in a wide range of fruits and vegetables including citrus fruit. Taking high dose vitamin C supplements means that any consumed over the amount the body can utilise is eliminated in our urine. Arguably there is little to be gained from taking very high dose vitamin C supplements since the excess cannot be stored or utilised.

Vitamin E

Vitamin E is a fat-soluble vitamin and is beneficial for a strong immune system, healthy skin and eyes. It helps to widen blood vessels and improve the circulation to the scalp, so improving hair growth. Sunflower seeds and almonds are particularly rich in vitamin E. As with all nuts and seeds, a small handful or cup of these is sufficient, especially if you are watching your weight. Eat seeds as a snack or sprinkle over salads.

Biotin

Biotin is a water-soluble B vitamin that plays a role in healthy hair and nails. When people have biotin deficiency (although rare) they will typically have brittle nails and hair loss. Biotin also plays a part in fat and sugar metabolism, helping to turn fuel into energy. There is a good supply of biotin in Swiss chard, carrots, whole grains and some nuts (see table opposite).

Zinc

Zinc is an essential mineral that is important for scalp health. Without it the scalp can be dry and flaky and hair can be brittle. It also needed for a healthy immune system .Oysters; lean beef and lean lamb are particularly rich in zinc.

Selenium

Selenium is a trace element. Trace elements are needed by the body in very small quantities for normal growth and development. Selenium works well alongside zinc to help in promoting hair growth. It can be used to reduce grey hair, hair loss and dandruff. Selenium works as an anti-inflammatory agent too and helps in skin conditions like psoriasis and eczema. Seafood, lean beef and lean lamb are the richest sources of selenium, although there are also good amounts in Brazil nuts. For most people it is generally safe at doses of 400mcg a day on a short-term basis but high doses and long term use should be avoided. However, selenium supplementation should be avoided in pregnant and breast feeding women and when taking certain medications. In particular, it may increase the effects of blood thinners (anticoagulants).

Supplements

There are many supplements on the market that are aimed at improving skin, hair and nail growth and it can be difficult to know how much difference they actually make. Although I did consume a diet containing lots of vitamins I did want to give my hair all the encouragement it could get. I also felt that after chemotherapy I was likely to be low in certain vitamins or minerals which are required for healthy hair growth such as zinc and selenium. The easiest way to replace these is with a healthy diet and additional supplements for maybe a month or two. Taking high dose or long term supplements especially for minerals and trace elements may actually do more harm than good and be expensive and unnecessary. Get advice from a nutritionist before buying them and if unsure just stick with healthy eating.

Enjoy a Healthy Diet for Healthy Skin, Hair and Nail Growth

Vitamin A/ Beta-carotene	Vitamin C	Vitamin E	Biotin	Zinc	Selenium
Liver/ Red meat /Poultry	Peppers	Sunflower seeds	Swiss Chard, Carrots	Sunflower seeds	Oysters
Dairy Produce	Tomatoes	Nuts Almonds	Nuts: Almonds, Walnuts, Hazelnuts	Nuts: Walnuts, Cashews, Pecans	Nuts ; Brazil Nuts, Walnuts
Sweet Potato	Sweet Potato	Broccoli, Spinach	Halibut	Oysters	Fish: Tuna, Halibut, Mackerel, Snapper
Pumpkin, Squash	Kiwi Fruit	Pumpkin, Squash	Whole Grains	Whole Grains	Whole Grains, wheat germ
Carrots	Strawberries	Avocados	Lentils	Lean Beef and Lamb	Lean Beef and Lamb
Dried Apricots	Citrus Fruit: Oranges, Lemons, Limes	Shrimp, Cod	Eggs		
Dark Green Leafy Veg	Dark Green Leafy Veg		Bananas		
Cos/Romaine Lettuce					

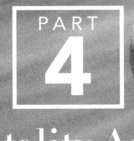

Vitality And Well-Being

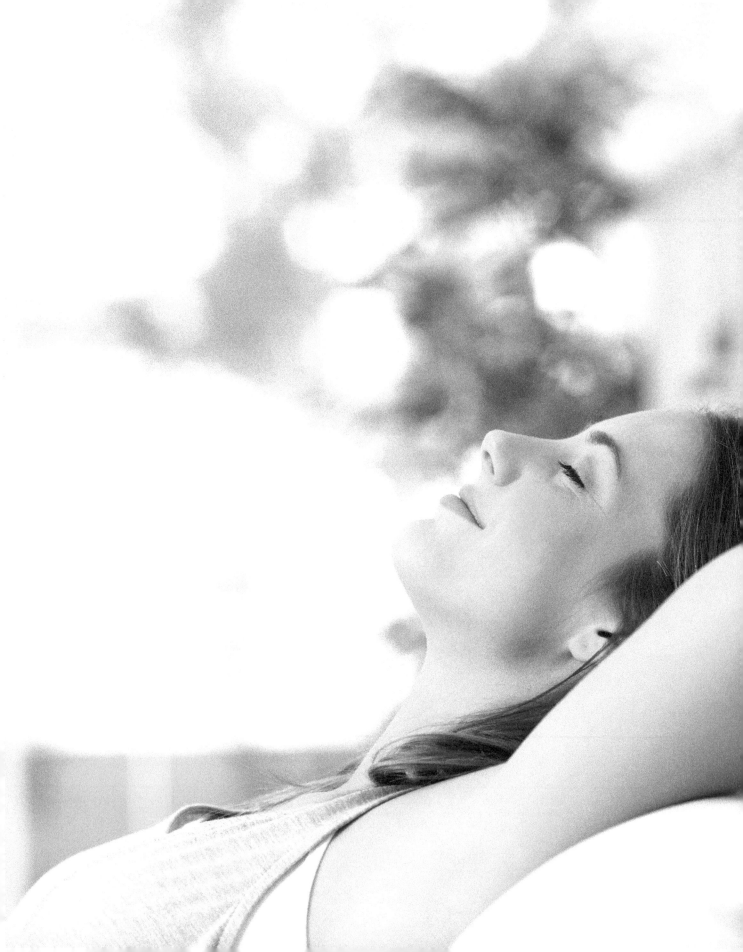

13

Cancer-Related Fatigue

The time will come when you have completed all of your treatment and, understandably, you are likely to feel incredibly relieved. When this day arrives you can start to think about moving on. However, for many breast cancer survivors the unfortunate reality is, despite your almighty efforts, you may just not have any 'oomph'. How you feel at the end of treatment will often depend on the extent of surgery and adjuvant therapies that you have had. Recovery may also be affected by any pre-existing health problems or if you have had any complications from surgery or your treatment. It can then become difficult and perhaps rather an anti-climax if you still don't feel that great and worries may then start to creep in.

What is now known is that Cancer-Related Fatigue (CRF) affects up to 90% of breast cancer survivors to some degree. The stress of dealing with the initial diagnosis, then upcoming investigations and imminent surgery can result in fatigue. Then there will be a few weeks spent recovering from surgery but also spent anticipating the following radiotherapy or chemotherapy. Women who have had radiotherapy often suffer with fatigue which can last several weeks or even months. After chemotherapy fatigue usually lasts at least six months to a year but it is not uncommon for it to last even longer, and some women never really get back to their pre-cancer levels of energy and fitness. Also women on hormonal therapies for receptor positive breast cancers may experience side effects of these medications that may contribute to fatigue.

As I advanced through my six cycles of chemotherapy, I was all too aware that my energy levels were draining away. By the end of the treatment I felt so grateful and relieved but by then I was also utterly exhausted. At this point I envisaged that it was going to take several months for me get back on my feet. I still faced a course of radiotherapy but I remember not feeling as daunted by that prospect, I was just pleased to put the chemotherapy behind me. As a General Practitioner I knew I couldn't rush back to work. I had been working as a locum GP prior to being diagnosed with breast cancer and knew that it wouldn't be feasible to return to work if I couldn't perform the myriad duties of a GP and keep up with the intense workload. As well as this I knew I had to feel not only physically robust, but also mentally strong enough to be able to support other people through their own difficulties. I proposed that six months should be ample time to recover sufficiently and so I set myself this timescale to get my life back on track.

I spent this time on trying to improve my fitness levels and looking after my two young boys. My family were still giving me a lot of support but I wanted to do more with the boys as it already felt like I had missed out on so much precious time. I was instantly reminded how hard it is to keep up with two young, very energetic children, however I was determined to get back to normal. So I pushed myself and kept going even when I knew I was struggling. The progress I made was very erratic but on the whole I felt that I was making a gradual improvement.

After the six months, just as I had intended, I returned to work. It appeared to go very well initially, although I did find it slightly disconcerting having to deal with my work colleague's kind attentions and remarks on my new appearance. Of course I knew that everyone meant well and that they were glad to see me back at work. I had been away for well over a year; a very trying year that I was never going to forget, and one which had left me looking and feeling considerably different. It suddenly seemed a monumental step; I felt rather conspicuous since I knew everyone knew that I had had cancer. However, after breaking the ice and everyone getting used to seeing me around again I soon started to feel at ease.

What I hadn't anticipated was that my body and immune system were not yet equipped for what I had planned. I was still too weak and my lowered immunity was not up to the job of defending me from the repeated exposure to bugs. I succumbed to one infection after another. This resulted in my energy levels plummeting again and it soon became a major challenge just looking after my two boys who were then aged four and six years . I wasn't able to juggle things the way I used to before my illness. Many nights, by the time I got into bed, I felt totally drained and irritable and yet I also found it difficult to get to sleep. It became a catch 22 situation as I knew that light exercise would help me to get stronger, but I just didn't have any energy to do any. After just one rather protracted month, I gave up work as my levels of fatigue meant I just could not continue.

It was deeply upsetting that, yet again, things had not unfolded as I had wished. I recognised that rather than just trying to push through it, I would need to adopt a different strategy in order to make better progress in my recovery. I started by researching how people with Chronic Fatigue Syndrome (CFS) manage their symptoms. I could identify many similarities between CFS and the difficulties I was experiencing with Cancer-Related Fatigue (CRF). I looked at the advice offered and it appeared to be relevant to my own situation so I thought it might be worth a try. Firstly I began to prioritise tasks rather than attempting to get everything done in one day. I also started to pace myself by staggering activities. I did this by giving myself more time to do things and planning my activities for the week.

Whenever I had done too much and was over-tired it would result in the same tell-tale signs, so I started to listen to my body more. I knew when I had done too much because when I got into bed at night my legs had a yawning ache all over and I just couldn't keep them still; I had developed Restless Legs Syndrome. I began to realise that rather than learning how to cope with this irritating symptom, it would be better to do less. As I listened to my body more, I started to gradually improve and not have quite as many bad days. I also found that having a 'power nap' in the afternoon helped me to get through the rest of the day without becoming as exhausted. I would have a nap whilst the boys were at school which gave me a much needed top up of energy before I went to collect them from school.

I found this pacing of activities helped, but I am quite certain that my real turning point occurred several months later when I started to pay closer attention to my diet. I had what I considered to be a healthy diet, but I made some further changes that really helped. I had read about the concept of detoxifying to remove a build-up of toxins from the body. After exploring this further and being inspired by some of the stories I read, I decided I would try a seven day juice detox. The idea of a detox is to remove toxins from the body but also to eliminate cravings and the dependence on caffeine as a pick me up, or sugar for an energy boost. The plan did involve a fair amount of shopping and preparation and I don't think I could have done this straight after finishing my treatment but by this point over nine months had passed.

I embarked on a seven day menu plan of nothing but freshly pressed juices consisting of lots of vegetables, with some fruit added to make the juices palatable, avocado to provide some healthy fats, and added super foods such as wheatgrass powder or spirulina. Initially I had some withdrawal effects due to the absence of caffeine and refined sugars. In particular I noticed headaches, sluggishness and cravings. I admit that this was difficult to begin with but I started to feel energised after the first 3-4 days. The juicing detox gave me a welcome energy boost; just what I needed. I decided to continue limiting my caffeine intake and intake of refined sugars to an occasional use. I felt happier and healthier eating plenty of healthy, unprocessed, home cooked food and this provided me with enough motivation to keep it going. I still juice regularly and try and have a juice every day and I also do a 2-3 day juice detox every few months.

What I am trying to highlight from my own experiences is that after treatment it isn't just a matter of getting back to normal, you are now entering a phase of recovery and recuperation. Being advised to get on with it, in reality or in your own mind will just add to any stress and anxiety that you might be experiencing. Often these pressures and thoughts come from within. Sometimes, it may feel like people are pressurising you or even being inconsiderate. After all you look much better and, let's face it; until you've been through it yourself you can't really fully comprehend how it can affect you. In most cases any negative comments are not intentional but just due to lack of awareness. If you are back at work you may find that you can just about manage to get through your working day but when you get home you have nothing left. Nothing left for socialising and your personal life. Fatigue for the majority does ease, but pushing too hard, too fast will only compound it and slow down the recovery process. You owe it to yourself and your family to explain that you are still suffering from fatigue or other side effects. You also need to discuss this with your doctor and your employer.

What Causes Cancer-Related Fatigue?

Chemotherapy and radiotherapy damage healthy cells as well as destroying cancer cells. This may leave the body with extra toxins and also now with the job of repairing the healthy cells that were damaged. Cells contain many smaller sub-units called 'mitochondria' which can be considered to be the energy producing 'powerhouses' of each cell. It is speculated by some that during cancer and its treatments that this cell damage also involves the mitochondria and that this damage may take some time to repair.

What Mitochondria Do

If we look at a mitochondrion in more detail we can see that it contains its own DNA and has a complex structure.

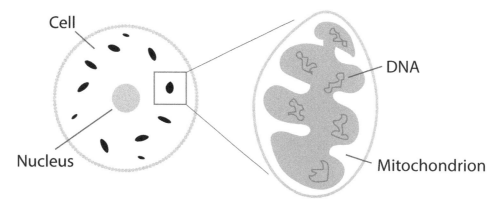

Cell

DNA

Nucleus

Mitochondrion

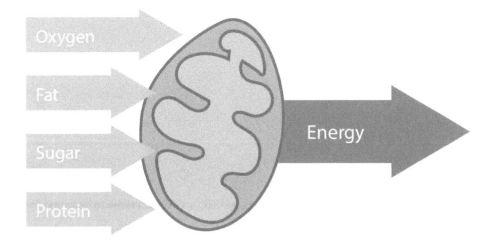

The above diagram shows how substances are taken from our diet then pass into cells then into their mitochondria where they are then are converted into the available energy for each cell. Impairment to healthy cells and in particular the function of mitochondria, combined with the stress our bodies have been under will all contribute to fatigue.

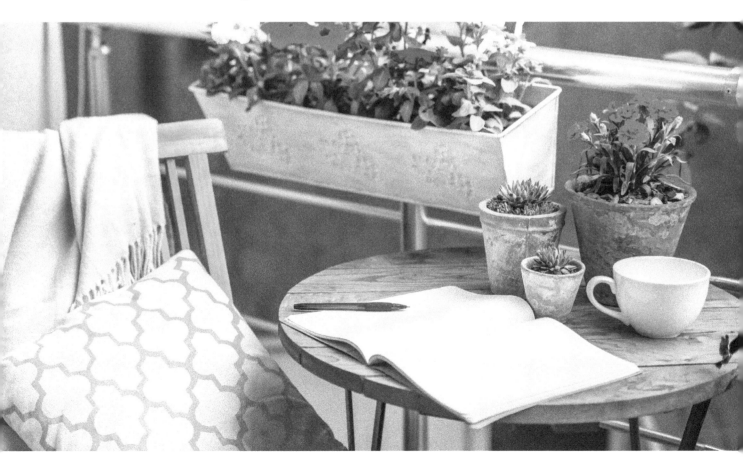

Symptoms of Cancer-Related (CRF)

The National Comprehensive Cancer Network defines Cancer-Related Fatigue as

> 'a distressing, persistent, subjective sense of physical, emotional and or cognitive tiredness or exhaustion related to cancer or cancer treatment that is not proportional to recent activity and interferes with normal functioning.'

Cancer-Related Fatigue is very similar to that of CFS. The fatigue in both of these conditions is present as a persistent symptom although there will be some fluctuations in energy levels with some good days and some bad days. There is likely to be more understanding and acceptance of Cancer-Related Fatigue since there is a much clearer cause and effect, however both conditions can be equally debilitating. Also the majority of people with CRF can expect that it will improve over time whereas those with CFS cannot be as reassured. Being aware that you will probably be affected by fatigue after treatment allows you to be more prepared and therefore you can manage it more successfully. The following symptoms are common in Cancer-Related Fatigue:

- Tiredness that makes normal daily activities difficult to complete.
- Sleeping or napping a lot
- Feeling weak and tired even after sleeping
- Mood changes
- Irritability and frustration at feeling tired
- Poor concentration
- Poor memory
- Heaviness of limbs and aches and pains
- Restless legs

Recovery

Prolonged cancer treatment, the lack of activity and reduced fitness levels may lead to a general de-conditioning of your body resulting in poor muscle tone and weakness. This in itself can make normal daily tasks harder to carry out. A vicious circle can also develop between fatigue which can lead to stress, a lowered immunity, low mood and poor sleep. Therefore tackling fatigue means addressing all of these issues as they all interact with each other as shown below.

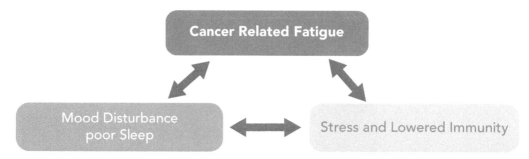

Treatable Causes

You will have had blood tests during your treatment and may have been told that these are all normal. However if you continue to experience fatigue I would advise you to discuss this with your GP or hospital doctors. Your GP can organise blood tests to rule out any treatable causes. If there are any underlying treatable causes then these need to be managed first of all as this should help to improve your symptoms. The table below shows the common blood tests that are used to investigate treatable causes of fatigue.

Common Blood Tests when you are Feeling 'Tired All the Time' (TATT)

TEST	RESULT	DIAGNOSIS	TREATMENT
Full Blood Count, Ferritin	Low count	Anaemia	Iron Supplements. Blood Transfusion if very low.
Thyroid Function Test	Underactive	Hypothyroidism	Levothyroxine tablets
B12 and Folate	Low level	B12 deficiency Folate deficiency	B12 Injection or B12/ Folate Supplements
Calcium	Low	Hypocalcaemia	Calcium tablets
Blood Sugar	High	Diabetes	Diet, Exercise, Medication

Other Symptoms Leading to Increased Fatigue

As well as any treatable causes identified by blood tests there may also be other treatable causes that can be identified by your symptoms. The symptoms of Cancer-Related Fatigue and lack of sleep overlap; both of these can cause headaches, poor concentration and poor memory. Therefore sleep disturbance from whatever cause will contribute to your levels of fatigue. There can be a number of factors that may affect your sleep and it can sometimes be difficult to separate these from each other as shown opposite.

Factors That Contribute to Poor Sleep and Fatigue

Pain

Depression

Anxiety

Side Effects of Medications

Restless Legs

Pain Management

Pain can contribute to fatigue and cause problems with sleep and also place limitations on exercising. Some pain after surgery is to be expected, but for most patients this should gradually ease over the first 1-3 months. Pain can sometimes last longer if you have had major surgery such as a mastectomy, axillary clearance or a flap reconstruction. Pain may also be related to lymphoedema or a stiff shoulder on the side that has been treated. Persistent pain may be related to nerve damage during surgery around the armpit and chest area. Nerve damage can cause neuropathic pain which tends to cause numbness and tingling, and sharp shooting pains.

Chemotherapy sometimes causes neuropathic pain which tends to affect peripheral nerves in the hands and feet; this is called peripheral neuropathy. Gabapentin and Pregablin are examples of medications that can specifically help with neuropathic pain and can also help with hot flushes. Pain management usually involves painkillers but further referral or management may be needed. For example, physiotherapy can be very helpful for dealing with pain from lymphoedema or a stiff painful shoulder. It is very important to speak to your doctors to try and get your pain management under control but if this proves to be difficult then a referral to a specialist pain clinic may be necessary.

Emotions after Cancer

To some extent, feeling low in mood or anxious after a cancer diagnosis and treatment is to be expected. After all, you have been through a hugely disruptive and worrying time. You may have surprised yourself by how 'strong' you have been so far. This may then make it difficult if this all changes after treatment ends and you suddenly find that you are no longer coping. Often the enormity and significance of a traumatic event only fully impacts on you after you have come through it. If stress or your emotions are affecting your ability to move on and causing significant symptoms then this needs to be dealt with. Speak to your GP or hospital team as soon as possible in order to avoid a downward spiral. They will be able to point you in the right direction for places to look for support and advice. Local support groups, relaxation therapies and psychological therapies can all be of great help. Medication may also be advised to help if your symptoms are more severe. These issues are dealt with in Chapter 15.

Side Effects of Breast Cancer Medications

Sometimes the side effects of medication or treatments can cause fatigue. Common problems that affect a large number of women after breast cancer treatment are hot flushes and night sweats. These are usually as a result of menopausal symptoms bought on by chemotherapy, hormonal therapy, Zoladex injections or removal of the ovaries. These symptoms are usually temporary but advice is needed on how to manage them (see Chapter 8).

Restless Legs Syndrome

Restless Leg Syndrome (RLS) a rather unusual neurological condition that causes a burning or throbbing sensation, or a heaviness in the legs, which causes an overwhelming desire to move the legs. It usually occurs at night and when resting so can make it difficult to get to sleep. The cause is usually unknown; however, it can be triggered by chemotherapy. It is not completely clear what causes it but some Neurologists think it has something to do with how the body uses dopamine. Dopamine is a chemical that plays a role in controlling muscle movement. If it is very troublesome seek help from your GP or oncologist. Otherwise RLS does generally tend to improve at the same pace as CRF does. In my case I found it was worse if I had overdone it that day and its severity seemed to correlate with my level of fatigue. Rubbing and stretching the legs helps and sometimes getting up and walking around the room can help to ease it. Avoid caffeine and alcohol if you have RLS as these can aggravate it.

Other Medical Problems

Other pre-existing health issues also need monitoring during and after cancer treatment. Your treatment may have had an adverse effect on conditions such as diabetes, high blood pressure and ischaemic heart disease. These health problems may require closer monitoring for a period of time as you try and get back to your previous state of health and hopefully even an improved one. These health problems may have become worse due to a lack of exercise, weight gain and the stress of the cancer and its treatment on your body.

General Management of Cancer Related Fatigue

Consider some simple strategies to help spread tasks out and prioritise which ones are more important.

You will need continued support from family, friends or carers.

Prioritise tasks for the best part of your day.

Avoid unnecessary tasks

Introduce regular gentle exercise as a priority for at least five days a week.

Eat a healthy, well balanced diet.

Limit alcohol

Use labour saving devices wherever possible.

Use lightweight vacuums

Don't overdo it on a good day.

Good sleep hygiene aids a restful sleep.

Sleep Hygiene

Issues leading to poor sleep need to be identified and good sleep hygiene rules applied. Good sleep hygiene means optimising the conditions leading up to bed time and during sleep. For most adults the optimum amount of sleep a day is eight hours. It is important to get enough rest but avoid sleeping too long or staying in bed all day. It is also worth trying to get into a routine of trying to achieve eight hours at night, but if this isn't enough for you try and sleep a bit longer. Often this is not practical due to other members of the household getting up for work, or if you have young children or it is just too light or too noisy. Ideally you should avoid napping, but if you can't get enough sleep at night then an early afternoon nap will help. Aim to start your nap before 3 pm and try not to nap for longer than 30 to 60 minutes. When you are not suffering Cancer-Related Fatigue, napping is generally not advised for good sleep hygiene but often this is not possible after cancer treatment. An early afternoon nap is preferable to nodding off in the late afternoon or early evening. The aim is to gradually reduce nap times or days that you need a nap as you improve. If you have had a particularly poor night's sleep then try not to respond to this by increasing your nap time as it is likely to affect your routine.

What Happens When We Are Asleep

While we are asleep our body and mind recharges and so we function better after a good night's sleep. Our body seems to respond naturally to day and night as if we have an inbuilt clock telling us what our waking and sleeping hours are.

Melatonin

Our natural wake and sleep cycle is in part due to a gland in the middle of the brain called the pineal gland. It responds to darkness by releasing a hormone called melatonin. Melatonin is released in the evening and remains raised overnight before levels drop again in the early morning. As you might imagine, melatonin levels can be affected by how much daylight there is. Some say an extended release of melatonin over the longer winter evenings and nights is responsible for low mood known as Seasonal Affective Disorder or SAD. Melatonin can be found naturally in some foods such as bananas, tomatoes and some grains such as: oats, rice, and barley so incorporating these foods into a light supper can help with sleep.

Sleep Cycles

It is not just the length of sleep that is important but, also the quality of sleep that counts. While we are asleep we have different patterns of sleep where our brains are more or less active. These are called REM (Rapid Eye Movement) and

Non-REM cycles respectively. During these phases our brains show different patterns of electrical activity that correlate with how deep we are sleeping. In the REM phase our brain is still relatively active and this is also thought to be the time when we are dreaming. It is easier to waken someone in REM sleep and they can often remember what they have been dreaming about. Non-REM sleep goes through three different phases that in total last about an hour. By the third stage we are in a deep sleep where our brain waves are slow and deep. It is harder to wake someone in non-REM sleep and we are less responsive to what is going on around us. REM and Non REM sleep cycles alternate throughout the night and this is important in order for us to wake up feeling rested.

Tips for a Good Night's Sleep

1. **Avoid Prolonged Daytime Naps.** Reduce the length of naps before reducing the amount of night-time sleep. Naps of 20-60 minutes should be enough to recharge your batteries or just help you get through the rest of the day. Napping for longer may mean you fall into a longer and deeper Non-REM sleep that will be harder to wake from and is then more likely to affect your sleep at night.

2. **Avoid Stimulants.** Avoid consuming stimulants such as caffeine, alcohol or nicotine close to bedtime. Caffeine should ideally be avoided from at least mid-afternoon as the effects of it last about five hours. Caffeine can be found in coffee, tea, cola, cocoa and some cold and flu remedies. Good alternatives to these are naturally caffeine-free teas such as redbush tea or herbal teas. If you drink more than 3-4 cups of coffee a day then try and cut down to about 1 -2 cups and have them in the morning.

3. **Avoid a Large Evening Meal.** In general try to avoid large, heavy and rich foods before bedtime. Instead try and eat small regular meals and snacks to maintain your energy levels. Include complex carbohydrates in your diet in order to provide a sustained release of energy rather than the peaks and troughs seen with refined sugars. Please refer to Chapter 17 for a further explanation of complex carbohydrates and sugars.

4. **Foods With Tryptophan May Help.** Tryptophan is an amino acid that helps to speed up the onset of sleep and improves sleep quality. You can get some extra tryptophan by having a small healthy supper of foods containing tryptophan. Examples of these include bananas, a turkey or chicken whole grain sandwich, poached or boiled eggs on toast, or a handful of almonds or pumpkin seeds.

5. **Gentle Exercise.** Any form of exercise will help with sleep and if you don't feel that you have the energy for it just try and build up very gradually. Practising yoga before bedtime can also help you to relax.

6. **Increase Your Exposure to Natural Daylight.** Going for a walk helps or just sitting outside in the garden, in a park or outside a café. Let plenty of natural light into your home.

7. Manage Stress. Exercise, yoga, relaxation therapies and Mindfulness meditation, all help reduce stress levels. It is worth getting in to a regular habit by practising one of these activities daily.

8. Have A Warm Bath Prior to Bed. A warm bath in the evening will help to relax your muscles. You can also have your bath by candle light and listen to some calming music, and perhaps add a few drops of lavender oil into your bath.

9. Read a Book. Don't watch television in bed at bed time. If you are finding it difficult to unwind then read a printed book using a soft bedside light .If you find it difficult to switch off then reading is a useful distraction.

10. Do not Use Tablet Devices at night. This is all too common these days but it is not conducive to a good night's sleep. The reason for this is that tablets emit 'blue light'. This light has been shown to suppress melatonin levels making it harder for us to get to sleep and also disturbing our REM and Non-REM sleep cycles.

11. Optimise Your Bedroom For Sleep. Make sure your bedroom and bed is comfortable and relaxing. Keep your bedroom cool and dark at night, if you wake up to use the bathroom or get a drink keep the lights low. Don't have the room cluttered and keep work and computers out of it. Try and minimise noise but if you are unable to then use ear plugs.

12. Set A Regular Bedtime and Wake Up Time. This will help you to establish a routine and get your melatonin and sleep cycles into a regular pattern.

What to do if you Wake Up?

Often you may be able to get off to sleep but then wake up in the early hours and find that you cannot get back to sleep. Practising mindfulness and breath and body meditations can really help to focus the mind and keep it quiet. Even taking a few deep breaths can be relaxing and a focus away from your thoughts. If you develop some relaxation techniques you will find that they become easier to utilise when you need them. See Chapter 16 for further information. If you can't stop thinking over problems, it is sometimes helpful to write them down on a piece of paper as if filing them away. This can help since you then know that you have noted down your thoughts and can ponder over them the next day.

If after twenty minutes you don't feel that you are drifting off then it may be worth getting out of bed. Try sitting in another room but keep the lights dim and do a relaxing activity or try to focus your mind with the use of relaxation techniques or by reading. When you feel drowsy then go back to your bed. Even if you cannot get back to sleep remember that you are resting so all is not lost. If you don't manage to get to sleep try and get up at the usual time the next morning and maintain your normal sleep routine.

Key to Success

Planning

Prioritising

Pacing

Graded Exercise Therapy

1. Plan ahead. Each week prepare a timetable or a list. Decide which essential tasks need to be done then plan around them, leave yourself plenty of time to achieve them so you do not have to rush. Try and spread these tasks out evenly over the week if possible. Planning also helps as you may find that your concentration is reduced and that you are more forgetful. If you are returning to work then a gradual phased return should be planned with your employer.

2. Prioritise. Decide which tasks are most important. So for example if cooking is the most important task for the day then it helps to prioritise it. Delegate or ask for help with more physical tasks that you may be struggling with such as shopping or vacuuming. Leave tasks that are not really necessary.

3. Make gentle exercise a priority each day. Start slowly with even a few minutes a day building up very slowly at a level you can continue moving forward with.

4. Pace Yourself Pacing is a way of balancing activity and rest to manage your reduced energy levels. Plan rests before and after activities. If you pace yourself your symptoms should actually stabilise and then start to gradually improve over time.

5. Break down chores or tasks into smaller chunks.

6. Spread these chunks over the course of the day. For example when you prepare a meal, you could peel and chop up the vegetables, marinate fish or meat earlier in the day. Sit on a chair or stool whilst you do so. Then you could cook later in the day. It is worth doubling up the amounts of some meals that you make so you don't have to prepare and cook food every day. You can freeze the extra meals which will allow you some days free from cooking for other tasks or to have a rest.

7. Avoid overdoing it, especially on a good day.

If you build up gradually on tasks you should find that you can slowly start to do more again. Generally, you will see an ongoing improvement so draw strength from that.

Graded Exercise Therapy

Exercise is an essential part of tackling Cancer-Related Fatigue. If you haven't been able to do as much as usual, then your muscles are likely to feel weaker and your general fitness levels are likely to be reduced too. I used to be able to run 10km in just under an hour. A couple of months after finishing treatment I struggled to even run for just a couple of minutes and when I did attempt my heart rate sky-rocketed. This was definitely the wrong approach.

There is a lot of evidence to show that exercise helps to reduce levels of fatigue and by looking at the evidence, this will hopefully give you the encouragement to make a start if you haven't done so already. A Cochrane Database Systematic Review, called 'The Effect of Exercise on Fatigue Associated with Cancer' was published in 2012. This review analysed the results of 56 studies with over 4,000 participants in total. Half of the studies had been carried out on breast cancer patients. The groups that exercised faired significantly better than the control groups that did not. The findings showed that aerobic exercise in particular is beneficial for individuals with Cancer-Related Fatigue both during and after cancer treatment.

A small randomised controlled trial published in 2012 also showed that yoga offers significant improvements in Cancer-Related Fatigue in breast cancer survivors. This study involved 31 breast cancer survivors that were randomly assigned to a twelve week Iyengar yoga intervention or a twelve week health education intervention. Health questionnaires completed at the beginning and end of the three month programme showed that the yoga group had a significant reduction in the severity of their fatigue compared to the other group. As well as the benefits for fatigue at least twenty studies have shown that physically active cancer survivors have a lower risk of recurrence and better long term survival than those that are inactive.

Approach

1. **Gentle exercise is the key** The amount of effort should be enough to increase your heart rate gently and slowly improve muscle strength but not really fast paced aerobic exercise where you are left breathless.

2. Check with your own GP or oncologist whether you are fit enough to start a gentle exercise programme. If so you should initially aim to work at 50-70% of your maximum heart rate, this can be approximately calculated using the formula below.

> Maximum Heart Rate (approx.) =
> 220 – your age

For e.g. in a 50 year old woman
MAX H.R = 220 - 50 = 180bpm
50-70 % MAX H.R = 90-126bpm

The table opposite shows how working at different intensities of exercise increases your heart rate and improves your fitness levels. You are just aiming to do some very light exercise initially and then build up on this gradually. It may be some time until it is wise or possible for you to exercise at a higher intensity but this is not important at this stage of recovery.

EFFORT	% HEART RATE	HEALTH BENEFITS
MAXIMUM	90-100%	High intensity for maximum performance and speed
HARD	80-90 %	Moderate intensity for improved fitness and cardiovascular benefits
MODERATE	70-80%	Light to moderate intensity. Fat burning zone
LIGHT	60-70%	Light intensity to gently bring your heart rate to 50-70% of your maximum
VERY LIGHT	50-60%	Aim for a heart rate of about 90-110 bpm if your resting pulse is between 60-70bpm

3. **Plan and prioritise exercise** along with other daily activities. Build it in to your daily routine.

4. To begin with find a level that you can manage fairly easily. Initially this may just be a few minutes of brisk walking. You may already be able to manage 10-20 minutes or more, so build on whatever your baseline level is.

5. Every two weeks try to increase the duration by a further 2-5 minutes.

6. Start at a slow pace and gradually build up the length of time to 30 minutes.

7. This can be split over the day if necessary e.g. 2 x 15 minute blocks.

8. Don't push harder on a good day as this may cause a burn out the next day.

9. When you can manage the stage you are at more comfortably, then you can start to work at a faster pace, at a higher resistance or for longer. Regular exercise will help to ease your fatigue as you increase your fitness and stamina.

Plan ahead, rest before and after exercise.

Make exercise a priority in your schedule

Find something you like.

Start gently

Progress gradually

The types of exercise listed on the next page are accessible for most people. Aerobic exercise improves your cardiovascular fitness levels and will also help to improve your muscle strength. Mind and body exercises have been shown to be particularly beneficial for cancer survivors as they also help with relaxation and as a way of managing stress.

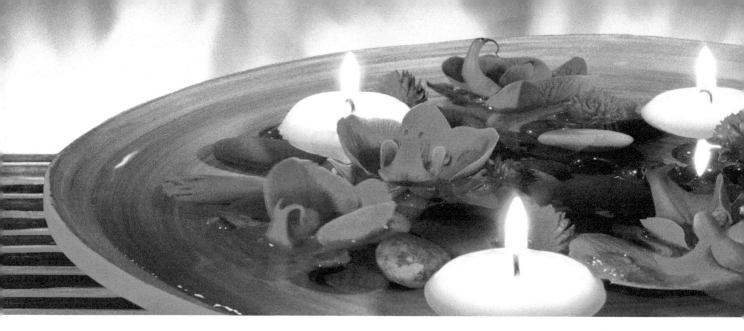

Gentle Aerobic Exercises	Mind and Body Exercises
Walking	Yoga
Swimming	Tai Chi
Stationary exercise bike	Pilates
Gardening	

Moving On from Cancer-Related Fatigue

You should expect fatigue to improve gradually but you may still need additional support as you set off on your road to recovery. Most importantly try to be kind to yourself and have some self-compassion. You now need to allow yourself a period for convalescence; this can range from just a few weeks to somewhat longer. During this time try and eat a healthy balanced diet that is easy to prepare. Get plenty of rest but try and prioritise some gentle exercise too. As you get your strength back, gradually increase the level and duration of exercise. You should try and go at a steady pace or you run the risk of going backwards not forwards. I learnt the hard way that pacing yourself is really important, especially on a good day.

How Does Stress Affect Us?

In our lives we all go through stressful times; these may include both happy occasions or sometimes difficult or challenging times. These are known as life events and include events such as marriage, starting a new job, moving home , birth of a child, divorce, the loss of someone close to you, and of course a cancer diagnosis. Life events may just cause stress in the period of time you are exposed to them or can have a much longer lasting impact. Being diagnosed with cancer can often be one of the most frightening and daunting times you will ever face. Getting your breast cancer diagnosis usually hits you like a bolt of lightning and then your life may feel like it has suddenly been turned upside down. Usually before you have had much time to take it on board you start your treatment which can sometimes be quite difficult and prolonged and leave you feeling weak and rather shell-shocked. As we persevere with the treatment most of us will focus on getting cured, surviving it all and eventually coming through the other end.

Thankfully the majority of breast cancer patients do survive and when we are approaching the end of our treatment most of us will be focusing on moving on with our lives. However for many of us completing treatment can be rather an anti-climax and this is often the time when we may start to worry. This may be about physical symptoms such as weakness, numbness and aches and pains and whether these symptoms are anything to be concerned about. You may be worried about returning to work and financial restraints. You may worry about what the future holds. Rather than becoming overwrought and allowing this to escalate into anxiety or depression it is helpful to acknowledge these worrying thoughts and concerns so that you can try and find the best ways to deal with them.

Your partner, family and friends may well offer you advice and support which

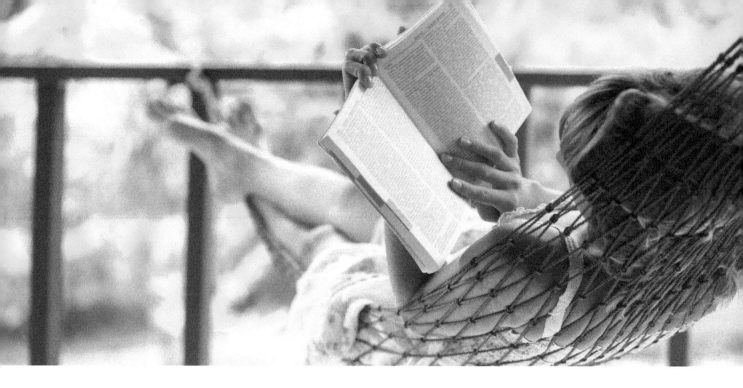

is often of great comfort. However, they have also had to deal with their own worries through your cancer diagnosis and may have struggled with knowing the best way to help you. They may struggle to find the right words or you may feel guilty that you are not now jumping for joy. Relationships with your partner, family and friends may have become strained or more dependent and you may all need to put in some extra time and effort to readjust and refocus.

To get through such trying times it often helps to express your feelings and for someone to listen carefully to what you have to say. This is where sharing your thoughts with a counsellor or with other people affected in a similar way can be invaluable. Talking openly about your feelings may not come naturally but in these settings you have an opportunity to express yourself at your own pace. You can often learn a lot by just listening and eventually you may feel able to share your own thoughts. If you are not coping very well this is a better

approach than just trying to put on a brave face. The problem with internalising your feelings is that you may just be suppressing your thoughts and emotions which may then surface at unexpected times. You may find that it doesn't take a lot for you to become very upset and burst into tears or suddenly become irritable and angry. Sometimes people try and block out upsetting thoughts by drinking too much alcohol, smoking or comfort eating but this will only lead to more health problems and now should be a time to try and live a healthier lifestyle.

Sometimes, despite talking things through, you may still not be handling things well and worries or thoughts can begin to preoccupy you or become heightened. This emotional state could then progress to an anxiety disorder or depression, so addressing your feelings and getting help early is very important in order to move forward in a positive way.

Getting Help

A couple of months after I finished my chemotherapy and radiotherapy, David and I had decided it would be a good idea to get away so that we could celebrate reaching this milestone. After all we had only been together for 14 months and for the majority of that time I was having treatment. It was going to be a special treat and we both looked forward to it with great anticipation. In the weeks leading up to the holiday I wanted to get toned up so I would look good for the beach, however, it didn't quite go to plan. Instead this became a frustrating and disappointing time since even light exercise now seemed such a chore and simply too much effort.

Trying on my bikinis was a stark reminder of how different my body looked. Not only was I trying to squeeze back into them, I was left wondering how I was going to hide the scars and lop-sidedness. It seemed that when I was in survival mode I had the ability 'to be mentally strong' and even laugh at myself and find the humour in many situations. Apart from the initial diagnosis I don't really remember crying, I can recollect being angry and frustrated but I had fight in me. This was now contrasted with me being fed up with how I looked and felt, struggling with fatigue and crying at the drop of a hat.

It seemed like, now, without the focus on treatment and the mental strength I had needed to get through it that I had started to unravel. Prior to going on holiday I remained reasonably optimistic that I would perk up and that it would be just the tonic I needed. Unfortunately, I was very wrong, it wasn't enough! The resort was beautiful but I still felt so tired all the time and my struggle with it must have emanated. David could see I was battling with my emotions and after further scrutiny I finally admitted that I had not been coping well for quite a while; I was hoping that the black cloud would just pass. We agreed it would be a good idea to see my own GP when we got back from our holiday. It didn't take too long to establish that I was suffering from depression and that it was obvious that at the core of this was my cancer diagnosis and treatment. After probing a little further the doctor and I both felt I would benefit from taking an antidepressant.

Looking back on this reflection really brings home to me how sometimes when your mood is flat and you feel devitalised that it can be difficult to admit it and seek help, even as a doctor. Not everyone goes through the same emotions or thoughts however if you can relate to some of this then it is better to share it. Seeking help was a major step in the right direction as it also meant I had begun to accept and confront how I was actually feeling rather than how I wanted to portray I was feeling. After a few weeks I started to get back on track and began feeling more positive. Although I was still suffering from fatigue I now had that little bit of motivation to do things and I was sleeping better; this meant that I could now manage some gentle exercise. Hence I began to re-build my strength and began to feel physically better. As well as this I began to think more about what I could do to help myself and how to get more support.

A Holistic Approach

I am continuing to learn that a holistic approach to good health involves nurturing our physical, emotional and spiritual selves in order to look after ourselves fully. In the Western World we are starting to realise that stress can negatively impact our health and that we need to start looking at our body as a whole. How we handle stress can have a major impact on our health. For example if stress pushes us towards making poor choices with our diet and alcohol, smoking and lack of exercise then it will have a negative impact on our health. Stress can also lead to anger, avoidance, anxiety and depression. Therefore learning techniques to lower stress levels and help us deal with stress has to be a positive thing.

Conversely are we less likely to get illnesses if we practise yoga, tai-chi or meditation? Practising mind and body exercises, learning relaxation techniques and meditation can really help you feel more energised and healthier as well as boosting your immunity and mental and physical resilience. Any form of exercise causes your body to release feel good chemicals called endorphins which also have a beneficial effect on your mood and your immune system. The immune system is at the core of creating an anti-cancer environment in our bodies. It protects us from pathogens, environmental toxins and potential cancer causing agents that can go on to damage cells and render them cancerous.

What is Stress?

Stress can be simply defined as a state of emotional tension or strain. We can all relate to being stressed on many occasions and we know that this is a normal part of life. When we are stressed it often feels like we are overwhelmed or feeling under pressure. It can be difficult to put it into words. Stress usually occurs in response to triggers. These stressors can come externally from our environment such as attending a job interview, speaking in public or dealing with a confrontation. Stress can also be caused by internal stressors that arise from our own thoughts such as when we worry or become anxious about something. Some stress is a good thing since it helps to keep us driven, motivated and excited. However, when stress is excessive and if it starts affecting your physical and mental health then it is bad for you.

Adrenaline and Cortisol

When we are stressed our bodies respond by releasing two very powerful hormones, adrenaline and cortisol. Under stress the body activates nerves that are connected to the adrenal glands (these glands sit on the kidneys) this results in the release of a hormone called adrenaline. Being stressed also stimulates the release of adrenocorticotropic hormone (ACTH) from the pituitary gland (sat at the base of the brain) which then also stimulates the adrenal glands, but this time they release another hormone called cortisol. This is shown opposite.

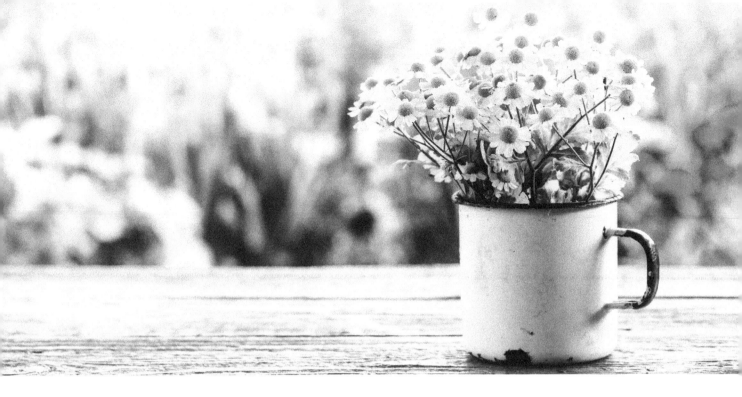

Adrenaline and Cortisol are released when we are stressed

Adrenaline

is released from the outer part of the adrenal gland, the cortex.

Cortisol

is released from the inner part of the adrenal gland, the medulla.

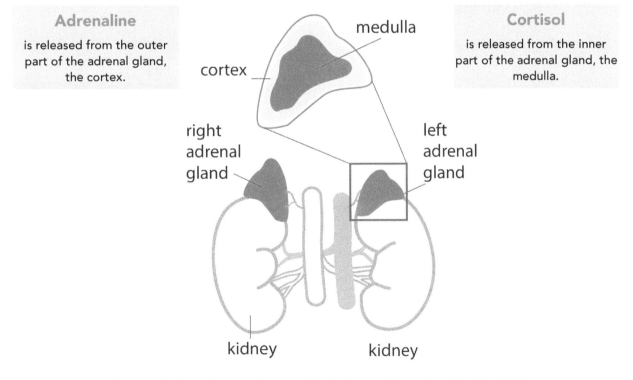

medulla

cortex

right
adrenal
gland

left
adrenal
gland

kidney   kidney

The release of adrenaline and cortisol both bring about the physiological responses and the physical feelings you experience when you are stressed. This is often known as the Fight or Flight response and these changes are intended to prepare the body for sudden action.

The Fight or Flight Response

The release of these two stress hormones results in an increase your body's heart rate and blood pressure so that the heart can pump more efficiently making you more ready for action; if you actually need to get away from danger or deal with a challenging situation then this is very helpful. At the same time non-essential functions are slowed down such as blood flow to the digestive system and a reduced immune system response.

Stress can vary in severity from milder but possibly chronic stress to acute very intense stress for example when you are in a frightening situation, having a panic attack or as a result of a phobia. The following diagram shows the common signs and symptoms you may experience when you are feeling stressed.

Below is a list of how our body reacts to stress.

Breathing rate increases

Heart rate increases

Blood pressure increases

Muscles become tense and ready for action

Blood sugar levels are increased

We become more alert

Digestive system slows down

Immune system slows down

THE SYMPTOMS OF STRESS

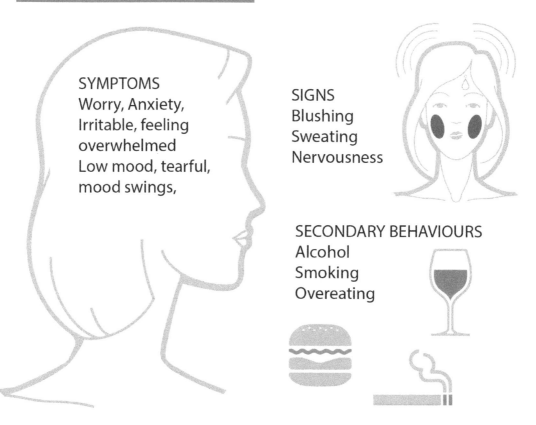

SYMPTOMS
Worry, Anxiety, Irritable, feeling overwhelmed
Low mood, tearful, mood swings,

SIGNS
Blushing
Sweating
Nervousness

SECONDARY BEHAVIOURS
Alcohol
Smoking
Overeating

Is Stress a Risk Factor for Cancer?

Considering the wide-ranging effects of stress there is an ongoing debate as to whether excessive stress contributes to cancer. Many believe it does but not all scientists back this view point. To research this area in humans is difficult because what is stressful for one individual is not necessarily for another; it is too subjective. For example flying in an aeroplane is fun and exciting for many but scary and terrifying for others especially those with a phobia of flying.

> Anecdotally many women do feel that the stress of a major life event did contribute to them developing breast cancer. In my own personal experience I believe that it could have been a factor since I had several very stressful years prior to being diagnosed with cancer. I separated from my partner in very difficult and untimely circumstances when I was pregnant with my second child. We were living in Australia and my first son was just 18 months old. After an extremely distressing six months and just five weeks after giving birth to my second child I returned back to England. Back in Manchester I moved in with my parents, I had a lot of support from my family but it did take time to rebuild my life. I am not saying that stress was the only factor that contributed to my cancer diagnosis but it was such a difficult few years that I do feel the ongoing stress did play a part.

Other women may consider that stressful events such as a divorce, bereavement or a child's illness may have contributed. It is impossible to be certain since we all get exposed to stressful life events yet we don't all get cancer? It is likely to be more about the person and how they deal with stress rather than just the stressful time or events themselves. We certainly shouldn't blame ourselves but stress and how we cope with it needs to be carefully considered alongside other factors as we move forward.

Studies on Stress and Breast Cancer Risk?

Since we cannot really create a standardised stressful situation most studies in humans have been on a retrospective or prospective basis. Retrospective studies on breast cancer and stress involve asking people diagnosed with breast cancer if they had had a period of stress or stressful events in the years leading up to their diagnosis. This can be very difficult to measure since past events and emotions can easily be forgotten and often only more recent events are recalled, this can lead to major flaws in the results.

One cohort of women from the extensive EPIC studies (see chapter 5) formed part of a follow up study to try and determine the effects stress on health outcomes. To remind you, these studies enlisted over half a million participants in total who were enrolled in 23 centres across ten European countries. This arm of the EPIC studies involved 11,467 women based in the Norfolk area (UK). At the outset the women were assessed by a questionnaire and on the basis of this, a measure of social adversity was made. The questions asked included whether they had had difficult circumstances in childhood or ongoing issues as adults and about any stressful life events over the preceding ten year period .They were then followed up to see if episodes of social adversity affected their likeliness to go on to develop breast cancer. The women were followed up in most cases for over a period of about nine years. Over that time frame 313 cases of breast cancer were identified. The results of the study showed that there did not seem to be any

association between social adversities and the development of breast cancer, and so the researchers concluded that there was no link with stress and the incidence of breast cancer.

However, as already mentioned stress is an extremely difficult entity to measure. Other studies have therefore attempted to measure stress and its effect on health in more objective ways than just using questionnaires. This has led to the evolution of a field of science called Psychoneuroimmunology which explores the complex interaction between our thought processes, our nervous system, immune system and physical health.

Psychoneuroimmunology

I first came across this word in Dr David Servan-Schreiber's excellent book, Anticancer: A New Way of Life, Chapter 9, (The Anticancer Mind), page 211. The science of Psychoneuroimmunology has been developed over the last thirty years and essentially explores the Mind-Body Connection. The word breaks down into three parts psycho, neuro and immunology. The first 'psycho' is to do with our psychology; essentially this is how we think and how this affects us and our ability to cope with life's hurdles. The second 'neuro' is to do with the release of adrenaline and cortisol and how our body responds to stress. The last immunology is how stress and these hormones then affect the function of our immune system.

Although some scientists do not believe there is a link between stress, the immune system and cancer, there are a number of studies that show that stress can affect

our health. One such study is a Japanese study published by Imai K and colleagues in 2000, in the Lancet. This was a prospective study involving 3625 Japanese participants. The study population was recruited between 1986 and 1990. They were given a questionnaire to complete about their lifestyle. Also and probably more crucially they had blood tests of some measurable immunological and biochemical markers of stress taken at the beginning of the study. They were then followed up for a period of about eleven years.

The blood tests that were taken reflected the level of Cytotoxic (toxic to cells) activity of the immune system in the study cohort. We now know that when we are stressed we produce a hormone called cortisol. Cortisol concentrates our body's effort on the Fight or Flight response at the expense of other activities that may not be essential for immediate survival. This includes lowering our immune responses in a number of ways that ultimately hinder cytotoxic activity. In the study period 154 cases of cancer occurred. It was found that people with low levels of these markers and therefore a low cytotoxic activity had an increased cancer risk. Whereas those people with a medium or high cytotoxic activity had a reduced risk of cancer. This study more clearly demonstrates that there is actually a strong relationship between our body's natural defences and our cancer risk.

As well as this there is indirect evidence that meditation and learning to not feel helpless can lower stress levels and the release of adrenaline and cortisol and so can help boost our immunity. I will explain a little more about the immune system since it is an integral part of our fight against cancer.

What is the Immune System?

Our immune system is a complex system that protects us from disease and potentially harmful substances. Our environment naturally contains millions of bacteria, viruses and other germs. If these enter our body then they can cause infections and illnesses. Our bodies are also exposed to potential cancer causing agents (carcinogens) that may be found in water, food and the environment. If a cell becomes abnormal and cancerous then it is usually destroyed by our immune system before it can multiply out of control and become a tumour. Your immune system is your body's defence against these invaders. It consists of our initial physical barriers to the environment, and then the action of white blood cells and the lymphatic system.

Natural Innate Immunity

Our immunity can be further generalised into our natural or acquired immunity. Our natural immunity is otherwise called innate immunity which means it is present from birth. There are a number of different components that make up this first line of defence against infections and carcinogens. An initial anatomical barrier exists and this is made up of our skin, fine hairs and mucus in our nasal passages and the good bacteria that are present in our gut flora as shown overleaf. This type of immunity gives us an immediate defence and fast response to invaders but doesn't give us future protection against the same invader.

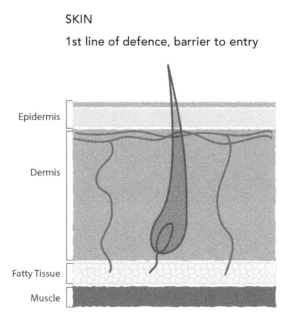

SKIN

1st line of defence, barrier to entry

Epidermis

Dermis

Fatty Tissue

Muscle

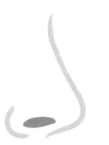
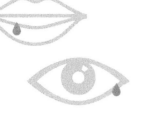
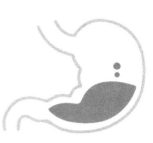
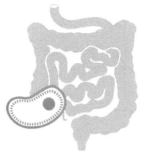

Nasal passages and
Upper airways
Mucous Lining Traps
dirt and Microbes

Saliva and Tears
antibacterial Enzymes

Stomach
Acid Ph destroys
harmful microbes

Bowels
Bacteria in normal gut flora
out compete bad bacteria

White Blood Cells

If infective organisms or carcinogens get past these initial protective barriers then a number of White Blood Cells come to the scene and respond quickly to the invasion in order to protect us. Luckily there are millions of these White Blood Cells (WBCs) in our blood stream and they come in various different forms as shown below. Each type of WBC plays a different role but they also work well together as a team; this allows for an increased and accelerated response as needed.

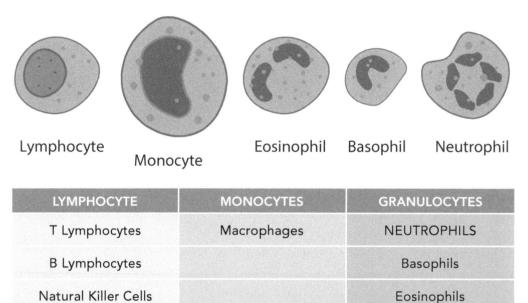

Lymphocyte   Monocyte   Eosinophil   Basophil   Neutrophil

LYMPHOCYTE	MONOCYTES	GRANULOCYTES
T Lymphocytes	Macrophages	NEUTROPHILS
B Lymphocytes		Basophils
Natural Killer Cells		Eosinophils
NK Cells can destroy infected cells and cancer cells. T and B Lymphocytes give us acquired immunity.	Macrophages and their precursor monocytes act as scavengers and destroy germs and toxins as they enter the body.	These WBCs can all destroy foreign cells such as bacteria, viruses and parasites

Macrophages

The initial attack to invaders is from WBCs called macrophages which circulate around the body and police it seeking out and destroying germs and toxins as they enter the body. They also act as scavengers and clear up cell debris and dead cells. They do this by engulfing them then finishing them off with the release of special chemicals. Just think of little Pac men.

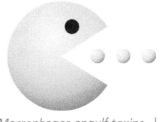

Macrophages engulf toxins, germs and cell debris

Natural Killer Cells (NK cells)

Natural Killer Cells are also part of our natural immunity. These WBCs are part of a subgroup of WBCs called lymphocytes and can seek out and destroy infected cells and cells that have undergone abnormal changes such as cancer cells. These target cells can be recognised because they have markers on their surface called antigens. The antigens are recognised by antibodies in our body which then attach to them. The presence of these unwanted cells also produces a localised inflammatory response which releases chemicals called cytokines.

The cytokine chemicals send a message out to other WBCs as well as NK cells; they also move towards the problematic area. Once they arrive, NK cells are able to recognise the cancer cells Antibody-Antigen arrangement. This marks out the infected or cancer cell for destruction by the NK cells as shown below. The NK cells now become activated and target the abnormal cell to bring about cell death.

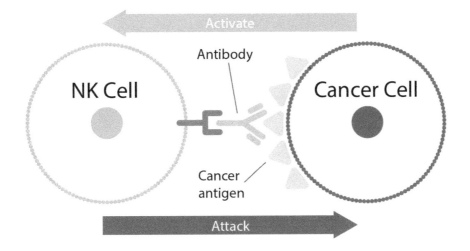

When NK Cells detect Antibodies that are attached to antigens on the surface of cancer cells they become activated and attack the cancer cells.

The activated NK cells destroy the infected or abnormal cell by releasing lethal proteins that create small holes in the cells surface which then leads to cell death (apoptosis). Hence NK cells are considered the major component of anticancer immunity and can rapidly remove cancer cells from the blood and possibly even from solid tumours. Luckily there are natural ways of improving the activity of our NK cells and also enhancing other aspects of our immune system which will therefore improve our cancer fighting ability. One such way is to give your immune system a boost by consuming a diet rich in antioxidants especially Vitamins C and E, and beta-carotene. (See Chapters 20 and 21)

Acquired Immunity

If the initial immune response doesn't succeed and our immune system does not manage to succeed in destroying an invading pathogen or an abnormal cell then this may result in illness or a single abnormal cell may develop further into a solid tumour. However, there is back-up and this is when the next prong of attack kicks in with a further reinforcement from large numbers of WBCs called B and T Lymphocytes. These WBCs will now also make their way to the target site. These lymphocytes form the next level of defence by making new antibodies to fight the infection or destroy an abnormal cell. In response to an infective agent antibodies will persist after the infection is cleared and will provide us with a future defence against the same infection in the future. This is called Acquired immunity.

Acquired immunity usually peaks after several days or weeks as shown below.

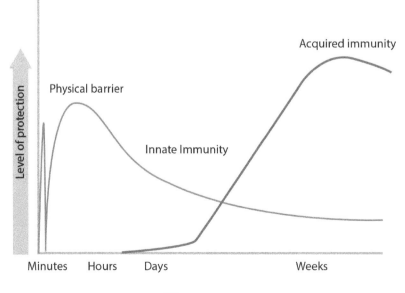

An example of this sort of long term protection can be demonstrated by considering an infection such as chicken pox. When you are infected with the chicken pox virus, this acquired immune response will produce antibodies that will persist in your body for a lifetime. These antibodies will be immediately available to attack the virus if you are exposed to it again. This makes it very unlikely for you to become infected with the same virus twice. However, this can occasionally happen especially if your immune system is suppressed.

The Lymphatic System

Most WBCs are produced in the lymphatic system as shown below. The lymphatic system includes a network of lymph vessels and about 600 lymph nodes that span across it. Within the chain of lymph nodes are clusters of them for example those found in your armpits, neck and groin.

Most WBCs are produced in the bone marrow, whereas B and T lymphocytes are also made in the spleen and lymph nodes. T lymphocytes mature further in the thymus gland. Our tonsils also form part of the lymphatic system and are made up of lymphoid tissue and help protect us from pathogens trying to enter the lungs or digestive tract. WBCs circulate around the body in the lymphatic system and blood stream.

The lymph nodes filter the lymph fluid as it flows through them. If there is an infection and therefore an increase in WBCs to the area, the local lymph nodes enlarge. This is because they now contain more WBCs and other cells from the immune system as they try to contain and fight the infection. These nodes will reduce in size again after the infection clears. When cancer spreads it often spreads initially to whichever lymph nodes are closest to it. If this happens the lymph nodes become enlarged but do not shrink in size. Therefore, after breast cancer it is important to remain vigilant and as part of regular breast self-examination it is also vital to check yourself for enlarged lymph nodes in the armpits, above the collar bones and along the breast bone.

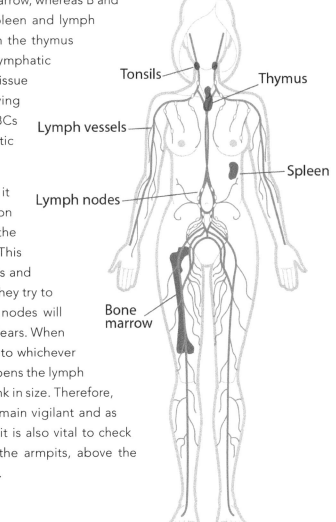

Tonsils
Thymus
Lymph vessels
Spleen
Lymph nodes
Bone marrow

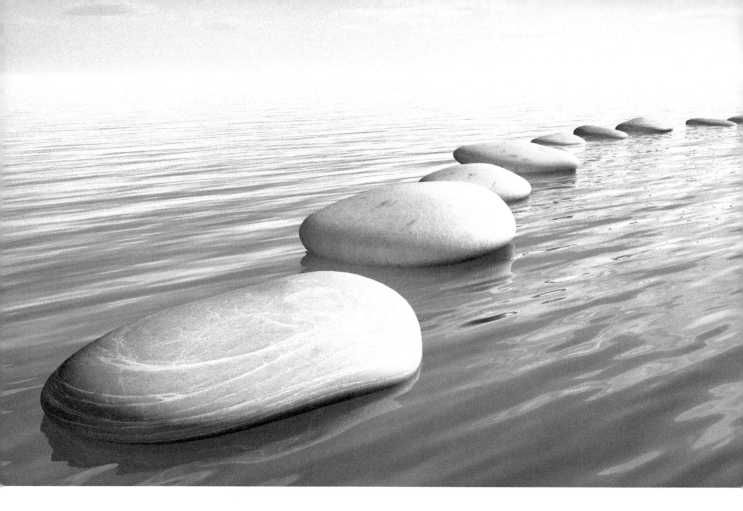

Summary

The mind-body-connection is certainly a complex and very powerful connection. How we react to stress can affect our immune system and our ability to fight off infections and cancer. Our ability to cope with stress may be reduced by Cancer-Related Fatigue, anxiety, depression and disturbed sleep creating a vicious circle as demonstrated in the chart below. This is why it is important to consider how you deal with your thoughts and emotions and start to learn techniques that may help. It may be difficult to know where to start and so I have discussed this in more detail in the next two chapters.

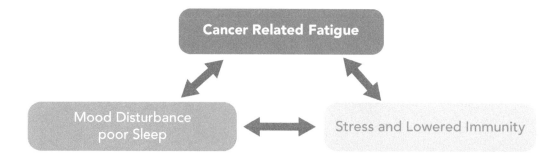

Cancer Related Fatigue

Mood Disturbance poor Sleep

Stress and Lowered Immunity

Dealing with Your Emotions

Going through cancer and its treatment can be a real rollercoaster of a ride and some days will inevitably be better than others. Chronic stress can have an impact on our health, but we can combat this if we learn how to lower levels of stress and how to cope with stress more effectively when it does arise. On a particularly trying day learning ways to deal with your emotions can often help to shift the negativity. A very accessible and effective method is the use of guided meditations. You Tube is a convenient online resource that can be used to find a large variety of meditations and so can be a very effective starting point. It takes regular practise before your ability to focus and fully relax develops so start with short meditations lasting around just five to ten minutes.

If stress is not managed effectively it can cause deleterious physical and emotional upset leading to problems such as restlessness, irritability, an anxiety state and/or depression as well as a dampened immune system. If you have tried lifestyle measures such as exercise, relaxation and mindfulness and have found that they are not helping or your emotional health is deteriorating then it is important to seek medical help; it is now more important than ever that you look after your emotional as well as physical health. There are differences in the ways anxiety and depression present, however, for many people these conditions overlap. The following is intended as a brief guide to help you recognise the signs.

Anxiety States

Being anxious or stressed prior to or during an important event such as taking an exam are very common. Usually the physical feelings subside after the stressful event. However if you have an anxiety state the triggers for these physical symptoms may be small or not even apparent and persist after the stressful event has passed. Below I have listed some of the feelings and thoughts you may experience if you are suffering from anxiety.

- Feeling tense
- Irritable and snappy
- Agitated and on edge
- Unable to relax which may result in poor sleep
- Reduced memory and concentration.
- Feeling that you might lose control
- Feeling people can notice your anxiety
- Feeling sick or faint
- Feeling you want to avoid/runaway from certain situations.

Anxiety can arise as a direct result of a past or currently stressful period of time and one that you have been unable to deal with or come to terms with fully. It may sometimes also be due to feeling you have a lack of control especially if you have been used to being in control or a much organised person. Sometimes being anxious can be partly due to your personality type, for example if you are an admitted 'worrier' and characteristically mull over things again and again or worry about making the right decisions or what the future might hold; this may then become exacerbated by a cancer diagnosis.

Being a breast cancer survivor means some of these factors are likely to apply. For most there will be some degree of anxiety along the way, which would be quite natural and to be expected. It becomes a problem however, if you feel like this most of the time or you are getting severe episodes of anxiety which are making it difficult for you to deal with everyday life. If you think that you are suffering from an anxiety state then it is important to seek help from your GP.

Panic Attacks

Panic attacks are different to an anxiety state but they can both occur in the same individual. Panic attacks often come out of the blue and cause an overwhelming fear or intense anxiety with lots of physical sensations and symptoms. You may feel fine most of the time but find certain situations trigger a panic attack. The trigger may be very obvious if you have a phobia such as a fear of spiders and then you are confronted with one. However attacks can also be triggered by less evident factors where perhaps something may have reminded you of a stressful situation. During a panic attack the body's response to stress is exaggerated. Typical signs and symptoms include those listed on the next page.

- Sweating

- Trembling

- Nausea

- Heart beat feeling irregular or fast i.e. 'palpitations'

- Numbness and tingling in the fingers and toes.

- Shortness of breath

- Hyperventilation (rapid shallow breathing)

- Tight chest

These attacks usually peak after about ten minutes. If they go on for longer than twenty minutes then it may be due to ongoing anxiety after the initial attack. The attacks can be very frightening to the person having the attack and people witnessing them and quite often are severe enough for people to seek urgent medical advice. During the attack some people may feel that they are having a heart attack but unlike a heart attack the physical sensations in a panic attack will completely disappear after the panic attack subsides. Panic attacks may feel frightening but will not cause you any physical harm.

Most people who suffer a panic attack will seek urgent medical advice at some point; this can allow medical problems that may be causing the symptoms to be ruled out. If nothing physical is diagnosed then this may be reassuring in itself but a medical review also allows an opportunity for you to be advised on breathing techniques. These can be utilised when you begin to recognise the early tell-tale signs to help regulate your breathing and stop the attacks from escalating.

Often when someone has a panic attack they will start to hyperventilate, the breathing becomes faster or deeper and this over breathing will cause light headedness, dizziness, weakness and a tingling sensation around your lips and in your fingers. If this happens then the simplest way to control your breathing is to take a deep breath in and then hold for a count of five (count in your head) and then let out a long, slow and full breath. Repeat this as needed and until the physical symptoms subside.

Panic Disorders

A panic disorder is a condition that is diagnosed when a person has recurrent panic attacks and often without an obvious trigger. In between attacks they still feel anxious and worried especially about having another panic attack, by definition this anxious feeling usually persists for at least a month after the attack. If you think you may have a panic disorder then it is very important to seek help from your GP. This is initially to exclude an underlying medical condition. If there isn't a physical condition then you should benefit from counselling or other talking therapies to help you overcome the disorder.

Depression

Feeling sad or fed up after a diagnosis of breast cancer is very common; often we find ways of coping and working through our feelings so that over a period of time our mood starts to lift. As we progress through treatment we may continue to have some bad days but hopefully some good days too. However, with depression the low mood becomes a persistent feeling and can affect your sleep, appetite, libido, motivation and ability to function. The depression can arise at any point, sometimes it may be when you are diagnosed, during your treatment or after your treatment is completed. With such a major life event even people who consider themselves as tough can succumb. It is common and figures suggest that up to a third of patients with a diagnosis of breast cancer may become clinically depressed at some point. Recognising the symptoms early is important because if you become severely depressed it can become difficult to find the momentum to then seek medical help.

Below is a list of some thoughts and feelings you may recognise if you or someone you know are suffering from depression.

Having little interest or pleasure in doing things, especially if it is something that you previously enjoyed.

Withdrawing from others and not socialising

Feeling low in mood or hopeless

Loss of libido/sexual dysfunction

Sleep disturbance i.e. trouble getting to sleep, waking in the early hours or sleeping too much

Loss of appetite or overeating

Trouble concentrating

Loss of interest in your appearance

Feeling bad about yourself

Feeling you have let yourself or your family down

Having negative thoughts

Feeling you may be better off dead

Thoughts of self harm

Suicidal thoughts

Some of the symptoms above are the same as those for Cancer-Related Fatigue and often the two overlap. Shared symptoms include problems concentrating or having a reduced interest in doing pleasurable things and socialising. Severe depression is more likely to result in having thoughts of harming yourself or suicidal thoughts and it is then essential to seek medical help as soon as possible.

Seek Help Early

Milder symptoms can often be managed by lifestyle changes, group support, talking therapies and learning techniques to help manage stress. If you think that some of these things are affecting you then you need to discuss them with your GP or hospital team. They should be able to refer you for support and/or counselling. If you are suffering from more severe anxiety or depression then your GP may recommend that you start medication. If medication is advised then you will be monitored regularly to check for any potential adverse side effects and to monitor your response and recovery to make sure that things progress in the right direction.

Below is a list of options that can help in the management of both anxiety and depression.

Reducing caffeine intake

Walking

Yoga

Any other form of exercise

Support groups

Talking therapies

Medication

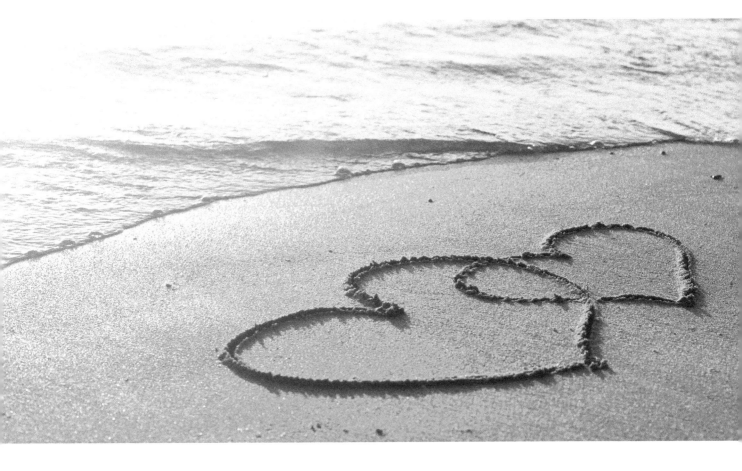

Lifestyle Choices

The management of anxiety, panic attacks and depression overlap to some degree. People will often have a mixture of symptoms and some general measures may help with any of these difficulties. More specific treatment options and medications can also help in each condition. As always, this involves a holistic approach and for many breast cancer survivors changes in lifestyle will be sufficient to alleviate symptoms. Therefore the initial step in treating anxiety, panic attacks and depression is to explore some simple lifestyle changes that may be of benefit to you.

Reducing Stimulants

As a starting point I recommend that you consider the adverse effects of your daily caffeine intake. Caffeine is present in tea, coffee, cola, energy drinks, chocolate, green tea, some cold or flu-remedies and weight loss pills. If you are feeling anxious or stressed caffeine can exacerbate these symptoms and make you feel even more restless or agitated. Therefore I would recommend restricting your intake to a couple of cups of coffee or tea per day (approximately 150 mg of caffeine). Caffeine can also cause an increase in the release of the hormone insulin which then causes a drop in blood sugar levels, energy and mood. This slump may then be followed by craving for more caffeine (or sugar) by making you feel you need more to give you a lift. Caffeine affects sleep if it is consumed later in the day since it takes at least five hours to eliminate half the amount from a single cup of coffee.

Many people underestimate or trivialise the potential effects of caffeine and only realise when they reduce or stop its intake. When people stop caffeine intake they may often experience noticeable withdrawal symptoms such as jitteriness, headaches, poor concentration, lethargy and strong cravings for caffeine. These symptoms usually take a few days to a week to pass in most people. During that time drink plenty of water, take simple painkillers such as paracetamol and get plenty of rest. If you are heavy consumer of caffeine (for example more than five cups of coffee per day) then it is wiser to wean off over a couple of weeks. After this phase has passed you should experience reduced anxiety levels, improved sleep and fewer fluctuations in energy levels.

Healthier options to caffeinated drinks are green tea and red bush tea. Swapping over to decaffeinated teas and coffees is a straightforward way to reduce your caffeine intake. It will certainly help but bear in mind that these drinks often still have some caffeine in them and will have had to undergo a chemical process to remove the caffeine from them. A healthier alternative is green tea; although this contains some caffeine it is much less than in coffee or black tea and it also has many anticancer health benefits. I recommend that you drink at least three cups of green tea daily and aim to consume your green tea before 3 pm so that it doesn't affect your sleep. The table below shows the amounts of caffeine in some commonly consumed beverages and in chocolate.

BEVERAGE/FOOD	VOLUME	AVERAGE AMOUNT OF CAFFEINE (MG)
Instant Coffee	240 ml = 1cup	60-100
Filter Coffee	240 ml	95-200
Espresso	30 ml = 1 shot	75-150
Tea	240 ml	50
Green Tea	240 ml	25-45
Cola	333 ml = 1 can	32
Diet Cola	333 ml	42
Energy drinks	250ml = 1 can	80
Dark Chocolate	25grams= 4 small squares	11
Milk Chocolate	25 grams	5

Another good alternative to regular tea is Rooibos otherwise known as Redbush tea. Redbush tea comes from a native bush found in the Western Cape Province of South Africa and is a naturally caffeine-free tea. It does taste quite different to your usual cuppa but most people I know that have swapped over to it, start to find it enjoyable after just a few days. As well as being caffeine-free Redbush tea also contains high levels of antioxidants and it aids the absorption of iron, unlike regular tea which reduces it. Herbal teas are also a good caffeine-free alternative and there are endless varieties so you should be able to find some that you like. Herbal teas that contain chamomile and/or lavender are particularly relaxing and are a useful aid for sleep.

Exercise

Physical exercise can help you look and feel better as well as being beneficial for your mental health. Doing regular exercise for at least thirty minutes a day can noticeably lift your mood. The key to sustaining it is finding something you enjoy. Even if you are feeling worn out, exercise will actually help to bolster your state of mind and raise your energy levels. You should always seek advice from your medical team before embarking on exercise since they know your individual case and any restrictions on exercise that may apply to you. You will gain increasing benefits to your mood as you gradually increase the amount of exercise that you do because more feel good chemicals called endorphins are released from the brain. As well as the immediate benefits of exercise, numerous studies have shown that physically active cancer survivors have a lower risk of recurrence and better survival rates than those that lead a sedentary life.

Walking is a great exercise and you can gradually build up your stamina and fitness levels by increasing your pace or gradient on which you walk and the amount of time spent doing it. Walking will help to reduce your stress levels and also improve your cardiovascular health. Walking outside also helps with your natural sleep-wake cycles by increasing your exposure to natural daylight. As well as benefits for stress reduction and improved sleeping patterns regular walking has been shown to reduce the risk of primary and secondary breast cancer.

A recent study by Agnes Fournier and others published in the American Association of Cancer Research in 2014 confirmed that walking is beneficial for lowering the risk of primary breast cancer. It gave rise to headlines in most of the national papers. The French team looked at almost 60,000 post-menopausal women who were followed up on average for eight to nine years. These women made up the French cohort of the large EPIC epidemiological studies. During that period 2,155 of the women went on to develop invasive breast cancer. However, women who had a good level of activity equivalent to four hours a week of brisk walking or two hours a week of more intense exercise had a ten per cent reduced risk of developing breast cancer. Of course this does not mean walking will stop women getting breast cancer but it is matter of reducing your risk. Walking for just over thirty minutes a day could do this. The other important finding was that exercise needed to be continued as those

who had become sedentary in the four years prior to the end of the study lost the protective factor from exercise.

Other studies have confirmed that walking has an even greater benefit in reducing the risk of secondary breast cancer. A large epidemiological study called the Nurses' Health Study was commenced in 1976 and involved a group of over 120,000 nurses from America who were aged between 30-55 years. They were given questionnaires to fill in looking at risk factors for cancer and cardiovascular disease. During the 14 year follow up period (1984 to 1998), 3,000 of them were diagnosed with stage I, II or III breast cancer. During that time their levels of physical activity and recurrence rates were also determined. (Women with more widespread disease were excluded as they were unlikely to be able to do much exercise.)

The researchers found that physical activity reduced the recurrence of breast cancer and was greatest for those that performed the equivalent to 3-5 hours of walking a week. The risk of breast cancer recurrence in this active group was reduced by 26-40 % compared to the group that exercised least. The benefits did not increase further for those women that exercised more intensely than this. The risk was particularly reduced for those women with stage III breast cancer and those that were hormone receptor positive.

Yoga is a form of exercise that certainly has many strings to its bow. It combines physical poses that strengthen and improve posture and flexibility, alongside relaxation through breathing and meditation. Yoga dates back thousands of years and has its origins in ancient Indian philosophy. It remains extremely popular since it allows people to gain better awareness and control of their bodies. The wide ranging benefits of yoga make it an ideal exercise whilst recovering from cancer treatment. The yoga poses are usually combined into a sequence to create a flowing movement from one pose to another which helps to energise and cleanse the body. The combination of breathing and meditative poses also improves relaxation and focuses the mind. After you have fully healed from surgery yoga can also help to stretch out scar tissue that may have become tight or restrictive and it can help improve lymph drainage if you are at risk of or have lymphoedema.

Many trials have been carried out to try and ascertain the benefits of yoga for cancer patients suffering with fatigue and low mood. One of the largest studies was published in the Journal BMC Cancer in 2012 by Buffart LM and colleagues. It was a systematic review of evidence from randomised control trials called 'Physical and Psychosocial Benefits of Yoga in Cancer Patients and Survivors'. 12 of the 13 RCTs that were included focused on patients with breast cancer. The review showed that there were large reductions in distress, anxiety and depression in the cancer survivors that had practiced yoga for at least 2-3 times per week. It also found that there were moderate improvements in their levels of fatigue.

A trial that was published in the Journal of Clinical Oncology 2014 by Kiecolt-Glaser JK and colleagues explored Yoga's impact on inflammation, mood, and fatigue in breast cancer survivors. This is the largest randomised trial on yoga that actually includes biological measures. The study involved 200 breast cancer survivors. The women were randomly chosen to either receive three months of yoga or be on a waiting list to receive it after the study period. The yoga group practised yoga twice a week for the twelve weeks whereas the control group did not do any yoga during this time. The participants were assessed on mood and energy levels by standardised questionnaires at the start of the trial. The significance of this trial was that women also had baseline blood tests to measure a number of cytokines (inflammatory markers) in their bloodstreams.

After the three month period all the measures were repeated. The two sets of results were then compared to see if there were any differences between the two groups. The women practising yoga had reduced levels of fatigue and improved vitality. This correlated with their blood results which showed that all four inflammatory cytokines were reduced by as much as 20%. Not surprisingly, all of these benefits were greater the more the yoga was practised. Certainly from this evidence I would agree with the study findings that for breast cancer survivors 'regular yoga practice could have substantial health benefits.'

If you have never practised yoga then it might seem a very unfamiliar or even daunting exercise to embark on, however yoga poses can be adjusted so that they are suitable for most people and at any age. You certainly do not need to be able to contort yourself into all sorts of convoluted positions. However if you have other health problems particularly high uncontrolled blood pressure, glaucoma, back problems or sciatica you will need to check with your doctor before you try yoga. If you are completely new to yoga try finding a local class for beginners; that way you can be guided through it to achieve the correct poses and techniques. Ask your local medical centre, library or friends for a recommendation. Inform the yoga instructor if you have any limitations due to surgery or treatment for example lymphoedema, back problems or other health problems.

When yoga is practised under the guidance of an instructor then poses can always be observed and modified or certain ones avoided if necessary. If there aren't any suitable classes and you are otherwise healthy then a yoga DVD for beginners is helpful since you can view the moves before trying them out. All the movements should be done slowly and smoothly, if the full pose is too difficult then avoid it or do a more basic version. Most postures will gradually become easier over time as your flexibility and strength improves. The other option is to get a good yoga book with lots of pictures and descriptions of how to carry out the poses. You can combine this with a look at how the poses are carried out in motion on You Tube or on the internet.

Support Groups

I attended a support group each week throughout the course of my treatment. It was a major part of my cancer journey and I am still so grateful that I was able to receive this care. It really helped to keep my spirits up along the way and also helped me to relax and feel normal. As a group not only did we receive mutual support, we were also taught some much appreciated techniques of relaxation and guided imagery. This helped us to achieve a relaxed state of mind and we were encouraged to try and use these techniques ourselves at home. Relaxing during guided sessions was hard initially, however as we progressed our ability to relax and switch off improved to the extent that often we would fall into a deep slumber.

Support groups for people going through cancer or after finishing treatment are such an invaluable resource and it would be ideal if this became a routine part of cancer care. Receiving some emotional support to deal with feelings such as fear, anxiety, sadness or despair can be of enormous assistance to both you and your family. In this type of setting you are able to join other people that have also been through a diagnosis of cancer. This can allow you the opportunity to share your concerns and feelings openly with others who are going through a similar experience. Sharing feelings in this way can provide a release of tension and comfort for each other. Support groups also provide a friendly environment in which to socialise without having to worry about your appearance or feeling that you have to put on a brave front. As well as this you can often gather information and pick up tips from each other about some of the practical ways of dealing with your treatment.

Your hospital doctor, GP or breast care nurse should be able to tell you which local groups are available .There are often waiting lists for support groups so it is worth getting your name onto a waiting list as soon as possible.

Talking Therapies

Talking therapies generally fall into two broad groups: counselling and Cognitive Behavioural Therapy (CBT). These types of psychological therapies have well proven long term benefits.

Counselling

After a cancer diagnosis, sometimes opening up to loved ones may not be easy, especially if you are subconsciously worrying about upsetting them. This is why it can often be less challenging to talk to someone that isn't personally involved. There is often such a rollercoaster of emotions; fear, sadness, hope, elation and after all the twists and turns on this ride you may feel disorientated, unsteady and fragile. Talking through fears with a trained therapist can help you to understand and come to terms with what you have been through and identify any ongoing concerns. As you open up you can often begin to learn what your underlying fears are. If these are then discussed and worked through it can help to reduce your levels of stress, worry and anxiety. This can subsequently help you to focus on your priorities and the best way forward.

Cognitive Behavioural Therapy (CBT)

Cognitive Behavioural Therapy (CBT) is a type of therapy that explores how you usually think (cognition), and then looks at the negative behaviour patterns you may have in response to these thoughts. CBT aims to rectify recurrent negative patterns of thinking and reduce unhelpful thoughts. Usually a number of hourly sessions are required over about 7-14 weeks to work through this process. Tasks or homework are usually given to you each week so that you can act on the advice in between each session.

Some conditions in particular are suited to CBT. These include generalised anxiety disorders where negative beliefs underlie the anxiety. CBT is also helpful for sufferers of panic disorders by helping people to recognise feelings that arise prior to a full blown panic attack. CBT can also be used to manage depression and conditions like agoraphobia and obsessive compulsive behaviour, and it can help with post-traumatic stress disorder where people often become trapped by their limiting beliefs and fears. Some people who suffer from cancer can experience post-traumatic stress. If access to CBT is an issue then computerised CBT courses are also available. Some people actually prefer this format since it is readily accessible and can be fitted in more easily with regular commitments. Others may find computerised CBT is just less daunting than arranging face to face meetings.

The Effects of Serotonin on Your Mood

Serotonin is a chemical that is mostly made in our brain and distributed throughout it but is also found in other areas of the body. This chemical acts as a neurotransmitter meaning it carries messages from one area of our brain to another. It plays a role in many different functions including psychological ones. Serotonin influences mood, appetite, sleep, memory and sexual desire. Usually when your mood is low then these other functions are affected too. When people are depressed their serotonin is depleted but it is not clear what the mechanism is and which comes first i.e. is it serotonin depletion that causes depression or depression that brings about the fall in serotonin. For whatever reason, when serotonin levels are low it can be very difficult to 'pull yourself together.' Antidepressants act to increase the serotonin levels back to normal so simply help on a physiological front. If you are feeling very depressed or anxious it is often beneficial to start on medication since you are likely to pick up a lot quicker and then be able to participate and get more benefit from talking therapies and other support networks.

Medication

Many people may perceive that doctors are too ready to dish out pills but that is not the case. Medication is not required for milder symptoms where changes in lifestyle, support groups, talking therapies and Mindfulness may be more beneficial. However, in reality if you are suffering with moderate or severe symptoms then it is likely that a period of time on antidepressants will help you over the hurdle. Once your symptoms are controlled then a further period of at least six months treatment is usually recommended. When weaning off antidepressants it is important to do so under the guidance of your GP and not abruptly as you may get withdrawal symptoms. They can usually be weaned down over just a few weeks. With all medications, your medical history, other medications and previous adverse drug effects will be taken into account on an individual basis.

Medications Used for Depression and Anxiety

There are a number of different antidepressant drugs. SSRIs and SNRIs are the ones most commonly used nowadays as they are generally well tolerated and have less potential dangerous side effects than older generations of antidepressants.

SSRIS (Selective Serotonin Reuptake Inhibitors)

SSRIS are amongst the most commonly used medications for treating anxiety and depression. These include Paroxetine, Fluoxetine (both not to be used with Tamoxifen) and Citalopram and Sertraline. Starting at a low dose and slowly working up to a therapeutic dose helps to minimise or avoid potential side effects; generally it takes two weeks on average to begin to feel an improvement in mood but sometimes longer. On commencing these medications it is important to be aware of common but short-lived side effects which include mild nausea, headaches and feeling a bit 'spaced out'. If any of these side effects do occur this is usually only for the first 3-5 days of treatment so it is important to try and persevere and get past this initial phase. After establishing whether the SSRI is helping the dose can be increased further in order to achieve the optimum benefit from it. Often a low dose works well but the final dose will depend on the level of symptoms. If one SSRI doesn't work for you then trying another is worthwhile.

SNRIS (Serotonin and Noradrenaline Reuptake Inhibitors)

SNRIs are another commonly used class of drugs used to treat anxiety and depression. SNRIs include medications called Venlafaxine and Duloxetine. These can also cause potential side effects however they don't interact with Tamoxifen so can be a good choice. Duloxetine works well for generalised anxiety disorders and depression but can also help with fatigue and/or chronic pain. Duloxetine is also used to treat patients with diabetic 'neuropathy' (i.e. numbness, tingling, altered sensation or pains in nerve endings in feet and hands). This can make it a useful drug that may also help with chemotherapy induced neuropathy. In the future duloxetine may well play an increasing role in post cancer care. It is started at a low dose of 30mg since it can cause nausea and headaches initially. These potential side effects usually settle by the end of the second week after which it is possible to increase the dose to a therapeutic dose of 60 to 120 mg per day. As discussed in chapter 7, SSRIs and SNRIs have also incidentally been shown to help with hot flushes.

Tricyclics

Tricyclic antidepressants are a class of antidepressants that have been around since the 1950s. Nowadays they only tend to be used if the newer class of antidepressant drugs aren't tolerated since they can have more potential side effects. Some of these drugs e.g. amitryptyline may also help with sleep and neuropathic pain. SSRIs are used as a first line treatment to treat panic disorder but if they don't work then tricyclics called imipramine and clomipramine can often be used effectively instead .

Mood Disturbance and Insomnia

If sleep problems are persistent then learning relaxation techniques and practising good sleep hygiene should help. If that doesn't help then you need to discuss it with your GP as it is often a sign of an untreated underlying anxiety or depression. Short term use of sleeping tablets is sometimes offered whilst other treatment is commenced and has a chance to take effect.

The most well-known sleeping tablets are called Benzodiazepines and these were first introduced in the 1960s and soon became the first line treatment for anxiety in the 1970s. These include drugs like Di-azepam (Valium) and Temazapam. They were shown to be effective in reducing anxiety but in the first decade after their widespread use it became clear that they created a problem with dependence. As a result, since the late 1980s the prescribing of these drugs declined substantially when both doctors and patients became aware of their major drawbacks. Physical and psychological dependence can occur even after just a few weeks of taking them. Now, because of the highlighted risks of dependence on sleeping tablets, if they are prescribed for insomnia they tend to be prescribed for just a few days.

Summary

If you have been suffering from anxiety or depression then making some changes to your lifestyle, talking things through and if necessary taking medication can all help. Besides these tried and tested methods it is worth trying to learn some new skills to help you with relaxation and reducing your levels of stress. These skills will stand you in good stead as you deal with the stresses and strains of life. I will discuss Mindfulness and relaxation techniques more fully in the following chapter.

The Mindfulness Approach

The quote opposite refers to the essence of a modern day style of meditation that is based on an ancient Buddhist practice called Mindfulness. I think it is easy to read the quote and then say, 'Yes that is

> 'Don't cry over the past. Don't stress about the future, it hasn't arrived. Live in the present and make it beautiful.'
>
> *(Anon)*

what I am going to do'. When I was learning about mindfulness this quote struck a chord because I realised that this was what I wanted to achieve but I just wasn't sure if it was at all possible. Sadly just saying the quote won't make it materialise but hopefully by practising mindfulness there is a way to actually learn how to live in the present and not stress about the future. I would imagine that most cancer survivors think, 'Right, I am going to make the most of my life now,' or 'This is my second innings'. However, it is all too easy to fall back into the old way of life. Getting back to 'normal' is desirable but ideally you want to try and be a healthier more in tune person so perhaps aiming for a slightly tweaked normal may be better.

What is Mindfulness?

Jon Kabat-Zinn, the author of several books on mindfulness, describes the process as learning 'moment to moment non-judgemental awareness'. Doing so has been shown to help people to reduce repeated and unhelpful negative thoughts and emotions. Although mindfulness has its origins in ancient Buddhist practice, the current approach does not link itself with any religion so can be used by people of any faith. This modern application of meditation has been shown to be effective in treating a variety of problems including chronic physical health problems, depression and anxiety. It can also be used in a more generalised way for all people to achieve improved concentration levels and emotional balance.

Over the past few decades mindfulness has grown in popularity worldwide and is now used for many purposes and in a wide variety of settings. For example it is used by professional sportsmen and women, business executives and large corporations like Google to help improve focus and performance. It is also being used in hospitals, schools and prisons to help people manage illness or stress. It is becoming increasingly popular as there is an increasing awareness that people need to look after their emotional as well as physical health to be able to deal with the pressures of our busy lives.

Mindfulness meditation is now recognised as a powerful tool that can teach you to accept negative thoughts and emotions instead of allowing them to take over; you can learn to recognise that these are just thoughts. It is not about saying you cannot feel sad or anxious. Instead it is about accepting these feelings and not worrying or over-analysing what you should or shouldn't do and not fixating on achieving a solution. This can give you a bit of breathing space that can aid relaxation and enhance your general well-being.

Mindfulness has also been developed and diversified in the last few decades so that variations of it can be used for more specific health issues. One of these particular uses is for people diagnosed with cancer. After a cancer diagnosis quite naturally people are often left with worries and fears that may become all-consuming and manifest as stress, anxiety, panic attacks or depression. Mindfulness is beginning to be offered more widely for cancer survivors to help them deal with these issues. It has other merits too such as helping people to manage postoperative or neuropathic pain after cancer. Another benefit is that it can be used to help improve confidence and self-esteem arising from body image issues that also affect so many cancer survivors.

The Origins of Mindfulness

Mindfulness has its origins in the ancient Buddhist practice of meditation. Buddhists have practiced meditation for over 2,500 years and there are many well-known and popular Buddhist leaders of our time including the current Dalai Lama (Tenzin Gyatso) and Thich Nhat Hanh. They have spread the teaching of Buddhism but have also have been important world peace activists. Thich Nhat Hanh has presented many lectures and written many books on mindfulness meditation and peace and is still very active and eloquent at the age of 87 years. As well as his writings about Buddhism he has also helped to make mindfulness meditation more relevant to our everyday lives.

Mindfulness began to gain increasing mainstream popularity about 40 years ago. This was in the late 1970s when it was developed into a Mindfulness Based Stress Reduction Programme by a scientist, Jon Kabat-Zinn. Jon is an American Professor of Medicine Emeritus (meaning he is retired

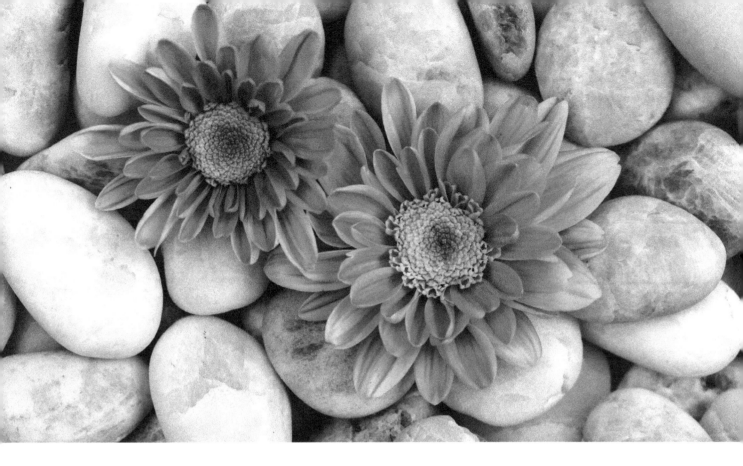

from practising) and he also has a PhD in Molecular Biology. Jon was first introduced to mindfulness meditation whilst he was a PhD student at Massachusetts Institute of Technology. He was interested in the concept since he already practised yoga and he was in tune with the connection between the mind, body and spirit. He went on to explore mindfulness meditation further and studied with some eminent Buddhist teachers including Thich Nhat Hanh. Jon Kabat-Zinn didn't become a Buddhist, but because he could see the many benefits of the practice he went on to incorporate the teachings of mindfulness into his own more scientific approach.

He first used mindfulness to treat people with chronic pain. Then in 1979 he successfully developed mindfulness teaching into a step by step eight week course called Mindfulness-Based Stress Reduction (MBSR). The course had the required, structured approach that made it possible to teach mindfulness effectively for a wide range of people.

After setting up and establishing the MBSR programme Jon also wrote several books which were published in the early 1990s. His books helped to make mindfulness even more popular and accepted by the Western world. His public profile was raised and then he went on to write a bestseller called Wherever You Go, There You Are. By providing people with a detailed, structured and easy to understand approach to learning mindfulness, he showed that the practice is accessible and beneficial to everyone independent of their faith or spiritual beliefs.

Mindfulness Based Cognitive Therapy (MBCT)

More recently, researchers including Zindel Segal, Professor Mark Williams and John Teasdale developed another programme based on the Mindfulness Based Stress Reduction (MBSR). Their research involved collaboration between three international research centres and helped them to develop a variation on the theme called Mindfulness Based Cognitive Therapy (MBCT). This eight week course also teaches mindfulness meditation but this time it was specifically aimed at treating people with recurrent bouts of depression.

It is recognised that people who are prone to relapsing into depression had a pattern of negative thoughts and 'ruminating' on these unhelpful, self-critical thoughts by asking themselves disparaging questions such as, 'What have I done wrong?' or 'Why am I such a failure?' The programme is designed to break the negative habits they have developed over a lifetime by teaching them how to let these thoughts pass by instead. The MBCT programme has been so successful that in recent years the NHS advisory body, NICE have updated their guidelines on Major Depressive Disorder. NICE recommend MBCT for people that may be currently well but who have had three or more episodes of depression in the past in order to prevent future relapses.

There are a number of Mindfulness Centres in the UK where extensive and rigorous research continues to take place on mindfulness in relation to other specific health problems. Some of these leading centres have been established for several decades and include those based at the Universities of Oxford, Exeter and Bangor. Their combined work has been at the forefront of the development of other variations of mindfulness programmes, for example Mindfulness for Reducing Anxiety, Mindfulness for Children and Mindfulness for Cancer Patients.

What Do Studies on Mindfulness and Cancer Show?

Another influential Mindfulness Teacher and researcher is Trish Bartley, she is based at Bangor University and has worked with cancer patients since 2001. She was at Bangor (Wales) University whilst the MBCT for depression trial was taking place. However, her work along with her colleague Ursula Bates has focused more on the development of the programme MBCT for Cancer Patients. She has used her general clinical expertise but, as a cancer survivor herself, she has also been able to call on her own experiences of the difficulties cancer sufferers and survivors face. Her book Mindfulness Based Cognitive Therapy for Cancer: Gently Turning Towards was published in 2012. The MBCT programme for cancer emphasises short practices that are simple to adopt so that cancer sufferers or survivors can turn to them easily and whenever they need to.

The results of several studies looking at the effects of mindfulness practised by breast cancer patients currently involve only relatively small numbers of women and take place over short durations of around 6 to 12 months. However even these studies show that the women involved gained considerable psychological benefits including better coping strategies, reduced anxiety and a reduced fear of recurrence.

In 2013 a five year Swedish study commenced and has recruited larger numbers of breast cancer survivors. The participants have been randomised so that some of them receive a self-instructing web based Mindfulness Based Stress Reduction (MBSR) programme and the remainder form a control group that do not receive MBSR. As well as involving more women than in previous studies, the women will be followed up for up to five years and they will be assessed at regular intervals along the way. If this study does show significant improvements to well-being then it may be able to provide sufficient evidence to make mindfulness a standard part of care for breast cancer patients. Due to my own experience of the benefits of mindfulness, it is in my opinion that it should be offered to all cancer patients and survivors.

Learning to be in the Moment

The underlying concept of mindfulness is developing skills that enable you to 'be in the moment'. This allows your brain to stop being in a 'doing' mode but instead allows some more time in its 'sensing' or 'being' mode. It may help to first look at the differences between these two states of mind as listed opposite.

Mindfulness quotes can also help you to understand the concept further and put it into context.

LESS DOING MODE	MORE BEING MODE
Remembering	Seeing
Day dreaming	Touching
Ruminating	Hearing
Planning	Smelling
Analysing	Tasting
Criticizing	
Comparing	
Problem- solving	

Let go of what you can't control. Channel all that energy into living fully in the now.

Karen Salmansohn

You can begin to appreciate the practise of mindfulness by breaking down some straightforward everyday tasks and focusing your mind on how you perform these by using your senses more. If you are unsure about mindfulness, or it all sounds rather vague, or not quite up your street, then there are some practical ways to introduce mindfulness into your everyday lives.

1. Waking Up To Autopilot

2. Learning to Breathe Deeply

3. Eating or Moving Mindfully

4. Being Grateful

Waking up to Autopilot

1

If you begin by firstly considering that a lot of what we actually do is done without conscious thought, for example eating, dressing and walking or driving somewhere that is on a regular route. Ask yourself, have you ever arrived at home or work and have no awareness of that journey? If the answer is yes, it is likely that your mind was on other things and you managed to get to where you needed because you were on autopilot. It is likely that you were thinking ahead, planning, analysing, judging or even worrying about something that has happened or might happen. We almost certainly spend hours of each day in autopilot.

> The best way to capture moments is to pay attention. This is how we cultivate mindfulness. Mindfulness means being awake. It means knowing what you are doing.
>
> *By Jon Kabat-Zinn*

If you can learn to sometimes focus on the task you are engaged with this can help you to do things with more purpose rather than just running through the motions. I am not suggesting that you never do things in autopilot but one way to grasp the essence of mindfulness is to just try doing something you normally do in autopilot and do it slowly and pay closer attention.

If you start by carrying out an everyday task mindfully then it can really help you to start experiencing the concept of being in the present moment. This can really be as straightforward as making a cup of tea, brushing your hair or putting on lipstick.

> Drink your tea reverently, as if it is the axis on which the world earth revolves- slowly, evenly, without rushing towards the future. Live the actual moment. Only this moment is life.

By Thich Nhat Hanh

2 Learning How to Breathe Deeply

Learning deep breathing and how your chest and body move as the air flows slowly in and out through your nostrils is an essential part of mindfulness. Deep breathing like this is also used in yoga. Your breath can be used as and when you need it to help you focus your mind. Increasing your awareness of your breath and body can aid relaxation and lower stress levels. You can practice this anywhere and at anytime, for example waiting in a queue or at a bus stop, sitting in a traffic jam, or at your desk at work. It can also be done more formally by sitting or lying down somewhere quiet and comfortable. You could try it now for a couple of minutes.

All you need to do for this is as follows:

> If sitting try not to lean back but maintain a straight spine and try and keep your head and neck relaxed.

> Lower your gaze or preferably close your eyes.

> Then start focusing on your breath as you take deep breaths in and out.

> When you breathe in deeply you should feel your abdomen and diaphragm rise and then fall back down as you breathe out.

> It can help to place a hand lightly on your chest and abdomen.

> Initially try counting in for a count of 3 and out for 5 to get used to the pace of breathing.

> Even taking a few deep breaths in this way can help to relax you if you notice yourself getting stressed or anxious.

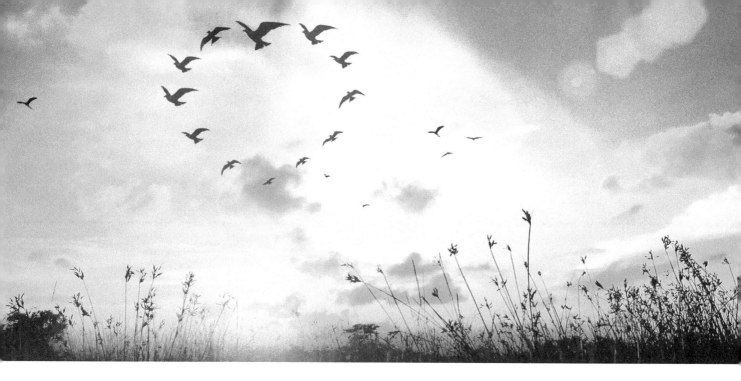

3 Eating or Moving Mindfully

If you try either eating or moving mindfully you can also experience how your senses are heightened and how you can then take more pleasure from these activities. Eating more mindfully in general can also be a good way to increase your awareness of when and how much you are eating. This can be a useful tool if you are trying to control your weight.

Try putting a single piece of fruit or chocolate in your mouth and really notice the texture, the smell, the feeling in your mouth, how your mouth moistens, how the food softens, how you chew it and how it really tastes.

Moving your body mindfully can also help you to savour the movements of your body; even a simple slow stretch from side to side or taking very slow, purposeful steps can really grab and intensify your senses and the awareness of your body. When you try doing things mindfully you start noticing so many things, colours, shadows, smells, tastes, textures and things that we just don't normally register. Your awareness is increased because you are using more of your senses.

I remember practising this very slow and mindful way of walking during the course I attended. By this stage we were in week four of the mindfulness programme so the group and I had got to know each other well enough to suggest practising this outside! After overcoming the initial embarrassment and amused gazes of passers-by we were able to appreciate taking in all the small movements of our feet and legs and notice how our mind and bodies connect and know exactly what to do.

Looking at beauty in the world is the first step of purifying the mind.

By Amit Ray

This next exercise is simply about appreciating what you have and being grateful for that. You can start by considering what you are grateful for and then write a list. No doubt family and friends will be prominent on it but a home, freedom, being able to drive; just about anything that you may take for granted but contributes to your happiness. Try and write a list of ten things you are grateful for and read the list just after waking up each morning. Put the list somewhere conspicuous where you will see it each morning or if you prefer last thing at night. Even this simple exercise can start your day off on a good note and with a smile. Just smiling can also lift your mood and illicit a warm response in other people too.

The Next Step: How to Learn Mindfulness

Many activities that relax you can bring you to a more mindful state, for example gardening, baking, painting, and playing music or even participating in exercise or sport, especially yoga or Tai Chi. With these activities you are usually absorbed in them so in effect are being mindful. However with mindfulness you can achieve a deeper relaxation and all you need to have with you is what you have with you at all times, that is your breath and body. Often mindfulness is described as a form of mental training since you are trying to retrain your thought patterns and this requires both patience and regular practice.

MBSR or MBCT Mindfulness Courses

Following an eight week Mindfulness Based Stress Reduction programme or a Mindfulness Based Cognitive Therapy programme teaches you how to practice the different mindfulness meditations and how and when they can be applied. Daily practice is encouraged to help improve general well-being and make you increasingly familiar with the meditations.

> You come to realise that thoughts come and go of their own accord; that you are not your thoughts. You can watch as they appear in your mind, seemingly from thin air, and watch again as they disappear, like a soap bubble bursting. You come to the profound understanding that thoughts and feelings (including negative ones) are transient.
>
> *Quoted from 'Mindfulness: A Practical Guide to Finding Peace in a Frantic World'.*
>
> *Chapter One, Page 5, by Professor Mark Williams and Dr Danny Penman.*

Although everyone can learn how to practise mindfulness, with repetition it becomes more easily accessible and relied on when you need it. If you find that the thoughts in your head are too difficult to ignore, then using guided mindfulness meditation is invaluable. The narrative guides you through the technique and at the right pace.

Personally, I found it extremely helpful to learn mindfulness on a course so I would certainly recommend taking a course if possible. If you are interested in doing so it can be helpful to get recommendations from health professionals or friends or you can look online for a nearby course. Courses are usually run in a small group setting and this helps people with similar difficulties to share their insights and support each other. Courses run over eight weeks with a two and a half to three hour workshop each week. The MBSR also includes one whole day session. During these weekly sessions you will focus on a particular part of the programme then your homework over the following week will involve practising what you have learnt. Once you have completed the course and are familiar with the meditations then you can successfully continue to practise them yourself at home.

Online Mindfulness Resources

An interactive course led by a trained mindfulness teacher helps to take you through the experience, the techniques and also helps to keep you on track. However not everyone may be able to afford to attend a course, may not be eligible for it on the NHS or through private health insurance or may be unable to find one nearby. If this is the case then there are still a number of other ways you can learn mindfulness very effectively. You can access online information for web-based courses and mindfulness apps can also be downloaded. Free meditations and other advice are also available on some websites, these include: www.franticworld.com, www.breathworks-mindfulness.org.uk and www.headspace.com.

There are also many online meditations you can access and many speakers on the subject. I would suggest you explore the teachings of Jon Kabat-Zinn, Professor Mark Williams or if you want a lighter take on it, Ruby Wax. The famous comedienne Ruby Wax is vocal about the virtues of mindfulness since it has helped her to overcome a cycle of recurrent bouts of depression. Mindfulness has been so influential for her that she has also written a book about it, *Sane New World: Taming the Mind*.

Mindfulness Books

There are many excellent books that can help you to learn mindfulness, in particular I found Professor Mark Williams and Dr Danny Penman's book, *Mindfulness: A Practical Guide to Finding Peace in a Frantic World* a very comprehensive resource. It introduces the concept of mindfulness and how and why it works and then takes you through an eight week step- by-step guide. You are advised to read a new chapter of the eight week programme each week and then focus on practising that particular area of mindfulness over the following week. The book includes a CD of the meditations which helps to make it an even clearer and more straightforward programme to follow.

Some of the Different Meditations Used

There are a number of different meditations used in mindfulness training. I have given you just a very brief outline of three of these to give you a little more idea of how they are used.

The Raisin Meditation

The Three Minute Breathing Space

The Body Scan Meditation

The Raisin Meditation

The raisin meditation is often used as an introduction to meditation and you will find that it will probably be described in more detail if you attend a course. It essentially involves really exploring a simple object such as a raisin by really looking, smelling, feeling, observing and tasting the raisin and fully experiencing the process over at least 5-10 minutes. Doing what sounds like such a simple task helps you to open up to the idea of focusing your mind and being fully in the moment.

> On the course I attended, after completing this meditation we were asked what we had noticed, and then to share this with other people in the group. The feedback from the group varied, some found it silly but most of us also enjoyed the experience. My reflection was simply that, 'it was the best raisin I had ever eaten!'

The Three Minute Breathing Space

I find that the Three Minute Breathing Space meditation is one of the most useful exercises in mindfulness. This short meditation can be very useful since people often find that when they are particularly busy or stressed that they just can't seem to find the time for longer meditations. This meditation involves spending just one minute on each of the following steps.

1. **Becoming aware.** Initially you are advised to focus on the thoughts, feelings and sensations you are experiencing right now. If you are stressed or worried then often these feelings are difficult ones such as fear or anxiety.

2. **Focusing Attention.** Then you are asked to redirect your attention to your breath as in the deep breathing section. Here you focus on how the air moves in and out and how your chest and abdomen move with each breath.

3. **Expanding Attention.** Finally you are asked to expand your focus from just your breath to the sensations of your body as a whole.

If you practice the three minute breathing space once or twice every day you will become very familiar with it. Then if you become aware of the tell-tale physical and emotional signs of feeling stressed, anxious or angry you can utilise it when you need it most. I find that this three minute exercise actually allows me to enjoy having that little bit of peace and quiet whilst taking this short breathing space.

The Body Scan Meditation

This is one of the slightly longer meditations, but even this only takes about ten to fifteen minutes. It is a very important meditation used in mindfulness to bring you greater awareness of your mind and body and as a result a deeper relaxation. It can be done either sitting or lying, however I prefer to lie down for this one. You begin by focusing on your breath and body. Once you have done this you begin to slowly bring your attention to one area of your body at a time. You notice how the awareness of that part of your body increases and the result of moving over the full body results in a deeper relaxation. I find this is a particularly useful meditation if I am tense or finding it difficult to get to sleep.

A General Approach

To learn mindfulness all you really need are patience, repetition of the meditations so you become increasingly familiar with them, and prioritising the time to do them. Ironically it is one of those practices that is needed the more stressed you are feeling but often this is exactly when you forget to use it or feel you don't have the time to fit it in. However, if you make a point of doing it even when you are very busy or stressed it can actually free up time by avoiding endless hours wasted on worrying, judging and analysing the problem. As well as the above, mindfulness teaches you to befriend yourself, and to be kind to yourself and others rather than judging or criticising yourself or others. I would say that this is similar to trying to be 'at peace with yourself'. Now I certainly don't expect you all to be saints but being a bit kinder to yourself and making and allowing this time for yourself does take a lot of the pressure off.

Other Ways to Relax

In addition to practising mindfulness there are many other ways to relax. Sleep is important to good health but having a rest and just relaxing is beneficial too. Setting aside some time each day to simply relax may seem difficult but on your road to recovery and for good health it is a habit worth cultivating. Having some relaxation time helps you to pace yourself and also reduces levels of stress hormones which in turn help to improve overall energy levels and boost your immunity. Any activity that helps you to relax and makes you feel good will do. Try doing something you enjoy such as reading a good book sat in your favourite armchair, watching a comedy, drawing, and gardening or just going for a gentle stroll; these can all be relaxing. However, it is sometimes easy to get distracted from these activities so that you don't stick to them or find yourself thinking about or doing something else. So learning other techniques of relaxation as well as mindfulness can help too.

Guided Visualisation

Visualisation is another very accessible tool that we can all use to achieve a deeper state of relaxation and emotional well-being. With visualisation the idea is to imagine you are somewhere peaceful and relaxing and then take yourself on a journey through that setting, whilst absorbed with all the finer details and sensations. You could imagine any setting, for example a sunny beach with the waves gently rolling and the wet sand between your toes, a fresh spring meadow, or a walk through a forest or some other peaceful enjoyable place that you like to visit. If you are feeling unwell you may also find it beneficial to visualise yourself looking well and moving with ease. You take yourself on a journey enjoying the surroundings, the noises, the colours and the feelings. With practise it becomes easier to do and for you to remain focused. This process should bring about the pleasurable feelings associated with the visualisation as if it was really happening. Your mind may wonder but just bring it back to where you were on your journey and carry on.

If you have tried this and are struggling to imagine somewhere relaxing or cannot stop your mind from straying then listening to a voice recording of a visualisation is really useful. There are CDs available or you can access guided visualisations online. In this way the scene is set; where you are and where your journey takes you will be described to you. The narrators soothing voice will help to slowly guide you through it. The background sounds of waves or birds help you imagine it all more readily. Your imagination is powerful and the more absorbed you become the greater the pleasurable feelings are. After listening to a guided visualisation a few times you should be able to find yourself getting into a deeper state of relaxation each time as you begin to familiarise yourself with the visualisation. If you are worried about falling asleep or if you have to be somewhere then it helps to set an alarm. Otherwise you are likely to be distracted by such worries and may not be able to relax fully.

Summary

Our mind is a powerful tool that is at our disposal and we can learn how to harness its power by learning mindfulness and relaxation. We all spend a lot of time using our mind in a doing mode rather than a being mode. However, with practise we can learn some simple techniques to help us relax and reduce our stress levels. You can bring some calmness into your life by trying these new approaches. Mindfulness is proven to work in many ways and as I mentioned, one day it will hopefully become a routine part of our care after cancer.

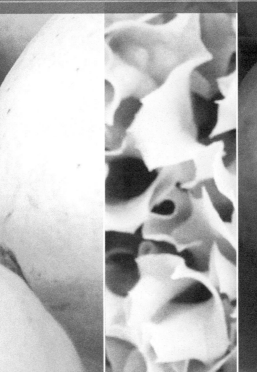

Eating for
Health ABC

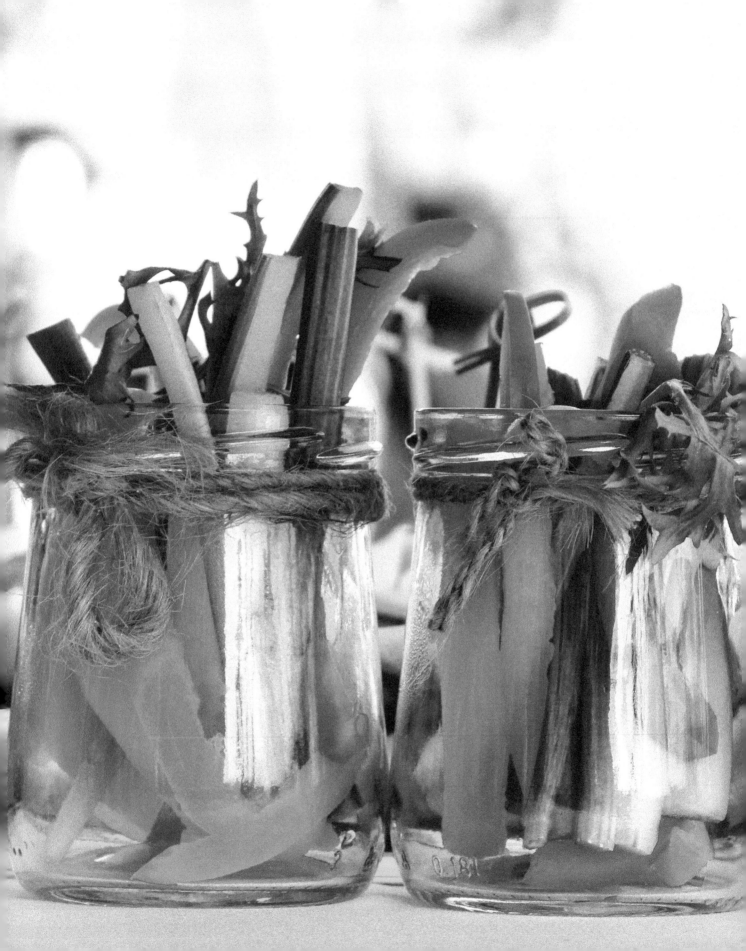

Eating for Health

Hippocrates (460-370 B.C.), the proclaimed Father of Western Medicine certainly deserves this prodigious title and his philosophy on food still

> 'Let medicine be thy food, let food be thy medicine.'
>
> *Hippocrates*

rings true today. Clearly, what we eat has a major influence on our health. We can derive many health benefits from our diet or conversely we can cause ill-health by eating unhealthy foods or by overeating. Processed foods laden with salt, sugars and unhealthy fats can often provide excess calories yet still leave us depleted of essential nutrients. So what I would like you to do, if you haven't done so already, is to start considering your diet with the mind-set of how you can optimise your nutrition. Ensuring a good intake of natural healthy foods containing essential nutrients, vitamins and cancer fighting antioxidants not only improves overall health but there is also now mounting evidence that it can also reduce the risk of breast cancer or its recurrence.

Eating tasty, nourishing food will also give your energy levels and immune system a welcome boost. If you make only a few small changes or food swaps to your diet each week you will soon be eating a much more wholesome diet. If this doesn't sound quite like what you are used to and you are already reaching for the biscuit tin then I will endeavour to show you how this can be achieved. If you have a family history of breast cancer then I would also suggest that you recommend the nutritional advice in this book to your relatives. This will enable them to make healthy choices about their diets and lifestyles that could help reduce their risk of breast cancer. In the group of women that have a known genetic predisposition, healthy lifestyle choices should be made alongside options for surveillance, medication and preventative surgery.

Changes in our Diet over the Years

Since the Second World War our eating habits have changed for the worse in many ways and these changes have gathered pace in the last 20-30 years. Globally there is an epidemic of obesity which is seen in both affluent societies and the less well off. In many countries including the UK, USA and Australia people generally do not face food shortages but are actually faced with an abundance of food and an overwhelming choice of food.

The major transformation seen in our diets is our increasing consumption of convenience foods which are often highly processed and contain hidden sugars and unhealthy fats. As well as being seen as more convenient, these processed foods are often cheaper than buying healthier options so that lower income families are actually more likely to consume more of them. Along with the changes to how food is manufactured there have been many agricultural advances that have also changed the way that food is produced.

Many of these dietary changes are now increasingly implicated as the major contributory factor for the steady rise in cancers as well as chronic diseases such as high blood pressure, heart disease and diabetes. The other trend that is now apparent is that although these diseases were once considered to affect people mostly in their old age, they are now affecting an increasing number of people at a younger and younger age. The table below summarises the major changes in our diet since WWII.

Changes to our diet

INCREASED	REDUCED
Consumption of refined sugars	Consumption of Fibre
Consumption of refined grains	Locally produced/Organic Foods
Consumption of unhealthy fats	Home cooked food
Takeaway meals and Fast food	
Consumption of excess alcohol	
Packaged and Processed Food	
Use of Pesticides	

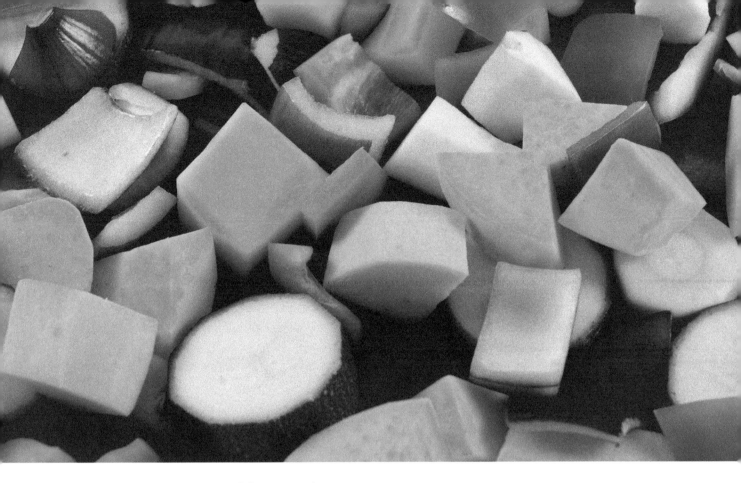

Maintaining a Healthy Weight

Maintaining a healthy weight is something that men and women may struggle with throughout their lives and now even more so if affected by fatigue, poor sleep, mood problems or physical symptoms that limit exercise. Most people are aware that it is important to try and maintain a healthy weight to reduce your risk of cardiovascular diseases such as heart attacks and strokes, and also late onset diabetes. However being overweight is also a risk factor for both primary breast cancer and its recurrence and it appears that this increased risk occurs particularly in postmenopausal women. This is because fatty tissue is the main source of oestrogen production in postmenopausal women so that having a higher body fat percentage after the menopause allows more oestrogen to be made. This oestrogen can then potentially stimulate oestrogen receptor positive breast cancer cells.

A general approach to achieving or maintaining a healthy weight is to consume predominantly high fibre, nutrient-rich whole foods and lean good quality protein as well as limiting the amounts of processed foods that you eat. You should find that eating in this way means that you feel satisfied with smaller portions of food and you remain so for longer. Eating wholesome foods helps to stabilise blood sugar levels which subsequently helps to reduce food cravings and this is pivotal for weight management.

Eating Less Sugar

The first step towards eating more healthily is cutting down the sugar in our diet. Do you remember some of the headlines about sugar in the UK Press at the start of 2014? Many of the headlines included the startling phrase 'Sugar is the new tobacco', coined by Simon Capewell, Professor of Clinical Epidemiology at the University of Liverpool. It wouldn't be surprising if you cannot recall it, since important news often becomes quickly forgotten as the next big story comes along. This quote aptly sums up the huge problem that sugar is causing to our health. Even if this particular headline has passed you by, on this occasion the message shouldn't have. The campaign against sugar is actually gathering momentum with government talk of a tax on foods and drinks containing added sugars being thrashed about.

The reason the concern has not gone away is that there are an ever increasing number of epidemiological studies that have investigated the connection between increased sugar consumption and the increasing levels of obesity and diseases linked to obesity (BMI > 30, See Chapter 4). The UK has the highest levels of obesity in Europe with as many as a third of children and two thirds of adults being overweight or obese. This growing body of evidence has resulted in the formation of a campaign group called Action on Sugar, which is attempting to tackle this major health problem. This group is made up of expert advisors from the UK and USA. By evaluating the evidence they have come up with an initial recommendation that the maximum daily amount of added 'free' sugar for adults should be just ten teaspoons of sugar. This has been lowered more recently to seven teaspoons (or sugar cubes) which is about 30g a day. This is supported by Public Health England and their very useful Change 4 Life app that allows you to scan barcodes on food labels and tells you how much sugar they contain.

As part of the campaign Action for Sugar have analysed many processed foods to determine the amounts of sugars in them, they have quantified the amounts as teaspoons of sugar since the idea of reducing number of teaspoons of sugar can make it easier for people to remember and relate to. You have to also remember that 'free' sugars do not refer solely to the teaspoons of sugar you or manufacturers might use in preparing food or drink but also to the sugar in fruit juices, honey and syrup.

Action for Sugars analysis of foods included processed foods that are considered to be healthy options such as cereal bars and yoghurts; however they were able to demonstrate that even the sugar contents of these were surprisingly high. These 'healthy snacks' can contain up to 4-7 teaspoons of sugar in just one serving. A can of Cola contains nine teaspoons and one Frappuccino can contain eleven teaspoons. In a bid to get the food industry to take notice, Action on Sugar published a list of foods they have analysed that contain large amounts of added sugar. By effectively naming and shaming many of these products they are hoping to bring about increased public awareness and encourage the food industry to voluntarily reduce the amounts of added sugars in their products.

The Chairman of Action on Sugar and co-author of the following commentary, Professor Graham Macgregor summarises the current state of affairs. (Action on Sugar-Lessons from UK Salt Reduction Programme, Lancet, 2014)

'We have known about the health risks of sugar for years and yet nothing has been done. We are calling the UK Government to reduce sugar in foods by any means necessary. We strongly urge the Department of Health and the Government to initiate a sugar reduction programme now by forcing the industry to slowly reduce the huge amount of sugar added by the food industry across the board, similar to salt. Unless they act now, obesity and diabetes are going to completely overwhelm the NHS.'

Action on Sugar have proposed a plan of action to the Department of Health, which aims to reduce the amounts of added sugars in food by an ambitious 40%, by the year 2020. This is certainly a target worth striving for and is similar to the effective campaign Consensus Action on Salt and Health (CASH). CASH was set up in 1996 in the UK, and was also chaired by Professor Graham McGregor. This campaign has achieved a reduction in salt added to processed foods in the UK by at least 20-30% in the last decade. The issue is that as a nation we are now beginning to realise that sugar is highly addictive but we have grown accustomed to it and are often consuming it unknowingly.

It will be interesting to see how this campaign evolves but as always we can make our own changes now by reducing the amounts of processed foods, fizzy drinks and fruit juices that we consume, this in itself may influence the food industry.

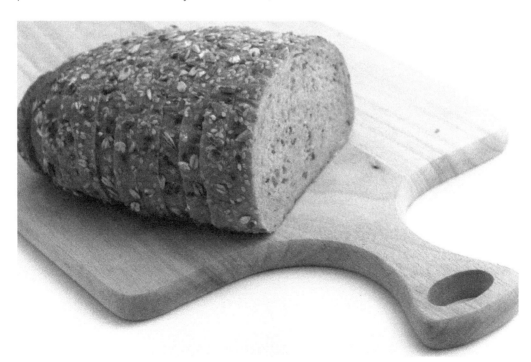

Sugars and Carbohydrates

In this quest to cut down on sugars in your diet it is also helpful to understand what sugars and carbohydrates are and where they are found in your diet. Generally sugar can be found naturally in many foods including fruit, vegetables, grains, beans and pulses. Sugars are also often added to many processed foods and may be present where you would least expect. Although all these sugars may taste the same, the way our bodies process them and use them is quite different.

Simple Sugars/Simple Carbohydrates

Simple sugars are either made up of a single sugar unit or are made up of two sugar units combined; these are called monosaccharides and disaccharides respectively. They can be considered to be the building blocks for much larger sugars called carbohydrates.

Monosaccharides

Monosaccharides are single units of sugars and include glucose, fructose and galactose. The most important monosaccharide is glucose since it is this sugar that circulates in your bloodstream and provides energy to your brain, muscles and other cells. Most other simple sugars or carbohydrates consumed in your diet are processed and converted into glucose within the body. This 'Blood Glucose' is also known as 'Blood Sugar' and these two terms are often used interchangeably. An integral part of how this blood glucose is then utilized is that the increase in circulating blood glucose that occurs after a meal brings about an insulin response. The insulin response triggers a further metabolic process that allows the glucose to move into cells and the cells can then use this glucose as fuel to make energy. It is the disturbance of this process that is implicated in the development of diabetes, as we shall see later on in this chapter.

Disaccharides

When two sugar units are combined they make a disaccharide, for example when glucose and fructose are combined they make sucrose, which is otherwise known as 'table sugar'. Sucrose is obtained from sugar cane or sugar beet and it can also be found naturally in fruits and vegetables.

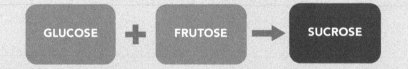

GLUCOSE **+** FRUTOSE **→** SUCROSE

When galactose and glucose are combined they make lactose which is the sugar found naturally in cow's milk. When two glucose units are combined they become maltose which can be found naturally in germinating seeds such as barley.

Sugars in Fruit

Sugars found in fruit and vegetables make them naturally sweet which means that they are appetizing for humans and animals. It is probably nature's way of telling us they are beneficial to consume since they are also nutritionally rich. Generally speaking eating plenty of fruit and vegetables is good for you because they are good sources of vitamins, minerals, antioxidants and fibre. Fruits and vegetables naturally contain either sucrose or fructose. Sweeter fruits tend to contain higher levels of sucrose and the amount of sucrose in fruit can increase rapidly as it ripens. In their natural state the sugars in fruit and vegetables are combined with fibre so they cannot be readily broken down, and there release is slowed down. Sugars are only present in relatively small quantities in vegetables and in some less sweet fruits such as tomatoes and avocados.

When juice is extracted from fruit although it may not be considered to be refined it is in a much more concentrated form so that the sugar is released into your bloodstream much more rapidly. To put this into context, it takes at least 4 5 medium sized oranges to make a small (250ml) glass of orange juice and drinking this probably won't satiate you. Whereas, consuming this number of whole oranges are likely to and in addition you are getting the added benefits of the fibre. For this reason in general it is important to restrict your intake of fruit juices and to eat the whole fruit instead.

Hidden Sugars

Most of the sugar we eat today is obscure since it is hidden in places we might not consider such as cereals, yoghurts, sauces and canned or packaged foods. Sugar is also abundant in sports and fizzy drinks as well as all the expected places like sweets, biscuits and cakes. It is important to look on food labels for sugars and the higher up they are on the list of ingredients correlates to a higher percentage of sugar. When you read the food labels to look for hidden sugars you also need to be aware of the many different names that can be given to sugars as shown in the table opposite.

This issue about added sugars has maintained a low profile over the past few decades whilst governments, doctors and dietitians have preached that the main bad

NAMES OF SUGARS	FOOD SOURCES
Granulated Sugar/ Sucrose	Cakes, Biscuits, Chocolate, Sweets , Cereals
Glucose / Dextrose	Packaged Foods, Fizzy drinks
Maltose	Savoury Sauces, Pasta Sauces, Salad dressings, Ketchup
Maltodextrin/ Dextrin	Food Additives, Batters and Food Coatings
STARCH (Corn-/ Potato-/ Modified Food Starch)	Cakes, cookies, crisps, noodles, soups
Corn syrup and high fructose corn syrup	Soft drinks, sports drinks, sweets, processed foods

guys in the war against obesity are the fats in our diet. As a result more and more 'healthier' low–fat versions of processed foods have appeared on our supermarket shelves. For this reason these hidden sugars have remained below our radar and the trend has been towards low- fat foods instead. However, if you start looking at the label of ingredients you will come to realise that many of these low-fat foods are actually high in sugar in one guise or another. The reason that sugars are added is that by removing the fat from food this also removes a lot of the taste, texture and consistency , so sugar is then required in these processed foods to make them more palatable and therefore marketable .

Refined Fructose

Refined fructose is another simple sugar that along with other refined sugars is often added to processed foods and drinks. A particularly harmful fructose exists in the form of high fructose corn syrup (HFCS). This HFCS is manufactured from hydrolysed corn starch and actually tastes sweeter than sucrose (table sugar) and it also blends more easily than sucrose into foods and drinks since it exists in a liquid form rather than as granules.

Currently, HFCS is manufactured and used much more widely in the USA than in Europe. This is predominantly because corn is so readily available in the USA that it is much cheaper to convert corn to HFCS compared to importing sucrose into the country. HFCS has almost certainly contributed to the higher levels of obesity, cardiovascular disease and diabetes in the USA. It is not just because HFCS is added to all sorts of foods and drinks but also because fructose is processed by the body in a way which can have further negative impacts on our health.

When fructose is absorbed it can only be metabolised by the liver and due to the different way fructose is metabolised it actually stimulates fat production, so large amounts of HFCS have an adverse effect on blood lipid levels and cardiovascular health. Its other drawback is that HFCS doesn't bring about an insulin response; an insulin response usually stimulates the release of another hormone called leptin. Leptin then sends a message to appetite receptors in the brain indicating that you are full. This feedback is missing with the consumption of HFCS so you are more likely to consume too much of it.

For some further insight I recommend that you watch a very detailed and eye opening analysis by Professor Robert Lustig on the use of HFCS, this can be viewed on You Tube. He is an eminent American Paediatric Endocrinologist who draws attention to the American Obesity crisis in his highly viewed lecture Sugar-The Bitter Truth.

Complex Carbohydrates

Monosaccharides are the building blocks for much larger structures called Complex Carbohydrates. When carbohydrates are broken down they can easily be processed into glucose and other monosaccharides to be used as energy. When sugars and carbohydrates are found naturally they are a good source of slowly released energy and have other benefits too.

Some Examples of Complex Carbohydrates
Green Vegetables
Starchy vegetables e.g. potatoes, sweet potatoes,
Beans, Lentils, Legumes
Nuts
Seeds

Benefits of Complex Carbohydrates
Good Source Of Energy
Good Source of Fibre
Good Source of Vitamins
Good Source of Antioxidants

Refined Carbohydrates

A general point worth considering is that both sugars and carbohydrates can exist in a refined form or in their natural unrefined state. Refined sugars and refined carbohydrates are made by extracting them or processing them from their natural state; in the production of white flour, white pasta and white rice the outer layer of the grain which contains the fibre and vitamins is removed. Subsequently these refined sugars and carbohydrates release energy much more quickly and when we eat them can cause rapid increases to blood glucose levels.

Unrefined Carbohydrates

Instead of these refined versions it is much more beneficial to eat the unrefined whole grains that retain the fibre and vitamins. These include brown rice, wild rice, wholemeal bread or wholemeal baked goods, whole-wheat pasta, buckwheat, rolled oats and quinoa. Whole grains are digested more slowly and gradually, giving a slower more steady release of glucose into the bloodstream. One other thing to be aware of on food labelling is that wheat flour is actually refined and is not the same as wholemeal flour; before I became aware of this, I for one presumed they were the same.

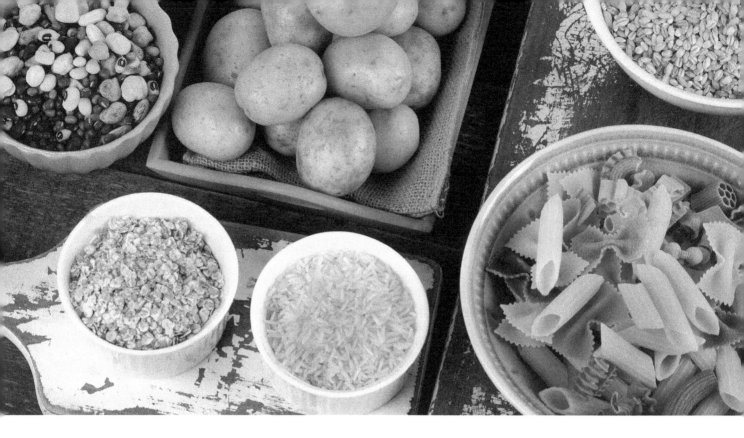

Glycaemic Index

Deciding which sugars or carbohydrates are good for you may not always be obvious so sometimes using tables that show the sugar load of certain foods can be helpful, these measures of sugar load include the Glycaemic Index (GI) and the Glycaemic Load (GL).

The Glycaemic Index is a numerical index that ranks foods and drinks on how quickly they can raise your blood sugar levels after consuming them. The GI of a food measures how high your blood sugar level rises after ingesting 50 grams of the carbohydrate. The GI of a food is given a figure between 0 and 100 with glucose having a GI of 100 and everything else is compared to this. Foods are considered to have a low GI the closer they are to 0 and have a high G.I if the GI is over 70.

| MORE of These | Low G.I = Slow Release | GI < 55 |
| LESS of These | High G.I = Fast release | GI >70 |

A food with a low G.I contains less sugar and brings about a more gradual and sustained increase in blood sugar levels; this also helps to keep you feeling fuller for longer. However, high G.I foods are digested quickly and cause spikes in blood sugar levels, this is then followed by a surge of insulin and subsequently a sharp drop in sugar levels.

Glycaemic load

Glycaemic load is a more accurate measure of how a food that contains carbohydrates actually affects your blood sugar and insulin levels since it also takes into account the average serving size. The reason this is important is that a 50g serving of carbohydrate from some foods would involve massive portions. For example the GI of carrots is about 70 which seems surprisingly high for a healthy food, however to actually consume 50 gram of carbohydrate from carrots you would need to need to eat over half a kg of them! This is because a high percentage of a carrot consists of water (88%) and only about 4.7% of carrots consist of sugars. Therefore eating 50g of a carbohydrate does not always give you a realistic idea of how people actually consume food. The same applies to watermelon which as the name suggests contains mainly water, so its G.I may be high but its glycaemic load is actually very low.

The Glycaemic load is calculated by using the formula

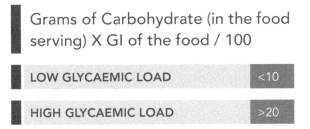

Grams of Carbohydrate (in the food serving) X GI of the food / 100

| LOW GLYCAEMIC LOAD | <10 |
| HIGH GLYCAEMIC LOAD | >20 |

Using this formula you could calculate the glycaemic load of foods yourself but this is still a bit difficult because to be able to do this you would need to know the amount of carbohydrate in a particular food serving. So, for example, if you were calculating the GL of a 30g (average size) slice of bread, you would not use 30g in the above formula but 14g which is the amount of carbohydrate in the slice of bread.

You can however find tables that do the calculations for you such as the Harvard medical school glycaemic index table.

http://www.health.harvard.edu/diseases-and-conditions/glycemic_index_and_glycemic_load_for_100_foods

The other consideration for how your diet affects your blood sugar levels is dependent on the complete meal. A meal consisting of whole grain carbohydrates consumed with healthy oils or fats and lean protein will release sugars in a much more gradual and sustained way and this food combination will also allow the vitamins and nutrients in the meal to be absorbed more effectively and efficiently. The table below helps to shows how swapping foods gives you foods that release sugar more slowly i.e. with either a lower GI or GL.

FOOD	ADDED BENEFITS OF WHOLE FOODS	SERVING SIZE	G.INDEX (<55 LOW)	G.LOAD (<10 LOW)
White bread		30g/1 slice	70	10
Wholegrain bread	High Fibre	30g	50	7
Cola		330ml (1 can)	63	21
Orange Juice	Vitamin C	250ml	50	12
White Rice		150g	89	43
Basmati Rice		150g	58	20
Brown Rice	High Fibre, Vitamin E	150g	50	16
Baked Potato (no skin)	Vit B6	150g (med sized)	98	26
Baked Potato (with skin)	Fibre, Vit C, Vit B6	150g (med sized)	76	23
Sweet Potato	B-Carotenoid	150g	70	22
Raw carrot	Fibre, Vitamin A, B- Carotenoid	1 large	92	1
Watermelon	Fibre, vitamins, lycopene	120g	72	4
Apple	Fibre, vitamin , antioxidants	1 medium	39	6.2

Healthy Carbohydrate Food Swaps

Baked Potato	Baked sweet potato , Baked Parsnips
White Polished Rice	Basmati Rice, Brown Rice, Wild Rice
White Bread, Wheat flour	Wholegrain Bread Multi-seed Wholemeal Bread
White Pasta	Wholemeal Pasta
Cous cous	Quinoa

Zero Calorie Sweeteners

I confess that I had never really questioned the idea of low fat, sugar free foods before I was diagnosed with breast cancer. If you are watching your weight surely this is the way forward? As a busy doctor and also trying to keep fit and healthy I often consumed diet colas, diet yoghurts, low fat sandwiches or meal replacements and due to my working patterns and long shifts I often resorted to ready meals. I managed to maintain a steady weight but I realise now I was going about it in the wrong way. Now having reconsidered my objectives I eat a much more varied, nutritious and balanced diet.

So whilst trying to avoid sugar, it might appear an obvious and simple solution to use a sweetener instead since these doesn't affect your blood sugar levels. Currently, the most common of these are the synthetic sweeteners, aspartame and saccharin. There is also another zero calorie sweetener called Stevia which is naturally derived from shrubs and herbs; it is very sweet but has no calories. Of these sweeteners I would certainly choose Stevia as the healthiest option.

If you are making a choice about sweeteners as an alternative to sugar then there are still some other considerations. Firstly sweeteners don't re-educate the taste buds or brain to reduce the desire for sweet things. Secondly artificial sweeteners are yet another group of chemicals that have entered our food chain and we cannot be 100% sure whether they are impacting our health. They were created so that people could continue their desire for sweet things but not gain weight. However, as a nation we are getting heavier and many overweight people will eat too much but feel they are compensating by having diet drinks and diet foods. The main objective is to retrain the palate and look for food that is nutritious as well as flavoursome.

Natural Sugars

Many 'healthier' recipes may advocate natural sugars as a suitable alternative to refined sugars such as sucrose. These natural sugars include.

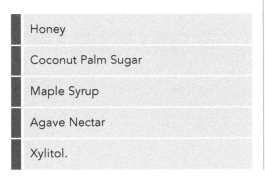

Honey

Coconut Palm Sugar

Maple Syrup

Agave Nectar

Xylitol.

Honey, coconut palm sugar and maple syrup contain small amounts of some vitamins and generally they are probably healthier since they have a lower glycaemic index than glucose. Agave Syrup is a well-known sugar alternative and has a glycaemic index of just 15-20 however it is made up of mainly fructose which isn't taken into account in its GI. As an alternative to sugar, agave can be added when baking since it blends in easily and its sweetness usually means that smaller quantities can be used in place of refined sugar. If you want to add a little sweetness to porridge oats or yoghurt then just a drizzle of honey or maple syrup should do.

Another alternative to refined sugar is Xylitol, this is a sugar alcohol that looks like normal sugar but it doesn't cause peaks in blood glucose so it doesn't stimulate insulin. It has a low glycaemic index of about 12 and about a third less calories than sucrose. It also does not cause tooth decay and when present in toothpaste or gum can actually prevent it. One of the reasons it doesn't cause peaks in blood glucose is that it is not completely absorbed in the digestive tract. Hence one potential drawback can be abdominal bloating and cramps, it can also have a laxative effect if too much is consumed. Another fact worth being aware of is that it is toxic to dogs even in very small quantities, so don't give dogs any treats containing Xylitol.

Healthier Baking

Desserts and cakes are a normal part of life, celebrations and socializing. Reducing the amounts of added sugars you get from processed foods and drinks means you can afford an occasional treat since you will be more aware of how much you are consuming and so find it easier to stay within recommended guidelines. Making baked goods yourself can also be a very good way of making healthier versions of the original recipe. Stevia, Xylitol or Agave can be suitable alternatives to sugar in many recipes and you can also use smaller quantities of these sugars than is suggested in the recipe by up to at least a third. This is similar to the process of reducing salt in foods; your palate soon adjusts so you don't need the same amounts as before to get the same hit on your taste buds. When you are baking, you should also consider the other main source of carbohydrates in the recipe, the flour. Perhaps try and use organic wholemeal flour or other wholegrain flours for baking bread or a mix of wholemeal and white in pizza dough or muffins.

How Sugar Stimulates Psychological Cravings

So the big question remains: is sugar the new tobacco? The comparisons between sugar and tobacco or other addictive drugs have been made because they can all lead to the same cycle of addiction. If you consider the different stages of addiction for any substance, you can see that sugar and addictive drugs have a lot of similarities. Essentially the cycle may be initiated by strong cravings for the substance which will often be followed by a loss of being able to control the urge for it; this then culminates in a relapse. These heightened desires can subsequently lead to bingeing on the substance and the health consequences that follow. This cycle of addiction is summed up in the diagram opposite.

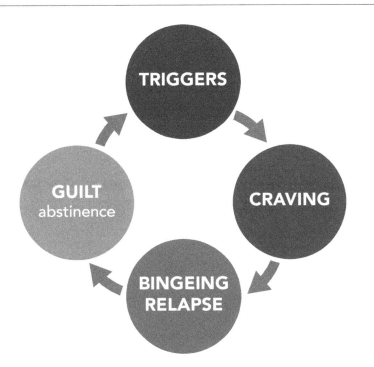

The reason that sugar can have such a strong effect on us is that as well as stimulating our taste buds, sugar stimulates the same neural pathways in the brain as drugs such as heroin and cocaine. Firstly if we consider sugar and then opiate drugs such as heroin and some prescribed analgesic drugs such as codeine or oxycodone; these substances all stimulate receptors in the brain called opioid receptors. The stimulation of opioid receptors can have a number of effects which include the relief from pain but they can also bring about a feeling of euphoria.

Sugar and the drug cocaine stimulate a different class of receptors in the brain called dopamine receptors. There are many neurological pathways in the brain that lead to a stimulation of these dopamine receptors, their stimulation results in the release of the chemical dopamine which acts as a feel good chemical. Dopamine triggers many psychological reward systems including motivation and pleasure.

Knowing that sugar stimulates both opioid receptors and the release of dopamine you can start to see why people can develop strong psychological cravings for sugar. This is why foods laden with sugar are often considered comfort foods and are intrinsically linked to emotional eating. Eating a lot of sugary food on a regular basis can lead to an excessive and repeated stimulation of opioid and dopamine receptors. If this continues then the desired effect starts to wear off and down regulate so that you actually develop a tolerance to sugar. Then the only way to achieve the same effect or 'high' is to consume even larger volumes of sugar.

How Sugar also Stimulates Physical Cravings

As well as the effects sugar has on your brain and your emotions, the consumption of sugar also stimulates a significant physical response. When we consume sugary foods in our diet, they have to be broken down and digested in the stomach before they pass into the small intestine (first part of the bowel) where the sugars can be absorbed into the bloodstream. The release of sugar into the bloodstream is then detected by an organ called the pancreas and in response the pancreas releases a hormone called insulin (as shown in the diagram below). This subsequent release of insulin prevents a sharp rise in blood sugar levels. This is very important since it helps us to maintain a stable environment for cells by keeping blood sugar levels within a narrow range of 4-8 mmol/L. The effect of insulin is therefore to provide our bodies with a regular supply of energy from the food we eat without allowing large increases in blood sugar levels that can be damaging to blood vessels and organs.

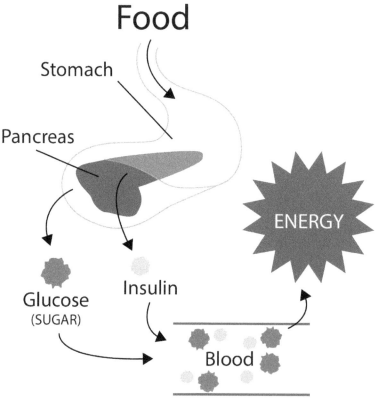

Food

Stomach

Pancreas

Glucose (SUGAR)

Insulin

ENERGY

Blood

Sugar leaves blood and enters cells for energy

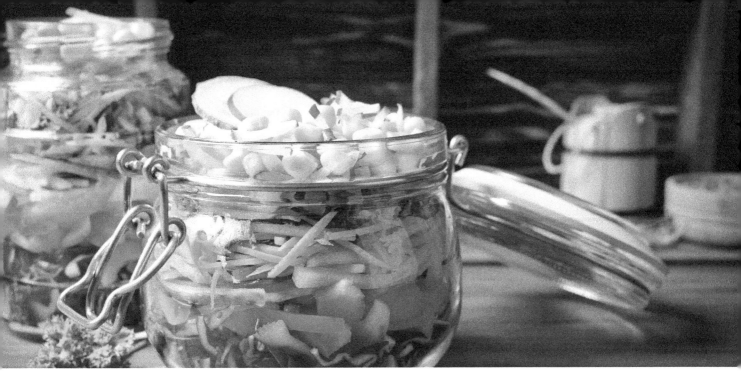

If we consume a lot of fast release (refined) sugar we get a large surge of insulin in response and this surge of insulin then results in your blood sugar levels dropping sharply. This peak and trough in sugar and insulin levels brings about strong physical cravings and the desire to have more of the sugary food as quickly as possible in order to relieve the cravings. The physical signs of sugar craving include hunger, lethargy, headaches and jitteriness. If you continue to eat a lot of refined sugar then this can wear out and overload this normal physiological process. Over time the body will then become less responsive to insulin and this mechanism leads to the development of Late Onset Diabetes. As a result, increased and more widely fluctuating blood sugar levels are seen in diabetics, who then become at an increased risk of damage to blood vessels and health complications affecting in particular the heart, kidneys and eyes.

Many people consider themselves as having a sweet tooth but it is more likely that they have just become addicted to sugar as I have depicted below. This creates a viscous circle that can be difficult to escape.

SUGAR ADDICTION			
YOU EAT SUGAR and get a release of energy and blood sugar	**DOPAMINE IS RELEASED BY THE BRAIN** making you feel good but also leads to craving for more and sugar addiction	**A SURGE OF INSULIN IS RELEASED** which causes a rapid drop in sugar levels	**LOW SUGAR LEVELS** Lethargy Hunger Headaches Jitteriness Craving more sugar

Does Cancer Thrive on Sugar?

There is a suggestion that based on the premise that cancer cells use up more sugar than non-cancerous cells that a very low sugar or very low carbohydrate diet will help starve the cancer. This theory is based on the knowledge that cancer cells are growing in an uncontrolled manner requiring more fuel and using more glucose than cells growing in a normal way. This theory that cancer strives on sugar has been further popularised because of the way a fairly new type of body scanner called 'Positon Emission Tomography' (PET) scan works.

PET Scans are used to get more detailed imaging of a cancer or to help locate where a cancer is. PET scans work by using a radioactive tracer injected into a vein followed by scanning the person to see where the tracer goes. Usually this tracer is a radioactive version of glucose. Since cancer cells use glucose more quickly, more of this radioactive version of glucose is also taken up by them and tiny particles called positrons are released. These positrons can then be detected by the scanner to locate where the cancer cells are. Based on this it has been postulated that if there is no sugar in the body the cancer cells will not have any fuel to help them grow.

However, it is not as simple as that since carbohydrates are essential for providing energy for proper brain and cell functioning. Unrefined carbohydrates are an excellent source of energy and are rich in fibre, vitamins and phytonutrients. Our bodies could not function properly for very long without carbohydrates and we would soon become deficient in essential vitamins and minerals. Very low carbohydrate diets are also likely to lead to an increased consumption of unhealthy fats which will carry their own risks.

What is actually really crucial is getting the energy from sugars and carbohydrates found naturally in foods and by cutting out refined sugars. It is a rather complex subject but I hope that the ideas discussed in this chapter will help you to find your own way of tackling the sugar crises. Following on from this, now that we are au fait with the facts about sugar let us not forget about the fats. Similarly the thing to be clear about is that fats can also be good or bad for us depending on the food source, the amounts consumed and whether or not they are processed fats.

The Good, the Bad and the Ugly

For as long as I can remember a low-fat diet has been touted as the healthiest diet and eating low-fat foods as the best way of keeping the weight off. Since fatty foods are calorie-rich and some of them in particular can raise blood cholesterol levels, consuming an excessive amount of fats is linked to weight gain and an increased risk of cardiovascular disease. Therefore many people believe that all fats must be bad; however, it is now becoming increasingly evident that this is not really the case. A certain amount of fats are actually required in our diet for good health and so what really matters is learning which the best types of fats to eat are.

The building blocks of fats are called fatty acids and as part of a healthy diet it is important to consume enough healthy 'essential' fatty acids. These are required for a number of important physiological processes. The reason a high-fat diet is linked to weight gain is that all fat is high in energy since 1 gram of fat provides 9 calories, whereas 1 gram of protein or carbohydrate only provides 4 calories. Therefore gram for gram fats do pack more than double the amount of calories into them compared with protein and carbohydrates.

Health problems especially heart disease and obesity can occur when excessive amounts of fat are eaten. The recommended amount of fat is approximately 20-25% of your daily food intake which is about 65g a day for the average women. However many people consume far more than this. A healthy diet involves keeping within this range and replacing unhealthy fats in your diet with healthy fats. These good fats are absolutely essential in your diet for a healthy heart and brain and for balancing your mood and energy levels as well as keeping you satiated for longer. Fats also allow you to absorb the fat-soluble vitamins i.e. vitamins A, D, E and K and other important nutrients such as beta-carotene and lycopene (see chapter 20).

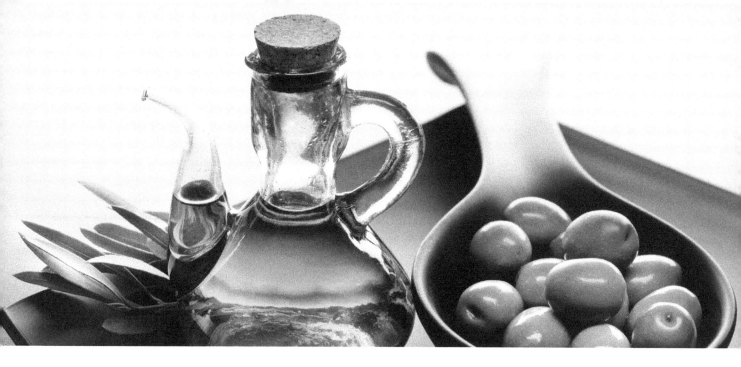

Good vs Bad Fats

The chemical bonds in different types of fats can differ in small ways that have a significant impact on how they are utilized by your body and whether they are beneficial or detrimental to your health. In general unsaturated fats are better for you and these are divided into two groups, Monounsaturated fats and Polyunsaturated fats. These unsaturated fats help to lower blood cholesterol. A property of unsaturated fats is that they are all liquid at room temperature. Hence a number plant based oils contain these unsaturated fats including olive oil and canola oil.

Trans-fats are the worst fats since they can increase blood cholesterol levels and increase your risk of heart disease and other health problems including cancer. Eating too much saturated fat will also have unwanted effects on cholesterol and the risk of heart disease. However trans-fats are particularly harmful since they produce free radicals which can damage cells. The table below breaks down the ways that you can change your balance of fats to make it a more desirable one.

GOOD FATS	FATS TO LIMIT	UGLY FATS
Monounsaturated (MUFA) Get most of your MUFA and your omega -3s from extra virgin olive oil, oily fish, avocados, nuts and seeds.	Saturated fats are mainly found in animal sources of food such as red meat, eggs and full fat dairy. Restrict daily intake to about 20 grams a day of the total of 65 grams of fat per day.	Trans-fats have been banned from margarines but can still be legally found in processed baked goods. On ingredient lists look for partially hydrogenated oils and avoid.
Polyunsaturated (PUFA) Omega 3 Fatty Acids Omega 6 Fatty Acids	Healthier sources of saturated fats include grass fed beef, organic butter and unrefined coconut oil.	

Monounsaturated Fats (MUFA)

Monounsaturated fats/fatty acids are found in a variety of oils and foods. These include olive oil, avocados, nuts and seeds. A typical Mediterranean diet contains foods that are rich in these mono-unsaturated fats and this is likely to contribute to the lower rates of obesity and cardiovascular disease seen in countries or individuals who consume a Mediterranean-style diet. This diet may contain relatively large amounts of fat but most will be derived from healthy extra virgin olive oil and oily fish. Simply replacing saturated and trans-fats with unsaturated fats can help to lower your blood cholesterol and your risk of heart disease.

It is also a good idea to consume your healthy fats alongside salads or vegetables since this will also allow you to absorb more of the fat-soluble vitamins, nutrients and antioxidants contained within the plant foods. There a number of key ways you can introduce more of these fats into your diet. For instance you can make homemade salad dressings or roast vegetables using extra virgin olive oil. Nuts and seeds are an excellent package of nutrients since they are made up of a combination of healthy unsaturated fats, complex carbohydrates, protein, fibre, calcium and vitamins. They lend themselves to being added to whole grain cereals or to salads and a handful of nuts or seeds also make a perfect snack.

Polyunsaturated Fats

Common sources of polyunsaturated fats are safflower, sunflower seeds, sesame seeds, corn, soya bean and their oils. These fats are also found in lots of nuts and other seeds. Polyunsaturated fats are divided into two types of Essential Fatty Acids: these are called Omega-3 and Omega-6 fatty acids. These fatty acids are said to be essential because we cannot make them in our bodies and they are required for many important physiological processes.

Omega-3 and omega-6 fatty acids are required for good cardiovascular and brain health as well as the health of our bones, joints, skin, hair and nails. Omega-3 fatty acids tend to reduce inflammation whereas some omega-6 fatty acids promote it.

Most diets contain plenty of omega-6 so more thought needs to go into consuming enough omega-3. A typical Western diet has a high ratio of omega-6: omega-3 by as much as 25:1 but we should be aiming for a ratio closer to 4:1 or even lower. Most of this omega-6 comes from meat which also has higher levels of saturated fats and from vegetable oils including sunflower oil and corn oil.

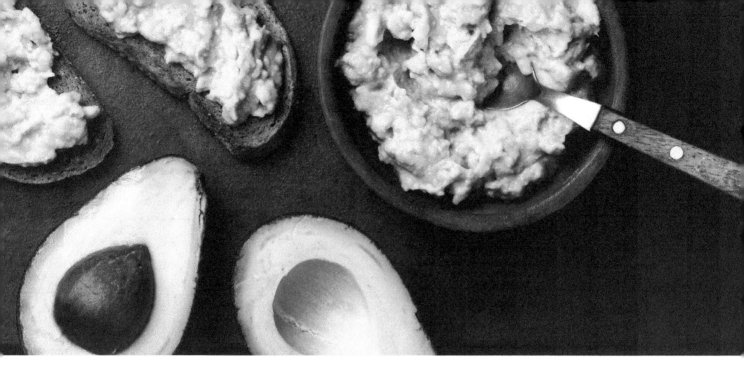

Omega-3 Fatty acids

The main dietary sources of omega-3 fatty acids are oily fish, nuts and seeds, grass-fed beef, soya beans and leafy green vegetables. Oily fish are particularly high in omega-3 fatty acids and are also a good source of high quality protein so you should try and eat oily fish at least 3 times a week. However, there is a concern that oily fish can contain traces of mercury so the benefits of eating more oily fish need to be balanced against the levels of mercury in them. Mercury is released into the air from industrial pollution and then released into rivers, rain water and into the ocean where fish can then absorb it. This is of particular concern for pregnant women and children under the age of twelve since mercury may harm the developing nervous system. However, by taking into consideration the mercury levels of different oily fish you can make sure that you are keeping well within safe limits.

Fish that live for a long time and those that are higher up in the food chains are the ones that absorb the most mercury. The Environment Protection Agency (EPA) in the UK currently advises against eating swordfish, shark and King Mackerel due to their very high mercury content. I think for most people it is not going to be a great hardship to limit their consumption of these fish. More commonly eaten fish that are low in mercury include salmon and canned light tuna in brine (otherwise commonly available as skipjack tuna). However since they do contain small amounts it is probably worth limiting salmon and tuna to 2-3 times a week, canned salmon has less mercury and more omega-3s than canned tuna. The other option is eating wild salmon which is very low in mercury (but is pricier). Small oily fish that are low in the food chain such as mackerel, sardines and anchovies contain hardly any mercury, so you can freely eat lots of these smaller oily fish.

Other very good sources of omega-3 fatty acids are milled linseed (otherwise known as flaxseed) or linseed oil, chia seeds, nuts (especially walnuts) and leafy green vegetables such as kale and spinach. Milled linseed or linseed oil should be stored in a sealed container in a cool dark place as air, heat and light damages these healthy fats. Once they are opened, they should be kept in the refrigerator in an opaque container in order to maintain their nutritional benefits. Linseed oil should not be used as cooking oil since its health benefits will be destroyed by the heat. Non-hydrogenated margarines (the concept of hydrogenation is discussed later in the section of trans-fats) are another source of monounsaturated or polyunsaturated fats. These margarines are soft and spreadable and made from polyunsaturated vegetable oils like sunflower oil, soya bean oil or safflower oil. All margarines and oils should be used sparingly since they are high in calories so using large amounts will contribute to weight gain.

Chia seeds are a small white, black or grey seed and are often described as a 'super food'. This is because they not only contain good quantities of omega-3s, they are also a good source of whole grain carbohydrates, protein, fiber, minerals (calcium, manganese and phosphorous) and antioxidants. Two table spoons of chia seeds contain as much omega-3s as a serving of salmon. This quantity can be easily added to your daily diet by sprinkling over cereals or salads, and adding to smoothies, or sprinkled into baking. When they are soaked in fluid they become more gelatinous which adds thickness to smoothies and this helps to keep you feeling fuller for longer. The table below summarizes some of the food sources that contain healthy fats.

HEALTHY FATS	FOOD SOURCES
Monounsaturated Fats	Olive Oil,
	Avocados,
	Nuts,
	Seeds
	Non- Hydrogenated Margarines
Polyunsaturated Omega 3 Fats	Oily Fish (Salmon, Mackerel, Sardines)
	Milled linseeds or linseed oil.
	Chia Seeds
	Free range eggs
	Walnuts
	Avocados
	Spinach
Polyunsaturated Omega 6 Fats	Nuts and Seeds
	Non-Hydrogenated Margarines

Saturated Fats

Commonly consumed saturated fats include the fats found naturally in red meat and full fat dairy products and as already mentioned an excessive amount of these fats can contribute to heart disease and cancer. The different chemical bonds in saturated fats make these fats solid at room temperature. The British Heart Foundation recommends that an average woman should eat no more than 20 grams of saturated fat per day, and that an average man no more than 30 grams per day. However, some foods that contain saturated fats have a more favorable composition and these include grass-fed beef (as discussed below), organic butter and unrefined coconut oil.

You can reduce your intake of saturated fats by avoiding any fatty processed meats like sausages, hot dogs, pepperoni and bacon and do not eat meat that has been burnt or char grilled as this can create carcinogens in the meat. You can also reduce the number of times you eat red meat to once or twice a week and use leaner cuts. As well as this try replacing red meat with skinless chicken, fish or legumes. You could also switch from whole milk and other full fat dairy to lower fat versions or dairy alternatives like soya milk and soya yoghurt, coconut milk, almond milk or rice milk. You are likely to be consuming too much saturated fat if you eat a lot of processed or fried foods so look on food labeling where possible for the amounts of saturated fats in these products.

Grass-Fed Beef

The animal feed that is consumed by beef cattle plays a major role in the nutrient composition of the beef that comes from them. British beef cattle are generally grass-fed on pastures for most of their lives then cattle are often brought indoors at the final stages of rearing to fatten them up or to simply avoid the cold winter months. However, a high percentage of the beef cattle in the USA are reared intensively in barns and fed with richer grain feed such as barley or corn rather than grass.

Research shows that both organic dairy and grass-fed beef where the cattle have a freedom to roam and forage have a healthier balance of fats in them. Organic milk contains more omega-3 fatty acids and less saturated fat; whilst grass-fed cattle contain more of a healthy fat called conjugated lineloic acid (CLA). In cell studies on tissue removed from breast cancer patients CLA is shown to increase the activity of a gene that helps suppress oestrogen-regulated tumours. Although the evidence in cells is encouraging further studies are needed in humans to see if CLA can have any role as a preventative or therapeutic agent. Food labeling makes it clear whether the beef is from cows that are 100% grass fed, it may also be labeled as free-range or organic and in most cases this means the same thing. Although 100% grass-fed beef contains healthier fats and is leaner, this beef is also considerably more expensive.

Trans-Fats

Trans-fats were first introduced in margarines as a healthier alternative to butter and lard and became popular in the 1960s to 1970s. The concept behind their origin was to replace the 'harmful' saturated fats found in butter and lard with a healthier version. Trans-fats are made by a process of partial hydrogenation of vegetable oils (which contain monounsaturated or poly-unsaturated fats). This process involves adding hydrogen to a vegetable oil which then solidifies the liquid oil at room temperature. Although extremely popular to begin with, it became clear in the 1990s that hydrogenated margarines were not actually heart friendly and ironically more problematic than saturated fats. Trans-fats raise the levels of bad cholesterol whilst lowering levels of good cholesterol.

With this knowledge trans-fats have been removed from margarines in Europe since 1996 and healthier versions that include olive oil or margarines that lower cholesterol have been introduced into the market. However what is quite alarming is that despite their restriction in margarines, trans-fats can still be legitimately added to baked manufactured goods such as biscuits, crackers and snack foods, and are also found in some fried foods and fast foods. They are used in baked goods because they enhance the large scale baking process and increase the shelf life and palatability of the finished products. Trans-fats are therefore still commonly found in foods and often without our knowledge. Government agencies and some food manufacturers have proposed reducing their use and some food manufacturers and suppliers have made a stance and have voluntarily agreed not to use them in their processed goods. However until this is established across the board, look on food labels for partially hydrogenated oils, these are trans-fats.

> As well as being bad for cardiovascular health, trans-fats (like refined sugars) also cause inflammation and increase free radical formation which increases the risk of cancer. This link between trans-fats and cancer has been investigated thoroughly.

The results of a USA epidemiological study published in the American Journal of Clinical Nutrition, May 2013 demonstrated this link clearly. The study was conducted by a team of researchers led by James N Kiage and Edmond Kabagambe based at the Department of Medicine, Vanderbilt Epidemiology Centre, in Nashville. The team recruited 18,000 men and women who were then followed up for seven years. Their findings showed that the individuals who consumed the highest amounts of trans-fats had an increased risk of death from any cause compared to those with the lowest trans-fat consumption; this included deaths due to an increased incidence of heart disease, strokes, diabetes and cancer.

E3N-EPIC Study of Trans-fats and Breast Cancer

The result of another large study which supports the links of trans-fats more specifically with breast cancer was led by Veronique Chajes and Colleagues in France. They published their results in the American Journal of Epidemiology, in 2008. They recruited 25,000 French women between 1995 and 1998 as part of the international EPIC studies. The women reported their dietary habits in a detailed questionnaire and also had blood samples taken to measure blood levels of trans-fats. This study led to conclusive evidence that diet questionnaires could be used as an objective measurement of fat consumption since the blood results correlated well with the diet reported. These women were then followed up until 2002 and during that time 363 of them were diagnosed with breast cancer.

Quite startling and convincing was the finding that those with the highest levels of trans- fatty acids were about twice as likely to get breast cancer as those with the lowest. From their dietary questionnaires it was clear that the women with high trans-fat levels were consuming them from processed foods.

The researchers advised that 'at this stage, we can only recommend limiting the consumption of processed foods, the source of industrially produced trans-fatty acids.

Blood Cholesterol

It is now common knowledge that high blood cholesterol levels are linked to an increased risk of cardiovascular disease. Too much fat in your diet can cause an increase in blood cholesterol levels. However, like fats you can also have good and bad cholesterol. The cholesterol in your blood is carried as either HDL (High Density Lipoprotein) or LDL (Low Density Lipoprotein). HDL Cholesterol actually has a beneficial effect and keeps arteries clean and therefore high levels of HDL cholesterol protect against heart attacks and strokes. Monounsaturated fats and omega-3 fatty acids increase the protective HDL cholesterol levels.

On the other hand, LDL cholesterol, otherwise known as 'bad' cholesterol causes a buildup of fatty deposits in arteries that can clog them and restrict blood flow to vital organs such as the heart or brain leading to heart attacks or strokes respectively.

Monounsaturated fats and omega-3 fatty acids increase HDL (good) cholesterol levels.

Saturated fats increase blood LDL (bad) cholesterol levels.

Trans-fats increase blood LDL (bad) cholesterol and also reduce the amounts of the protective HDL cholesterol.

The table below summarizes where saturated and trans-fats are found. Foods containing saturated fats should be restricted and trans-fats avoided completely.

RESTRICTED FATS	FOOD SOURCE
Reduce Saturated Fats Mainly in Red meat and Dairy	Fatty Cuts of Meat.
	Sausages, Bacon, Skin from Chicken
	Full-Fat Dairy Products
	Cheese,
	Butter, Lard
	Palm oil.
	Some processed savoury snacks
AVOID Trans Fats Foods made with 'partially hydrogenated vegetable oils' i.e. Processed Baked and Fried foods	Fried foods (e.g. French fries, fried chicken, chicken nuggets)
	Processed snack foods (e.g. Crackers, Crisps)
	Processed Ready Meals
	Some cakes, biscuits, pastries and bread.

Changes in Farming and the Food Industry

There have been many agricultural advances over the past few decades that have succeeded in yielding higher crop harvests and increased meat production. Increased productivity requires land to be more intensively farmed which leads to nutrient-poor soil; this reduces the nutrient composition of the crops that are produced. In addition to this, the now widespread use of fertilizers and pesticides results in an increased exposure to potentially harmful chemicals that enter the food chain.

Some farm animals and in particular poultry are often reared in much more crowded conditions nowadays. These cramped conditions are more likely to lead to an increased incidence of infections and the increased requirements for antibiotics to stop these infections from spreading amongst livestock. These farming conditions and the way animals are fed can also affect the nutrient quality of the meat we eat.

Hormones in Meat

In the last two decades there has been a major concern regarding the potential use of hormones in cows and whether this contributes to the risk of hormonally driven diseases. The use of hormones in dairy cows was instigated in order to increase their milk production and in beef cows to stimulate their growth and so to increase their value. However as well as the concern regarding the use of these hormones and whether they affect humans, these hormones are known to increase the incidence of health problems in the cows. In particular there is an increase incidence of udder infections (mastitis) and reduced fertility and lameness. The increased incidence of mastitis as a result of hormone use leads to the much higher requirement of antibiotic treatment in these infected animals.

Synthetic Hormones Similar to Oestrogen, Progesterone and Testosterone

Most beef cattle in the USA are given hormone implants that are natural or synthetic versions of oestrogen, progesterone and testosterone. These sex hormones are used to increase the productivity of farms by promoting faster growth of their cows. Hormones have been utilized in beef cattle since the 1950s and then increasingly over the following decades. In the USA the Food and Drug Association (FDA) advise that the measurable levels of these hormones are so low that they are safe. However the EU has banned their use since 1998 and also bans the import of beef containing added hormones. These bans took place around the time of the European Mad Cow Disease crisis. At that time we were faced with the devastating media images of funeral pyres of the cattle being destroyed; this was a necessary response to contain the infection. The British public at that time were paying much closer attention to how farm animals were reared and this may have added further pressure not to allow the use of these added hormones.

Recombinant Bovine Growth Hormone

Recombinant Bovine Growth Hormone (rBGH) is a synthetic hormone used in the USA since 1993. The FDA approved the introduction of rBGH for use in dairy cattle to increase their milk production. The synthetically made rBGH stimulates an increase in the cows own Insulin-like Growth Factor (IGF-1) which results in an increased milk production by 10-15%. The concern is whether these added growth hormones enter the milk and other dairy products such as cheese and butter. Studies show that rBGH does not appear to enter the dairy produce. However IGF-1 levels are increased to the higher end of a normal range.

IGF-1 is a natural hormone and is involved in normal growth and development during childhood. In adults increased levels of IGF-1 are found in people that have central obesity (i.e. large amounts of fat around the abdomen and stomach). Central obesity affects sugar metabolism which leads to increased blood sugar levels and subsequently an increased release of insulin. However, over time the body becomes resistant to these high insulin levels and this leads to Late-Onset Diabetes. It is this insulin resistance that also results in an increase in the growth factor, IGF-1. This is of concern as there have been many studies that show a link between increased levels of IGF-1 and an increased risk of cancer especially of the breast and prostate. It can be hard to separate the affects of IGF-1 from other contributory risk factors for cancer; however cell studies support this link since they show that IGF-1 stimulates oestrogen receptors.

The American Cancer Society, however, believe that the scientific evidence doesn't show a risk from using rBGH since studies do not seem to indicate an increased cancer incidence in milk drinkers. However the use of rBGH has never been permitted in the EU, Australia, New Zealand or Canada. Nowadays the use of rBGH in America is also being reduced due to public demand and less than 20% of dairy cattle are now injected with rBGH. Milk Cartons actively promote the fact that they are hormone-free and this is yet another good example of how consumer pressure can lead to a change when consumers feel strongly that there is something amiss.

Antibiotics in Animal Produce

There has also been increased scrutiny over the widespread use of antibiotics in farming and whether this contributes to antibiotic resistance, not just in animals but in humans too. This is something that we really need to limit as we are seeing more and more resistance to antibiotics and the emergence of hospital 'superbugs' which are notoriously difficult to treat. In general, it seems clear that a more judicious use of antibiotics should be encouraged in animals and humans, and the widespread use in intensively farmed animals should be restricted.

It is reported that in the EU antibiotics are only used in farming when they are required rather than routinely or as a preventative measure. However, the likelihood is that in situations where animals are reared in very close proximity, when one animal becomes infected, the infection could spread quickly so the more widespread use of antibiotics is required. Further regulations are being put in place to restrict the use of certain antibiotics where resistance to them in humans is already high or where there aren't any suitable alternatives available if needed to treat human infections.

Animal Welfare

Compared with dairy cattle reared using organic methods, non-organic dairy cattle are fed on mainly cereal based foods and housed in cramped conditions. This farming method means the cows are much more prone to infections especially of their udders (mastitis) and the requirement for antibiotics. Organic dairy cows in comparison feed mainly on grass or forage and are free to be outside except for the very cold spells and the pastures they roam on are not sprayed with pesticides.

Organic dairy products do tend to cost more than non-organic, but a switch to such products is probably one of the most important food choices you can make. These items are now available at more budget supermarkets and so are becoming more affordable for everyone. Organic meat remains expensive so it may be a better ploy to eat the meat you can afford but less often, and if you are eating less meat maybe you can budget for grass-fed or organic meat. There are fewer differences in the rearing practices adopted for the production of organic and non-organic lambs compared with those used for cows. In general all lambs are free range since they get to graze and roam freely on grassy banks and are a well-recognized site in the UK and many other countries.

Poultry farming probably involves the most intense and cramped conditions of all meat producing practices, so infections tend to spread very quickly and mass antibiotic use is more likely to be required. Free-range eggs and chicken cost more but free range hens do get a bit more room to peck around in and have outdoor access. There appears to considerable variation in the practices adopted by free range poultry farms and the conditions may vary from one farm to the next. Having experienced raising 'chucks' in Australia I am sure that what often happens in reality is that this outdoor access is often blocked by bossier birds in the pecking order. The other welfare issue is that birds in cramped conditions often become distressed and end up pecking each other; they may routinely have their beaks clipped to avoid this. Organic poultry are raised without the use of antibiotics and fed on pesticide-free feed (unlike free-range or cage chickens). These organically reared chickens will also have much greater freedom to move around than those that are reared non-organically, but the consequence of the more humane environment is that it will also cost considerably more to buy the organic produce in the shops.

The main objective regarding the food you eat is to be informed so you can choose healthier options. Meat and dairy are a good source of fats and protein but shouldn't be the only source. I suggest cutting down on processed foods and reducing the amount of meat and full fat non-organic dairy you consume. This will help to reduce saturated fats in your diet and to limit the amounts of unwanted antibiotic residues you are likely to consume from animal sources of protein. Instead you can get plenty of healthy fats and good quality protein from fish and plant based foods as discussed further in the next chapter.

Protein Sources and Optimal Nutrition

In order to achieve a balanced diet it is also important to consume sufficient protein. Protein is made from building blocks called amino acids which are essential for the repair and renewal of our cells. There are twenty different amino acid building blocks that can combine in many different ways to make up a huge variety of proteins. Nine of these are called 'essential' since they can only come directly from food. The remaining eleven 'non-essential' amino acids can actually be made in our bodies and therefore do not necessarily need to be provided from our diet.

Proteins are an essential component of all body tissues, especially our muscles and they are also important since enzymes are made of proteins and these allow many metabolic processes to occur. These and the other main roles of proteins are listed below.

The Many Roles of Proteins

1. Muscles

Proteins make up the bulk of our muscles; if we do not eat enough protein our muscles soon become weak and begin to waste away.

2. Collagen

Collagen is a structural protein found in many tissues giving them strength and elasticity and acts like a cement, holding cells together. There are different types of collagen and in total they make up 30% of the body's total protein content. Your skin, blood vessels, tendons, ligaments, bones and teeth all contain collagen.

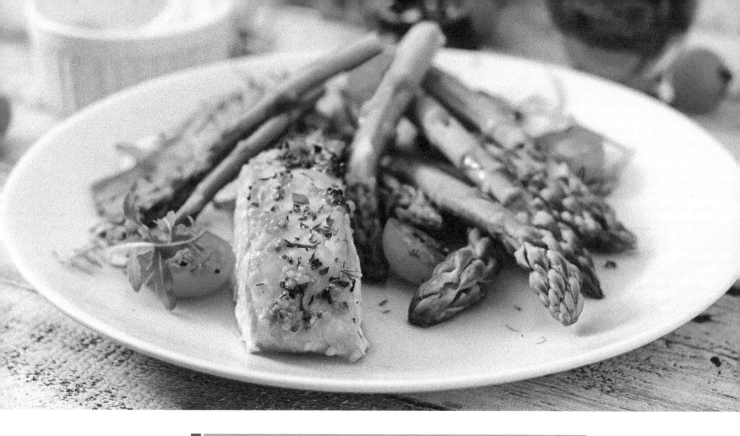

3. Keratin

This structural protein gives strength to our skin, hair and nails.

4. Enzymes

These proteins are involved in aiding many chemical reactions and metabolic processes in our body including digestion and removing waste products from the body.

5. Antibodies

These proteins are an essential part of your immune system and the way your body fights infections.

6. Hormones

Hormones are proteins that act as chemical messengers between different areas of the body.

7. DNA

Proteins make up part of the structure of your hereditary code, your DNA.

8. Haemoglobin

In red blood cells a transport protein combines with iron to form haemoglobin. This important protein structure is crucial to us since it is able to transport oxygen from the lungs to other areas of the body.

How Much Protein do we Need?

The amount of protein each person needs for optimum health will depend on their body weight and whether they have increased physical demands such as intense exercise or pregnancy. An average sized woman will need about 45-50 grams of protein a day but this will increase by at least a further 10 grams if she is active. An average 70 kg man requires about 55 grams of protein a day and again this will be increased further if physically active.

Another added benefit of protein consumption is that protein takes longer to digest than carbohydrates and so meals containing protein can help you to feel fuller for longer. If you are underweight it is important to add extra protein into your diet in order to rebuild and repair your muscles and gain strength.

The table below shows food portions that contain good quantities of protein and if you look at the plant based sources you will see that it is reasonably easy to achieve the 45-55 grams of protein recommended for an average woman or man respectively without eating animal produce. The conversions provided in the table between ounces and grams provide a rough estimate of the equivalent weight.

FOOD SOURCE	PORTION SIZE	AMOUNT OF PROTEIN GRAMS
Steak	6 oz (170g)	42g
Chicken breast	4 oz (115g)	36g
Salmon steak	4 oz (115g)	26g
Sardines	100g small tin	25g
Greek yoghurt	170g =1 tub	17g
Cow's milk/soya milk	1cup	8g
Medium sized egg	1	6g
Tofu	½ cup	20g
Wholemeal Bread	60g (2 slices)	7g
Cooked quinoa	Cup	8 g
Cooked beans	Cup /half a can	7-10g
Nuts/seeds	Small handful	6-8g

Animal Sources of Protein

MEAT
CHICKEN
FISH
DAIRY
EGGS

Foods that contain all the essential amino acids are called 'high quality proteins' Animal sources contain all of the essential amino acids in a single food, and so people often view these as the most important foods for ensuring an adequate protein intake. These sources include

Meat, Poultry and Fish

However some of these animal sources of protein are also high in saturated fats and cholesterol. A 240g (roughly 8 oz) steak contains around 40 grams of protein or even more depending on the cut and is also a good source of iron but it may also contain 24 grams of saturated fat. Fish and chicken are naturally low-fat sources of animal protein and so can be consumed on a more regular basis than red meat. A salmon steak (120g) contains 23 grams of protein and a small chicken breast about 30 grams. Oily fish are a good source of protein and have the added benefits of omega-3 fatty acids.

Dairy

Dairy products are a good source of high quality protein and essential vitamins and minerals such as calcium, phosphorous, and vitamins A, D and some B vitamins. However cheese, butter and full fat milk are also high in saturated fats. For this reason it is important to limit the amount of cheese you eat, use butter occasionally or sparsely and use low-fat dairy products where possible. Organic dairy food is also preferable to the non-organic variety as the cows are not exposed to antibiotics or feeds where pesticides have been used. A good alternative to dairy produce is unsweetened soya milk or yoghurt which contains the same quantities of protein as dairy items but is naturally low in fat and also contain omega-3 fatty acids and fibre. A cup of cow's milk or soya milk both contains about eight grams of protein.

Eggs

Eggs are another source of high quality protein containing all the essential amino acids and they are also a relatively inexpensive source of protein. A single medium egg contains about six grams of protein. It has been shown that free range eggs and organic eggs are nutritionally superior to cage eggs and nowadays free range eggs are widely available and affordable. Several years ago it was advised that the number of eggs that we consume per week should be limited since they also contain cholesterol and therefore eating too many would raise blood cholesterol levels. Most recent research has actually shown that this is not the case since most of the fats in eggs are monounsaturated or polyunsaturated fats so the overall effect is beneficial.

Eggs also have many other nutritional benefits: they contain several B Vitamins i.e. B2, B6, B12 and folate, fat-soluble vitamins (vitamins A, D, E and K) and trace nutrients Zinc, Selenium, Copper and Choline. It is pretty hard to think of any other food that provides such a good balance of healthy fats, good quality protein and such an abundance of vitamins and nutrients.

Plant-based Sources of Protein

WHOLE GRAINS

LEGUMES
(Beans, Lentils , Peas)

SEEDS

VEGETABLES

SOYA

Even though most plant based foods do not contain all the essential amino acids in a single food, eating a variety of legumes such as beans or lentils alongside whole grains can just as effectively provide you with all the essential amino acids you need.

Looking at the table below of essential and non-essential amino acids you can begin to see how plant based foods that may be missing an essential amino acid can complement each other in a meal and together make a high quality protein. Most beans for example are low in an essential amino acid called methionine but high in lysine, whereas whole grains have the reverse and are high in methionine but low in lysine.

An increasingly popular plant based food that you may have heard of is 'Quinoa'; this is a type of complex carbohydrate that has edible seeds that can be cooked like rice. However, it is high in protein and

ESSENTIAL AMINO ACIDS	NON-ESSENTIAL AMINO ACIDS
Histidine	Alanine
Isoleucine	Arginine
Leucine	Asparagine
Lysine	Aspartic Acid
Methionine	Cysteine
Phenylalanine	Glutamic acid
Threonine	Glutamine
Tryptophan	Glycine
Valine	Proline
	Serine
	Tyrosine

contains all of the nine essential amino acids. One cup of quinoa can provide eight grams of protein and this is one of the reasons it is becoming more widely available and popularized as a health food; especially as an excellent protein source for vegetarians and vegans. Quinoa is also high in fibre and contains minerals (manganese, magnesium, phosphorous, and iron) and B vitamins.

Beans, peas and lentils are all naturally high in protein and fibre, very low in fat and rich in antioxidants. If you currently rely mainly on animal food sources for protein then I suggest that you start to replace two to three of your main meals each week with a bean or pulse based dish instead, eat these alongside whole grains and plenty of vegetables. Beans come in many different varieties including, for example adzuki beans, black beans, butter beans, cannellini beans and kidney beans. Lentils and peas come in many varieties too and all these plant based foods can be made into a huge variety of dips, dhals and curries or added to soups and salads.

Nuts and seeds are another excellent source of protein and also contain healthy fats, vitamins and antioxidants. However they should be consumed in moderation because they are energy dense. One to two handfuls a day is usually sufficient to contribute to your intake of healthy fats and protein. One small handful of nuts and seeds will provide you with approximately 6-8 grams of protein.

What about Soya?

Another high protein, low-fat, plant based food is soya. Soya is derived from soya bean pods and it can be made into a number of different soya products. A commonly used derivative is tofu which can come in a firm or soft consistency. Tofu doesn't have a very distinctive flavour but it absorbs the flavours from herbs and spices well so is very versatile and because of its texture it can be used as a meat substitute. Fermented soya foods include tofu, miso, tempeh and edamame beans. This process of fermenting the soya breaks down the soya and removes phytic acid which makes it easier to digest and absorb the beneficial nutrients within the soya beans. There is a debate however whether soya is beneficial or harmful to women that are at risk of or who have had a breast cancer diagnosis.

Phyto-oestrogens

The controversy surrounding soya and breast cancer is mainly due to the fact soya products contain Phyto-oestrogens, the prefix 'phyto' meaning plant. However, the important thing to understand is that phyto-oestrogens are not the same as female oestrogen although they do have a similar chemical structure. There have been a number of epidemiological studies comparing soya intake and its effect on health in countries that consume a lot of soya and those that don't. In countries like China and Japan which have a high soya consumption women have negligible menopausal symptoms and much lower rates of breast cancer. The women generally consume soya in their diet over their entire lifespan but will have other beneficial dietary and lifestyle differences that may play a part in their reduced risk. These additional differences include their much lower consumption of meat and dairy products and they are also less likely to smoke and drink alcohol than women in the UK, USA and Australia.

Soya's most active phyto-oestrogens are isoflavones called genistein and daidzein. These isoflavones have a mild oestrogenic effect and although this is at least 100 times lower than naturally occurring oestrogen it may explain their mild benefit in alleviating menopausal symptoms. These isoflavones also have health benefits due to their considerable antioxidant effects which help to protect us against harmful free radicals and angiogenesis (see chapter 20). Most Japanese women will consume approximately 2-3 servings of fermented soya per day, which provides between 25-50 mg of isoflavones per day; whereas in America even those with the highest consumption only consume a mere 2-3 mg of isoflavones per day.

The wide discrepancy in the levels of soya consumption in the UK and USA compared with parts of Asia make it difficult to make meaningful comparisons about the effects of soya on health. This means that the results of studies on soya and breast cancer are often conflicting because they are not comparing like for like and also many other favourable dietary and lifestyle factors in China may contribute. Outside of Asia most people consume soya as soya milk and meat-like substitutes. You will also often see soya in the list of ingredients for processed foods but in this guise it is being used as a cheap ingredient to simply bulk out the product. Soya isoflavones are destroyed by this industrial processing so the soya has no health benefits in this processed form.

Evidence for Benefits of Soya and Breast Cancer Survival

A major study called *The Shangai Breast Cancer Survival* study has investigated the role of nutrition and risk of breast cancer recurrence. In 2009 a paper on the effects of soya was published in the well renowned *Journal of the American Medical Association (JAMA)*. The paper is titled 'Soy Food Intake and Breast Cancer Survival' and was led by researcher Shu XO and others, based at Vanderbilt Epidemiology Centre in Nashville. The team recruited almost 5000 breast cancer survivors in China and then followed them up looking at their levels of soya consumption and disease recurrence or deaths. Most were followed up for about 4 years from 2002 to 2006. They found that the higher their consumption of soya, then the better the outcomes for both hormone receptor positive and hormone receptor negative disease and that this was the case for women whether they took Tamoxifen or not. The four year recurrence rate was reduced from 11.2% to 8 % i.e. a relative risk reduction of 30 %.

Another paper that supports this finding was a 2013 systematic review of 131 studies examining the safety of soya in patients with or at risk of breast cancer. This was published in the peer reviewed *PLOS One Journal*. The study was led by a team in Ontario, Canada. Based on the results of long term observational studies they could not find any evidence of harm from soya relating to breast cancer. They commented that soya did not seem to have any significant oestrogenic activity in humans and, 'soy intake consistent with that of a traditional Japanese diet (2-3 daily servings, containing 25-50mg isoflavones) may be protective against breast cancer and its recurrence'. High dose supplements of isoflavones i.e. >100mg per day were not recommended as there is insufficient evidence to confirm that they are safe.

How Do Isoflavones Work?

Isoflavones bind to oestrogen receptors in the same way that SERMS such as Tamoxifen do and therefore they too can block oestrogen from binding to the oestrogen receptors. This stops oestrogen from subsequently stimulating the cells (see Chapter 8). Soya seems to be particularly protective when started prior to breast development and the differentiation of breast cells since it reduces women's exposure to their own natural oestrogen. It also has a protective influence on breast development producing less dense (lower risk) breast tissue.

Phyto-oestrogens are also present in other plant based sources of protein such as linseeds and legumes. These are also safe for women with a history of breast cancer since cell studies show they reduce breast cancer cell proliferation. Another question raised about soya is whether it can reduce the potency of Tamoxifen; however a number of studies show that soya actually works synergistically with Tamoxifen i.e. the two cooperate with each other to improve the ability of Tamoxifen to block breast cancer receptors from oestrogen.

Conclusion on Soya

Soya in moderation is a safe and healthy, low-fat protein. The soya in Japanese diets generally consists of fermented unprocessed forms of soya like tofu, miso, tempeh and edamame beams. Soya milk may not be as high in antioxidant isoflavones but if you do drink soya milk look for unsweetened whole soya bean milks. You do not have to eat soya but if you do so, eat it in moderation, this is equal to about 1 to 3 servings a day. I suggest that you avoid high dose supplements and processed soya seen as 'soya protein' on the food label. Processed soya is more likely to be in meat-like soya products or soya junk food. Also avoid genetically modified (GMO) soya since we cannot be sure at this stage what long term effects this method of production will have; the labelling of soya products will tell you if they are organic and/or Non-GMO products.

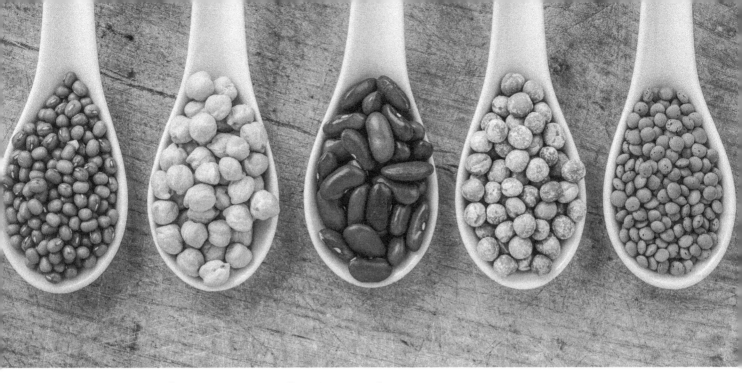

Is it Worth Paying Extra for Organic?

Another debate surrounding the food that we eat is whether organic food is better for you and worth the additional cost. In 2009 the Food Standards Agency (FSA) in the UK concluded that there was no significant benefit in terms of nutrition from organic food compared to non-organic. This was based on a review of 46 studies looking at organic crops, dairy products and meat. Since then many more studies on this subject have been carried out and a more up to date review of available good quality evidence now shows that organic crops are certainly better for you.

This more extensive Newcastle (UK) University led analysis took place in collaboration with a number of experts from other European countries and the USA. These experts analyzed 343 studies which compared organic and non-organic crops. The study was published in The British Journal of Nutrition, Sept 2014. Professor Leifert, the Professor of Ecological Agriculture at

Newcastle University who led the study comments that 'more data is available to us now than five years ago' and that these studies contradict the FSA (2009) findings.

Organic food is desirable for a number of reasons and the title of the study says it all, namely 'Higher antioxidant and lower cadmium concentrations and lower incidence of pesticide residues in organically grown crops.' This systematic review showed that the amount of different antioxidants in each organic crop was increased by as much as 19-69% compared to non-organic crops. However, overall this amounted to just 1-2 servings of fruit or vegetables per day. Results also showed that the presence of pesticide residues was four times less than in non-organic crops. There was significantly less of the toxic heavy metal cadmium in organic produce by 48% lower on average. However, the levels still remained very low in non-organic produce. These findings are not surprising really since I presume that most people would expect that organic food to contain more nutrients and fewer pesticides.

For most people, the major reluctance in purchasing organic produce is due to the cost, this makes it an unfeasible choice for many. However, I would suggest trying to switch to organic for some of the produce you buy. Look for local Farmers markets where you can buy locally grown, therefore fresher and also often organic produce. It is also worthwhile looking for seasonal organic produce since the cost of organic food varies considerably over the year and tends to be noticeably cheaper when the produce is in season.

Some fruits and vegetables may be sprayed more often with pesticides so will have more residues; further information is available on the environmental working group website www.ewg.org . Pears and apples feature high on the list along with soft citrus fruits. Washing fruit and vegetables thoroughly helps reduce the amounts of residues and with soft citrus fruits avoid using the rind/peel since most of the pesticides are in the peel. Some organic produce is reasonably priced so more affordable and available e.g. carrots, spinach, potatoes and flour. I would also try and shift to organic milk and other organic dairy products if possible.

Main Differences between Organic and Non-Organic Crops

Clearly the benefits of fruit and vegetables will always outweigh any risk from the pesticide residues but it is still sensible to wash off as much as possible. People often claim to prefer the taste of organic produce and in part this is likely to be because it is picked when it is ripe and so has developed more flavour. Organic crops are also grown from soil of better quality that is not depleted of nutrients compared with non-organic farming in which the soil usually requires improvement and this will be achieved by the use of artificial fertilizers.

ORGANIC	CONVENTIALLY GROWN
More Expensive	Cheaper
Can be more difficult to source.	Available Everywhere
Significantly Less Pesticide Residues	May Last Longer If Treated With Pesticides
Increased Nutrient Composition	
Better Animal Welfare	
Better For The Environment	
No Antibiotics Used In Meat Or Poultry	
Tastes Better	

AVOID / REDUCE	ALTERNATIVE
Non-Organic Full Fat Dairy Products	Low Fat Organic Milk or fortified dairy substitute's e.g. almond milk, coconut milk, rice milk or soya milk. Organic cheese and low fat organic yoghurt or soya yoghurt
Fatty Red Meat Processed meats	Lean cuts, Grass-fed Beef
	Beans and Pulses
	Oily Fish, Chicken
Cut down on butter and margarines	Small amounts organic butter , unrefined coconut oil or non-hydrogenated margarines
Refined sugars	Eat less sweet things. As an alternative use Xylitol, Stevia or Coconut Sugar in baking or add a small drizzle of honey, maple syrup or agave nectar to sweeten.
Processed foods with trans fats and added sugars	Home cooked foods
Saturated fats in meat and processed foods	Healthy fats as in oily fish, Avocados, olive oil and linseed oil.
High fat , high sugar snacks	Nuts, seeds, popcorn, fruit, crudités with hummus/guacamole/salsa dips.
High fat, high sugar dressings	Olive oil/Flaxseed oil homemade salad dressings

Optimal Nutritional Plan ABC

Now you have a clearer understanding of the foods you should be eating you may be wondering how you actually incorporate this knowledge into your everyday life. Eating a healthy well balanced diet is essential and if you can afford some changes then do so with things that will have the most impact. It is as simple as avoiding some foods and swapping to the healthier alternatives, as shown above. Eating more home cooked meals instead of processed foods will also make a major difference.

Healthy Plate

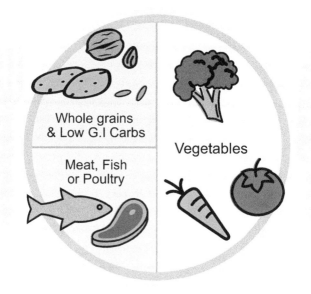

A balanced diet is key to staying healthy.
You should look at you plate as a great way
of checking that half consists of vegetables
and the other half is split between whole grains
naturally low-fat proteins and healthy fats.

Basic Principles

When you are buying packaged, pre-pre-pared food then it is worthwhile looking at the ingredient list to try and buy things without the added sugars, sweeteners, fla-vourings, thickeners, colouring or additives wherever possible. The main objective is to eat more fresh home cooked foods as opposed to processed foods. If we are aiming to eat more healthily then there is no reason that it cannot be homemade fast food too. For example, it doesn't take long to throw together a salad, or toss some vegetables in a tray with olive oil and roast them. While this is going on some chicken or fish can be poached, baked or grilled with some garlic, herbs and spices.

The main objective is eating a healthy, well balanced diet with lots of nutrient dense foods such as whole grains, legumes, nuts, seeds, fruit and vegetables together with some good quality protein and a moderate amount of healthy fats. As well as the added nutritional benefits of plant based foods, these foods are also rich in cancer fighting antioxidants as discussed in the next chapter.

MOVING ON AFTER BREAST CANCER

Antioxidants and How They Work

Antioxidants are natural compounds that can be obtained from many different food sources. Most people know that they are of benefit to their health but may not be exactly sure what they are or how they work. Without a real understanding of how they work they may appear to be just another health fad.

Free radicals are produced in our bodies every day and can be harmful to cells and cell structures if present in excess. Antioxidants can neutralise these free radicals to make them harmless. I will explain how antioxidants achieve this but if chemistry or biology are not your forté then feel free to skip to 'Benefits of a Plant Based Diet' found later on in this chapter. However by going into a little more detail hopefully I can help you to understand more about the importance of dietary antioxidants.

What Are Metabolic Processes?

Metabolic processes are a collection of chemical reactions that take place in our cells; these processes occur constantly and are essential to the maintenance of life. There are two categories of metabolic processes: anabolic and catabolic. The main roles of anabolic metabolic processes are for building or storing. For example, anabolic processes will be involved in supporting the growth of new cells, maintaining our body's tissues and helping us to store energy from food for future use. This energy is stored predominantly in the liver, muscles or fatty tissue.

Catabolic processes have the opposite role and act to break down and convert the building blocks of carbohydrates, fats and proteins from our diet into energy. This cannot take place in one easy step but requires a series of different chemical reactions to occur one after the other in order to achieve this. Free radicals are by-products of these metabolic processes. The chemical reactions that make up a metabolic process are aided by enzymes. Enzymes regulate and speed up the reactions and drive them in the desired direction. The activity of the enzymes is influenced by the cell's environment and also by signals sent from other cells.

Free Radicals

So we now know that free radicals are produced naturally by our bodies every day as a normal by-product of our cell's energy production and other metabolic processes. A free radical is defined as any single 'atom' or 'molecule' that has an unpaired 'electron'. Free radicals can have a positive or detrimental effect depending on the quantities present. In normal amounts they are useful since they act as messengers between cells. However, when there is an excess of free radicals they can start to play havoc and cause damage to cells and their structures. Antioxidants help to neutralise the free radicals by providing a spare electron, and when they do so the free radical is no longer harmful. The diagram below helps to demonstrate the main components of atoms and molecules.

█ Atoms and Molecules

Atoms are made up of a central body called a nucleus and this contains positively charged particles called protons and particles which carry no charge called neutrons. In an orbit around the nucleus are negatively charged particles called electrons. An atom contains the same number of protons and electrons, so that their positive and negative charges are balanced and negate each other. When atoms join together they become a molecule. For example two atoms of hydrogen (H2) can join together with one atom of oxygen (O) to make water, otherwise commonly known as H_2O.

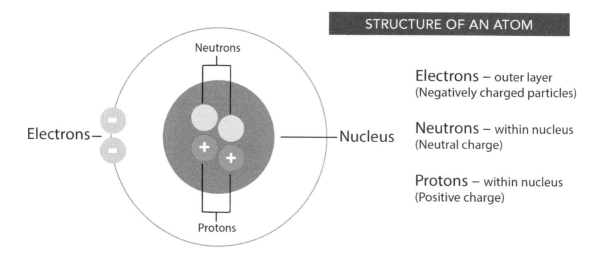

STRUCTURE OF AN ATOM

Neutrons

Electrons —

Nucleus

Protons

Electrons – outer layer
(Negatively charged particles)

Neutrons – within nucleus
(Neutral charge)

Protons – within nucleus
(Positive charge)

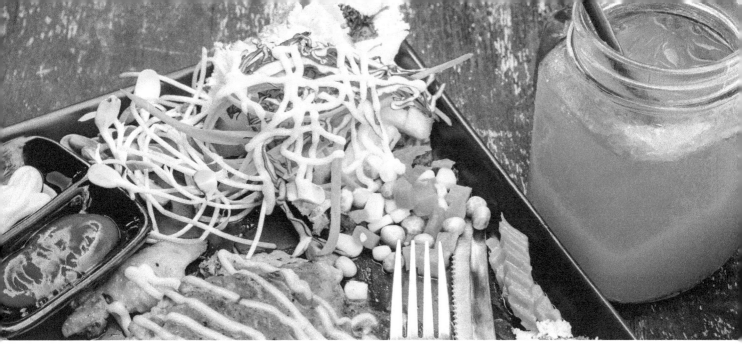

When the negatively charged electrons are not paired up the atom or molecule now shows the features of a free radical. This free radical is now very unstable and can whizz around causing damage to important molecules and structures such as cell membranes (the outer wall of a cell), mitochondria (energy producing powerhouse of a cell) and DNA. Some cancers may be triggered by this damage to cell DNA.

Increased numbers of free radicals are formed during inflammatory processes which occur when our immune system is defending the body against infection, environmental toxins and other harmful substances. Exposure to cigarette smoke and excess alcohol can both increase free radical formation as can the excessive consumption of refined sugars and trans-fatty acids.

Reactive Oxygen Species

There are many different types of free radicals but the most harmful ones are produced during a process called oxidation in which our cells interact with oxygen. These free radical products are known as Reactive Oxygen Species (ROS). They are formed naturally in any animal that breathes oxygen. Their presence can be beneficial when kept in check since a normal amount of ROS helps to send messages between our cells and they are also involved in gene expression and cell death. Some cells that are part of the immune system also rely on

ROS to help them attack harmful invaders.

However increased levels of ROS are produced in response to environmental stress or pollutants and this can be harmful. Too many ROS cause 'Oxidative Stress' and damage to cells. Cancer cells exhibit an increased growth rate and energy use and so continue to produce increased amounts of ROS. This can create a vicious cycle and perpetuate the whole process, creating further oxidative stress. ROS include substances that you may recognise the names of, such as Superoxide, Hydrogen peroxide and Nitric Oxide.

Antioxidants vs Free Radicals

As we have already seen, free radicals are not necessarily a bad thing. However, an overload of free radicals can contribute to a multitude of health problems. These include accelerated ageing and degenerative diseases such as arthritis and osteoporosis, and chronic health conditions such as heart disease, lung disease, dementia and cancer. Our bodies can repair some of the damage done by free radicals but unfortunately with advancing age we become less efficient at doing so. Therefore as we get older it becomes even more important to pay closer attention to our diet and consume more antioxidant-rich foods.

HOW AN ANTIOXIDANT CAN NEUTRALISE A FREE RADICAL

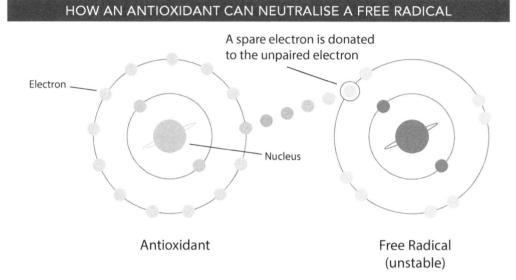

A spare electron is donated to the unpaired electron

Electron

Nucleus

Antioxidant

Free Radical (unstable)

An antioxidant is a very helpful molecule since it is stable and can donate an electron to a free radical and thereby neutralise the free radical (as shown above). This then prevents the free radical from causing potential damage to our cells.

Stages of Cancer Cell Growth

There are different mechanisms by which antioxidants and other plant nutrients can help to protect us against cancer. This can be demonstrated by looking more closely at the stages of cancer cell growth.

Cells in our bodies have a natural lifespan ranging between just a few days and several years after which they usually die; they are then replaced by new healthy cells. For example, red blood cells circulating in our bloodstream and carrying oxygen to different areas of our body have a life span of about 120 days, whereas cells lining our stomach only survive for about 5 days. Abnormal or aging cells are usually removed and destroyed by our immune system. For cancer cells to form and increase in numbers they must undergo the following three stages of abnormal change and behaviour, Initiation, Promotion and Proliferation.

1 Initiation

The initiation stage involves an abnormality occurring to cell DNA; this is called a mutation. The initiation of cancer cells may occur in response to carcinogens (cancer promoting substances) or free radicals. When normal cells undergo mutations into cancer cells then these cells develop the ability to evade normal cell signalling and therefore escape cell death. The cancer cell is also able to divide and grow uncontrollably.

2 Promotion

The environment surrounding these abnormal cancer cells will affect whether these initiated cancer cells are able to survive. The cancer cells have to avoid the initial response from your immune system which aims to destroy and remove them. Cells from the immune system come to the site where the cancer cells are and in the process of trying to destroy the cancer cells they release inflammatory chemicals such as cytokines. The growth of cancer cells may actually be encouraged by the presence of excessive inflammatory chemicals and the inflammatory environment can also promote the formation of new blood vessels called angiogenesis. These vessels bring oxygen and nutrients to the area.

As well as this, breast cancer growth can also be promoted by oestrogen and/or progesterone hormones in hormone receptor positive cancers.

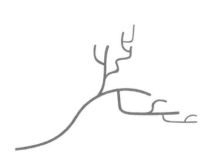

Before angiogenesis

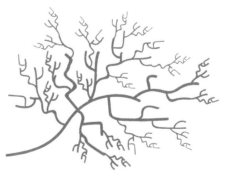

After angiogenesis

3 Proliferation

Once formed these cancer cells continue to increase in numbers exponentially by dividing; in effect they keep doubling up from 2 to 4, 8, 16, 32, 64, and 128 and so on. This stage is called Proliferation. When observed under a microscope cancer cells are often seen to become more abnormal in appearance as they proliferate; this allows them to avoid normal inhibitory mechanisms even further.

Below is a summary of these stages of cancer cell growth and proliferation.

	INITIATION MUTATION OCCURS TO CELL DNA	2	PROMOTION	3	PROLIFERATION
1	Exposure to Carcinogens		Inflammation		Unresponsive To Normal Inhibitory Mechanisms
	Tobacco		Inflammation at the site of the tumour encourages cell growth and angiogenesis		Cell Death (apoptosis)
	Excess alcohol				Activity of Natural Killer Cells
	Excess UV Radiation				Removal of cancer promoters by liver enzymes
	Pollutants				
	Cell Damage		Oestrogen/Progesterone		Angiogenesis
	Free Radicals		Promotes growth of hormone receptor positive breast cancers.		The formation of new blood vessels which bring nutrients and oxygen to the cancer cells.
	Reactive Oxygen Species				

HOW CANCER CELLS DIVIDE AND GROW ABNORMALLY

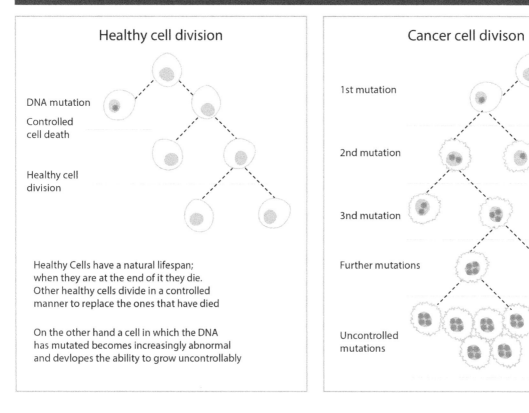

Healthy cell division

DNA mutation

Controlled cell death

Healthy cell division

Healthy Cells have a natural lifespan; when they are at the end of it they die. Other healthy cells divide in a controlled manner to replace the ones that have died

On the other hand a cell in which the DNA has mutated becomes increasingly abnormal and devlopes the ability to grow uncontrollably

Cancer cell divison

1st mutation

2nd mutation

3nd mutation

Further mutations

Uncontrolled mutations

Classifications of Antioxidants

Antioxidants play a very important role in our overall health and exist in four main categories (as shown in the table below). Intrinsically our bodies contain a number of antioxidant enzymes that are produced by the liver. However we can also obtain additional antioxidants from food; these dietary antioxidants can be found in the form of antioxidant vitamins, trace minerals (co-factors) and a large variety of Phytonutrients otherwise called Phytochemicals. The prefix 'phyto' simply means plant.

There are more than twenty five thousand different antioxidant phytonutrients which are found in the huge variety of edible plant sources. Each individual plant can contain several hundred phytonutrients and the way that they are naturally packaged together (compared to a supplement form) enhances our ability to absorb them. However, if you have a vitamin or trace element deficiency then the short term use of supplements can be beneficial. Always get advice on the use of supplements from your GP or a qualified nutritionist who will take into consideration your overall health and any medications you are taking.

This table shows the four different categories of antioxidants. Enzymes are made in our body whereas the other antioxidants come from our diet.

ANTIOXIDANT ENZYMES	ANTIOXIDANT CO-FACTORS	ANTIOXIDANT VITAMINS	ANTIOXIDANT PHYTONUTRIENTS
Superoxide Dismutase		Vitamin A	Polyphenols
Catalase	Copper	Vitamin C	Sulphur Compounds
Glutathione Peroxidase	Iron	Vitamin E	Terpenes
Glutathione Reductase	Manganese		
	Selenium		
	Zinc		

1 Antioxidant Enzymes

Humans have a sophisticated defence mechanism consisting of a number of antioxidant enzymes produced by the liver that can remove reactive oxygen species (ROS). These are the particularly harmful radicals we discussed earlier. For example, if we are faced with an excess of a ROS called superoxide, then the enzyme Superoxide Dismutase (SOD) can start to neutralise it. The initial reaction is followed by the actions of two other antioxidant enzymes; they are either Catalase or Glutathione Peroxidise. The end result is that the harmful superoxide is basically converted to water and oxygen.

Glutathione is an important water soluble antioxidant that can move freely within cells. It has a simple structure that can attract and mop up

ROS. However when glutathione interacts with ROS it becomes oxidised and temporarily becomes a free radical itself. However the antioxidant enzyme Glutathione Reductase can protect cells from damage by changing the glutathione back into its original and stable form.

Antioxidant Co-Factors

2

Antioxidant enzymes require the co-factors listed below to be maximally effective and efficient. These co-factors are trace minerals and can be found in a number of animal and plant food sources. Insufficient dietary intake of these trace minerals could compromise the effectiveness of our antioxidant enzymes. Intake is more likely to be inadequate in the elderly both due to poor consumption but also decreased absorption associated with aging.

Copper
Beans, pulses, lentils, nuts, seeds, whole grains

Manganese
Seafood, lean meat, milk, nuts, widespread in plant foods

Iron
Meat, poultry, egg yolks, dark green vegetables, fortified cereals

Selenium
Oysters, lean beef or lamb, Brazil nuts, walnuts , whole grains

Zinc
Oysters, Walnuts, cashew nuts, sunflower seeds, chickpeas, tempeh

Antioxidant Vitamins

3

These vitamins have antioxidant effects and they also give your immune system a boost. I have previously discussed Vitamins A, C and E at the end of chapter 12 (Looking good, Feeling Good) since they are also beneficial for healthy hair, skin and nails.

Vitamin A
Vitamin C
Vitamin E

Vitamin A

Vitamin A is a fat-soluble vitamin and as such it can be stored in the liver and fatty tissue in the body to be used at times of shortage. Vitamin A exerts an antioxidant effect by neutralising free radicals. It also enhances the function of white blood cells and is needed for the growth and repair of all tissues and to promote wound healing. It also encourages healthy skin and hair, and maintains healthy mucous membranes in our nostrils and upper airways which act as a protective initial barrier from external invaders.

Good sources of vitamin A are animal foods, including cow's liver, red meat, poultry and dairy. Animal produce can provide good amounts of other beneficial nutrients especially iron, zinc and omega-3 fatty acids. As well as being present in the above foods vitamin A can also be obtained in the form of a precursor that is converted to vitamin A in the body. The most common of these is beta-carotene found in bright orange fruits and vegetables and in dark green vegetables. This means that sufficient vitamin A can easily be derived without eating any animal based produce.

Vitamin A deficiency is very rare in affluent societies but an accumulation can be harmful and so consuming vitamin A rich foods every day or high dose vitamin A supplements is unnecessary. This is particularly important for pregnant women since too much vitamin A can harm the developing foetus.

Vitamin C

Vitamin C is a water soluble vitamin and so it can exert its antioxidant effects widely within cells since they consist mostly of water. However it cannot be stored in the body and therefore a regular intake is required from your diet. Vitamin C can donate electrons and so it exerts its antioxidant effect by stabilising free radicals and reactive oxygen species. Vitamin C also boosts our immunity and has an anti-inflammatory effect. It is also required to make collagen, this protein is found in many tissues.

Vitamin C is found in a wide range of fruit and vegetables including oranges, berries, peppers, broccoli, leafy greens and tomatoes. It is easily damaged by light, air or heat and so foods containing vitamin C will retain more of it when they are eaten raw or lightly steamed or lightly stir fried. A deficiency of Vitamin C leads to dry split hair, dry skin, bleeding gums, lowered immunity and at worse scurvy. Scurvy is a disease that used to plague sailors when at sea for months on end without access to any fresh fruit or vegetables. This resulted in them having swollen bleeding gums and wounds that would not heal.

Vitamin E

Vitamin E is another fat-soluble vitamin and as such can also be stored in the body which is helpful at times of low supply. Vitamin E acts as an antioxidant against free radicals. Vitamin E is also involved in red blood cell production and helps to stop blood from clotting. It also modulates a number of different functions of the immune system such as promoting the development of mature T lymphocytes as part of our acquired immunity (see chapter 14), its different actions result in a stronger immune system. As well as these other important roles Vitamin E is also protective against neurological diseases such as Alzheimer's Dementia. Good sources of vitamin E are vegetable oils, fortified cereals, sunflower seeds, almonds and green leafy vegetables.

Vitamin E deficiency in developed countries is very rare and is usually due to some underlying problem with fat metabolism. It is quite common in malnourished adults and children in poor countries. Vitamin E deficiency may lead to anaemia (i.e. a low haemoglobin count), poor immunity and problems with the nervous system.

4   Antioxidant Phytonutrients

Phytonutrients are nutrients that are mostly found in fruit and vegetables. However they can also be derived from other plant based foods including whole grains, legumes, nuts, seeds and tea. We can boost our immunity and defences against carcinogens by harnessing the power of naturally occurring phytonutrients. I have listed below some of the different ways in which phytonutrients can exert an effect.

Phytonutrients PROMOTE

1. Activity of Natural Killer Cells (see chapter 14)
2. Cancer cell death (apoptosis)
3. The activity of liver enzymes that remove toxins from the body

Phytonutrients INHIBIT

1. Cell damage from free radicals (antioxidant effect)
2. Cell proliferation
3. Inflammation
4. Angiogenesis

In plant based foods a variety of phytonutrients will be present in a single food source and as an added bonus they also exist alongside antioxidant vitamins and trace minerals. The main groups of antioxidant phytonutrients are Polyphenols, Terpenes and Sulphur compounds.

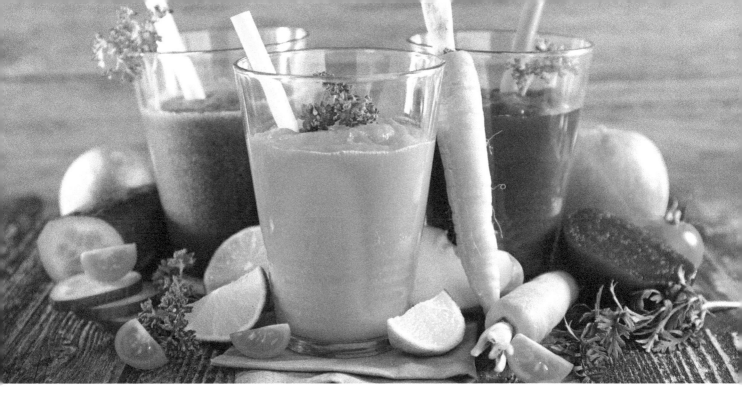

Polyphenols

Polyphenols are a group of large antioxidant molecules that derive their name from the fact that they all contain a large number of phenol rings. Polyphenols are broadly divided into four main groups dependent on their structure and these groups are named Flavonoids, Lignans, Stillbenes and Phenolic acids.

I have mentioned polyphenol antioxidants separately since there are many thousands of them that exist in nature. They are found in abundance in many plant based foods where their presence helps the plant to protect itself from UV radiation and attack by pathogens such as bacteria, fungi and parasites. Their large structure makes them ideal for absorbing and neutralising free radicals. Polyphenols all act as antioxidants and also block the action of some enzymes that cause inflammation and promote cancer growth.

Below is a list of the main groups of phytonutrient antioxidants and some of the antioxidants within each group. It is not an exhaustive list by any means but will hopefully give you an idea that all antioxidants are not the same.

POLYPHENOLS	TERPENES	SULPHUR COMPOUNDS
Flavonoids	Caretonoids	Sulphides
Lignans	Beta-Carotene	Isothiocyanates
Stilbenes	Cryptoxanthins	
Phenolic Acids		

Benefits of a Plant Based Diet

One of the most influential books I have read that has encouraged me to improve my diet is the bestselling book, The China Study, written by T.Colin Campbell PhD. and his son Thomas M.Campbell MD. The book outlines the findings of this huge epidemiological study. It was first published in 2005 and has since sold over a million copies.

The China study was a very impressive initiative and undertaking which involved collaboration between researchers in China and the USA. The detailed study explored the relationship between dietary habits and disease and mortality. It commenced in 1983 and continued over the following twenty years. At the outset 50 families were selected from two villages in each of 65 rural counties in China. Dietary questionnaires and blood tests were used to gather information and then this information was reviewed alongside death rates in the different counties. What they found was that as the consumption of animal based foods rose so did levels of blood cholesterol and the incidence of Western diseases including heart disease and cancer. They concluded that 'there are virtually no nutrients in animal-based foods that are not better provided by plants'.

Colin Campbell grew up on a farm that produced beef and dairy produce and consequently he had a relatively high consumption of animal fats throughout his childhood and early adult years. However, since orchestrating *The China Study* he firmly advocates a plant based diet. An informative TV documentary *Forks over Knives* outlines the research of both Dr Campbell and another advocate of a plant based diet called Dr Caldwell Esselstyn. The programme has been screened in the USA, Canada, China and the UK as well as being previously available on Netflix.

Dr Esselstyn's early career was as a well-respected surgeon and he was also the head of the Breast Cancer Task Force at the world renowned Cleveland Clinic, in the USA. As a surgeon he specialised in endocrine disease and breast disease. He has many professional accolades but can also boast an USA Olympic gold medal for team rowing in 1956! His research includes a follow up study spanning over twenty tears exploring the links between dietary habits and heart disease. His bestselling book, *Prevent and Reverse Heart Disease* summarises this study.

The filmmakers of *Forks over Knives* trace the similar childhood backgrounds of Campbell and Esselstyn. They then go on to unravel how both of them through separate and lengthy research come to the same conclusions regarding the excessive consumption of meat, processed foods and dairy produce and their links with many chronic health diseases such as heart disease, diabetes and cancer. The concerns raised by the doctors is that many animal based foods are relatively high in saturated fats and many processed foods contain large amounts of saturated fats, trans-fats and free sugars. Trans-fats and free sugars can lead to the increased production of harmful free radicals. Conversely plant based foods contain lots of antioxidants so they actually have a protective role in the body against the free radicals. The doctors also conclude that a mainly plant based diet is not only protective to your health but it is also cheaper, lower in calories and better for the environment.

Dr Campbell demonstrates his findings from his extensive work in China showing that rural communities had practically none of the cardiovascular diseases or cancers seen in the Western world. However, as communities gained wealth and ate more meat this pattern of disease changed for the worse. Dr Esselstyn's work included the use of detailed medical images (angiograms) of the narrowed coronary arteries of patients with severe heart disease. He was able to demonstrate irrefutably that the abnormal

appearances of these arteries could be reversed by simply consuming a plant based diet.

The programme follows the doctors' stories and also features a number of patients who each have a number of chronic medical conditions. The patients explain what conditions they suffer from and the difficulties they face every day because of their diseases and their futile attempts to improve their own health. Their journeys are followed as they are placed on a plant based diet. Watching how they overcome many personal challenges and begin to look and feel so much better as well as reversing some of their health problems offers striking and compelling evidence that hugely supports the doctor's advice.

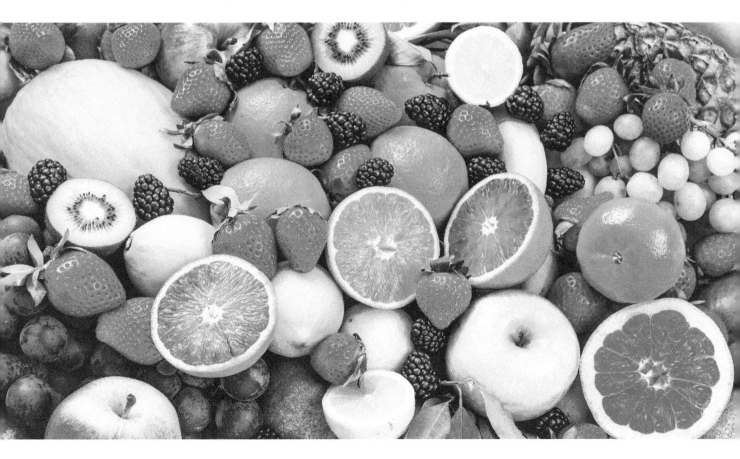

Commonly Consumed Phytonutrients

As it becomes clearer that plant based foods are nutrient-dense you can see why it is important to include as many of them as possible in your daily diet. For ease of future reference I will now list some well-known and particularly beneficial phytonutrients in alphabetical order.

Allium Sulphur Compounds

> Allium sulphur compounds are found in onions, shallots, leeks, chives and garlic; they have been shown to be particularly protective against heart disease and cancers of the digestive tract such as stomach and bowel cancer.

These vegetables and herbs contain compounds that have many health benefits including lowering blood cholesterol levels, regulation of blood sugar levels and lowering blood pressure. Their antioxidant properties come from the sulphur and the polyphenols they contain which also have anti-inflammatory properties and promote cancer cell death (apoptosis).

Anthocyanins

> Anthocyanins are a group of flavonoid polyphenols seen in many deeply coloured pink, red, blue and purple fruits and vegetables. They are particularly concentrated in berries.

Blueberries and raspberries contain the most followed by strawberries and cranberries. These antioxidants can also be found in plums, purple grapes, cherries, beetroot and aubergine. The antioxidant effects of anthocyanins include reducing the production of inflammatory chemicals and an ability to neutralise free radicals.

Beta-Carotene

> Beta-carotene belongs to the large family of carotenoids and acts as a precursor that can be converted in the body to vitamin A. It is found in fruit and vegetables that have an orange colour such as apricots, mangoes, carrots, pumpkin and squash.

Beta-carotene can also be found in green leafy vegetables such as kale, spinach and parsley where the orange colour is masked by chlorophyll. The absorption of beta-carotene is improved if it is eaten alongside dietary fats since it is fat-soluble. We require vitamin A for healthy mucous membranes, skin, hair, good vision and a healthy immune system. Beta-carotene is an excellent pre-cursor of Vitamin A since the body only converts as much as it requires. The remaining beta-carotene acts as an antioxidant and protects the body from free radicals.

Catechins

Catechins are part of the flavonoid polyphenol group and are found in many types of fruit, especially apricots.

A catechin called 'Epigallocatechin-3-Gallate' (EGCG) is the catechin most strongly associated with cancer prevention and is found in abundance in green tea (see next chapter).

Cryptoxanthins

Cryptoxanthins are closely related to beta-carotene and also act as a precursor to vitamin A. They are found in orange rind, red peppers, papaya, pumpkin and mangoes.

Cryptoxanthins can also neutralise free radicals and switch on genes that protect against cell damage and help repair oxidative damage to DNA. They are a fat-soluble chemical like beta-carotene and Vitamin A so also need to be consumed along with dietary fats in order to be absorbed effectively.

Ellagic Acid

Ellagic acid is a flavonoid antioxidant found in many fruits, especially berries, and it is also present in nuts.

Ellagic acid can bind with chemicals or toxins that are cancer promoting to prevent damage from them, and it also halts cancer cell division and promotes cancer cell death.

Flavonols

These are the most widely found flavonoids and are present in onions, leeks, curly kale, broccoli, tomatoes and blueberries. They are also found in many other fruits.

In these foods the flavonols tend to accumulate just beneath the surface since they require exposure to sunlight to synthesize them. This means that smaller fruit with a high skin to flesh ratio such as small cherry tomatoes contain more flavanols than larger salad tomatoes. Similarly, the green outer, more exposed leaves of a head of cabbage contain more flavonols than the lighter inner leaves. Like other phytonutrients in the flavonoid group they play many different roles and are mostly known for their anti-inflammatory and antioxidant effects. They also play an important role in cardiovascular health and in supporting the nervous system.

Indoles

Indoles are phytochemicals with a unique structure that are found in cruciferous vegetables. These vegetables include bok choy, broccoli, kale, cauliflower and spinach.

Indoles have been shown to promote the production and activity of enzymes that remove toxins and protect cell DNA. A particular indole called indole-3-carbinol has been shown to interfere with the structure of oestrogen making the oestrogen less able to stimulate oestrogen receptor positive breast cancers.

Isoflavones

Isoflavones are a type of flavonoid found in soya and legumes.

They can bind to oestrogen receptors and have very mild pseudo-oestrogenic effect; however they stop the more potent oestrogen from binding to oestrogen receptors in the same way as Tamoxifen does and they do not hamper the actions of Tamoxifen or Aromatase Inhibitors.

Isothiocyanates

Isothiocyanates are sulphur containing phytonutrients that are found in cruciferous vegetables.

They promote a number of anti-cancer mechanisms including cancer cell death, reducing oxidative stress and increasing the activity of enzymes that are able to remove carcinogens. A vast amount of research has been undertaken using cell and animal studies in which isothiocyanates have been found to be highly effective at preventing or reducing cancerous changes when cells or animals are exposed to carcinogens. Epidemiological studies looking at a population's diet and disease outcomes back these findings.

Lignans

Lignans are antioxidant compounds that are found in plant cell walls. The richest dietary source of lignans by far is linseed (otherwise known as flaxseed) followed by sesame seeds.

Some other seeds and grains contain small amounts of lignans too; however the concentrations of lignans in linseed are hundreds of times higher. Lignans act as antioxidants, have anti-inflammatory properties, help to control blood pressure and also bind to oestrogen receptors stopping oestrogen from doing so. Lignans can also block the action of aromatase enzymes to reduce the peripheral formation of oestrogen seen mainly in fatty tissue.

Lycopene

This antioxidant comes from the carotenoid family and has a number of cancer fighting properties. It gives fruit and vegetables their vibrant red colour.

It can be found in watermelons and pink grapefruit (avoid grapefruit if taking Tamoxifen or statins) but it exists in its highest concentrations in tomatoes. Interestingly, unlike vegetables and other fruit that retain most of their nutrients when raw, tomatoes actually need to be cooked first to release their nutrients.

Resveratrol

Resveratrol is the most widely seen polyphenol antioxidant found in the skins and seeds of grapes and raisins, wine (especially red wine) and also in cocoa and dark chocolate.

Resveratrol has a number of prongs of attack on cancer cells. It inhibits cancer cells from forming and it can prevent those that do form from proliferating. One glass of red wine a day contains sufficient resveratrol and a number of other polyphenols to have a beneficial effect. However, once consumption increases beyond this and certainly beyond recommended safe drink limits (see chapter 4) then the harm from red wine outweighs any benefit.

Variety is the Spice of Life

Plant based foods often contain many different antioxidants whereas some may have an abundance of just a few. Antioxidants usually confer a colour to the food, so eating fruit and vegetables with a variety of colours will provide you with a good selection of antioxidants. In the next chapter I will discuss some foods that have been found to be particularly beneficial for fighting breast cancer. As with all studies on nutrition a lot of information is gathered from cell and animal studies and from prospective studies comparing nutrition and health outcomes in different populations or within populations. More evidence is gathering all the time for the many benefits of a healthy diet including long term health outcomes; but the benefits are also more immediate with a healthier appearance, improved weight control, increased vitality and a stronger immune system.

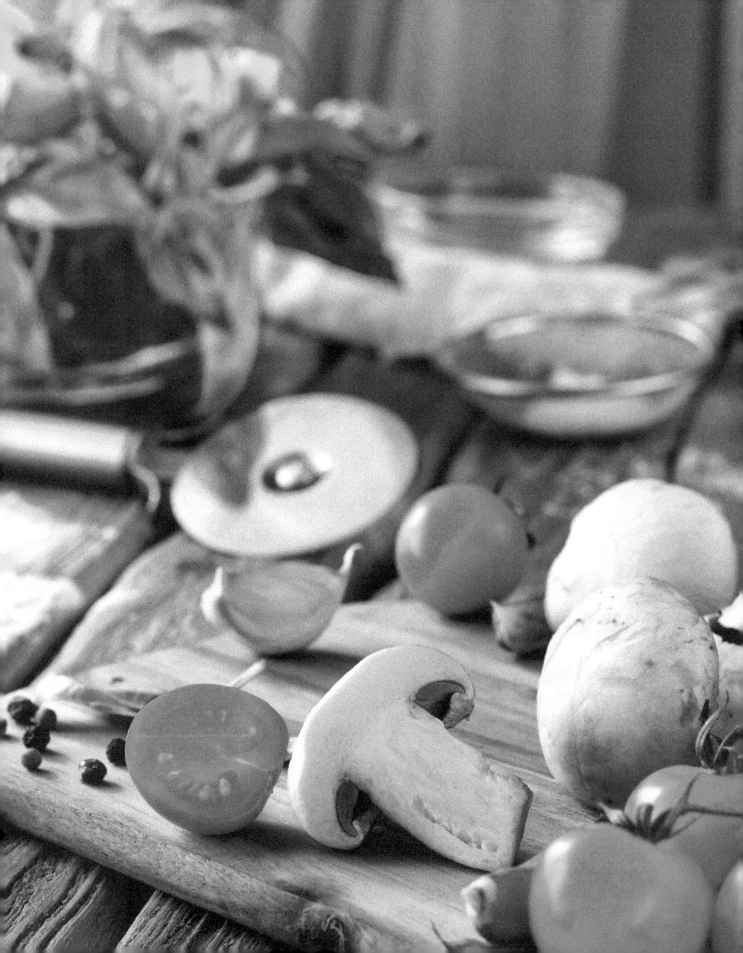

The Best Foods for Fighting Breast Cancer

There are many foods that contain antioxidants and promote good health and well-being but some in particular are linked to a protective role against the development of breast cancer. This is shown from the results of studies that explore how diet can influence a person's risk of developing breast cancer and some more specifically at secondary breast cancer.

Studies exploring the risk of breast cancer recurrence recruit breast cancer survivors. The researchers then gather information on the women's diet by asking questions using a standardised food questionnaire. Then, over the following years they monitor the health outcomes of the survivors. The purpose of this is to see if there are any noticeable differences in the diets of those women who do or do not go on to develop a recurrence of their breast cancer. This allows researchers to ascertain if there are any particularly protective or harmful foods or drinks that should be advised or avoided respectively. Studies which also take blood or urine samples as a quantitative measure of the amounts of vitamins or other antioxidants not just consumed but actually absorbed into the body, provide additional strength to a study.

The 10 Best Foods to Help Fight Breast Cancer

1	GREEN TEA
2	TURMERIC
3	CRUCIFEROUS VEGETABLES
4	YELLOW/ORANGE VEGETABLES and FRUITS
5	BERRIES
6	TOMATOES
7	BEETROOT
8	MUSHROOMS
9	ALLIUM VEGETABLES
10	LINSEED

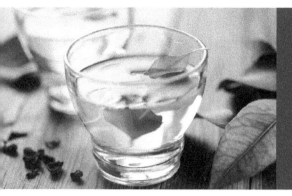

Green Tea

Epidemiological studies show that those nations and individuals that consume the most green tea have the lowest breast cancer rates and lowest levels of breast cancer recurrence.

Drinking tea is a pleasurable and regular part of most people's daily routine. As well as being enjoyable and almost universally popular, tea can also be beneficial to our health. 'Having a cuppa' also allows a moment to pause whilst we enjoy its soothing benefits. Green tea and black tea both contain antioxidants; however green tea contains significantly more antioxidants than black tea and so has more health benefits. Both of these teas come from the same plant but by taking green tea and subjecting it to a fermentation process the green tea changes colour to now become black tea. Since green tea does not undergo this process it not only retains its colour it also preserves a lot more of its polyphenol antioxidants called catechins.

Green tea has particularly high concentrations of the catechin *Epigallocatechin-3-Gallate (EGCG) which is a very powerful antioxidant and is strongly linked to cancer prevention.*

Epidemiological studies show that those nations and individuals that consume the most green tea have the lowest breast cancer rates and lowest levels of breast cancer recurrence.

In animal and cell studies green tea has been shown to suppress angiogenesis (see chapter 20); without the formation of these new blood vessels cancer cells cannot receive the nutrients and oxygen they require to grow. EGCG also inhibits the proliferation and growth of breast cancer cells and it has a detoxifying effect by activating enzymes in the liver which help to remove potential carcinogens from the body.

As part of a healthy lifestyle it is worth getting into the habit of drinking at least three cups of green tea a day, but do bear in mind that green tea does contain some caffeine. However, the amount of caffeine in a cup of green tea is only about a quarter of that found in coffee and about half of that found in black tea; so ideally you should try to consume your green tea between waking and mid-afternoon so that it doesn't affect your sleep.

The other important fact to be aware of is that all green teas do not provide the same amount of catechins. This can vary greatly depending on where the tea is grown, how it is harvested and how it is subsequently processed. In the excellent book, *Foods to Fight Cancer* written by Professor Richard Béliveau and Dr Denis Gingras there is a list of Chinese and

Japanese tea regions and the EGCG concentrations of the green teas from those regions. Overall, Japanese green teas were found to contain substantially more than the Chinese ones with Sencha-uchiyama containing the highest. However, they all fair well, so I recommend that you find a green tea you like and also make sure you store and brew it properly so that you don't destroy its health promoting benefits.

The catechins in green tea can be destroyed by air, heat and light and therefore green tea should be stored in an airtight and lightproof container to help retain the catechins. It is preferable to brew fresh green tea leaves rather than teabags. To avoid destroying the catechins it also essential that you do not brew green tea with boiling water: instead allow the boiled water to cool for a minute or two before adding it to the tea.

> If you do not enjoy the taste of green tea you could try drinking green tea with a slice of lemon or some fresh mint. This can smooth out the flavour; also the vitamin C in lemon and mint can actually help you to absorb more of the catechins. Alternatively try a flavoured green tea or combine green tea with a herbal tea that you enjoy.

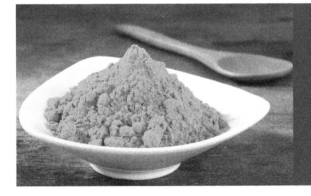

Turmeric

Many studies support the anti-cancer properties of curcumin and the effects are due to a combination of actions which include its anti-inflammatory nature. Cell studies also show that curcumin can slow down or halt the growth of breast cancer cells, promote cancer cell death and also inhibit angiogenesis.

The spice called turmeric has a distinctive mustard-yellow colour and is used widely in Asian cooking. Besides its culinary use it has also been used in Ayurvedic (Ancient Indian medicine) and Chinese medicine for many centuries as a natural anti-inflammatory agent and in the prevention or treatment of cancer. Curcumin is the major active component of turmeric and there have been quite extensive studies looking at the effects of curcumin on cancer cells in the lab and the incidence of cancers in animals exposed to carcinogens with or without concomitant curcumin.

Many studies support the anti-cancer properties of curcumin and the effects are due to a combination of actions which include its anti-inflammatory nature. Cell studies also show that curcumin can slow down or halt the growth of breast cancer cells, promote cancer cell death and also inhibit angiogenesis.

Studies in humans have only included small numbers of people so far but do show some benefits. As seen with other studies on the impact of nutrition we can find further observational evidence when we look at cancer rates in nations that consume regular amounts of turmeric in their diet and those that don't. One important finding is that the absorption of curcumin from the stomach can be very low, however this can be increased by over a thousand times by consuming it with black pepper (active ingredient piperine).

A particularly interesting study was published in the journal, *Cancer Prevention Research in* 2014 by Dr R.Gupta and colleagues. This explored the well-recognised issues relating to curcumin's beneficial anti-cancer properties but its relatively poor absorption. Using rats as an animal model they found an alternative way of delivering good amounts of curcumin to the site of tumours. Instead of adding it to their diet they used a capsular implant of curcumin that was inserted at the tumour site. In this experiment they found that the curcumin implant reduced the size of the tumour by 30%. Although we are a long way of exploring this in humans it does go some way towards demonstrating the cancer fighting properties of curcumin.

The way turmeric is used in cooking will greatly enhance its absorption into the body. A combination of turmeric, healthy oils and black pepper helps the body to be able to absorb the most curcumin from the digestive tract and into the bloodstream. Turmeric is a spice that can be added to curries but can be overpowering if too much is added. A teaspoon is usually sufficient for most lentil, bean, tofu, fish or chicken curries or dishes. Due to its strong colour turmeric can also stain clothes and kitchen surfaces so be careful to avoid this.

A good way to use turmeric is in the spice base for any curry dish. To make a curry begin by lightly sautéing an onion in some olive oil, then add finely chopped garlic and ginger and stir for 1-2 minutes then remove from the heat. Add your choice of spices including a teaspoon of turmeric and a few generous twists of ground black peppercorns then return to a medium heat and stir through for about 1-2 minutes. Allow enough time to just heat through the spices and release their aroma but ensure you don't overheat and burn the spices. Tomatoes, which are also very beneficial for your health, can be added at this point.

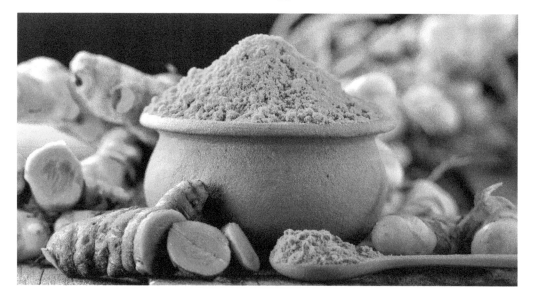

MOVING ON AFTER BREAST CANCER

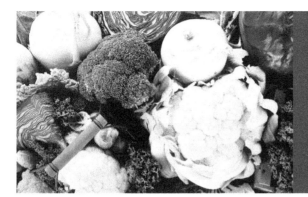

Cruciferous Vegetables

The study found that Chinese women consuming the most cruciferous vegetables were the least likely to have a breast cancer recurrence.

I was unfamiliar with the word 'cruciferous' prior to investigating potential cancer fighting foods but broadly speaking they are vegetables from the cabbage family and some dark green vegetables. They are a diverse group of vegetables which include plants whose leaves or flowers branch from a stem to vaguely resemble a crucifer (cross) and whose leaves, stems and roots can be cooked and eaten.

The following are some commonly consumed cruciferous vegetables

- Bok Choy (Pak Choi)
- Broccoli
- Brussel Sprouts
- Cabbage
- Cauliflower
- Turnip greens
- Radishes
- Rocket
- Kale
- Watercress

All cruciferous vegetable are rich in a number of nutrients including vitamins C, E and K, iron and beta-carotene.

In addition to these they contain a group of substances which contain sulphur called glucosinolate compounds; these glucosinolates give cruciferous vegetables their flavour and aroma.

Glucosinolates are only converted into their active antioxidants when the plant cells are broken down. This means that the vegetables need to be chopped or blended, chewed and digested before the antioxidants are released. The most studied glucosinolates are isothiocyanates and indole-3-carbinol. Both of these powerful antioxidants have been found to inhibit the development of a number of cancers including breast cancer in animal studies and there is also good evidence from epidemiological studies that they offer this protective role. These vegetables often contain other antioxidant vitamins and antioxidant polyphenols, for example kale and broccoli also contain beta carotene, flavonols and lignans.

Isothiocyanates and indole antioxidants in cruciferous vegetables pack a powerful punch since they act on many anti-cancer pathways which include the following:

| Anti-inflammatory |
| Anti-oestrogenic effects |
| They induce enzymes that inactivate carcinogens and ROS |
| Inhibit angiogenesis |
| Inhibit migration of tumour cells (as in metastatic breast cancer) |
| Promote apoptosis (cell death) |

As always, studies looking at dietary questionnaires and health outcomes can be difficult to interpret and often provide conflicting results or no evidence of benefits. The reason behind this may be that often the people who consume a healthy diet, with a good amount of cruciferous vegetables, will have other healthy dietary habits that are contributing to better outcomes too. Rather than comparing countries with high dietary intake of vegetables such as China against those with lower consumption it may be better to compare the different levels of consumption of individuals within those countries that already consume a lot of vegetables.

The Shangai Breast Cancer Survival Study (as mentioned in Chapter 20) investigated the role of cruciferous vegetables and breast cancer survival in almost 5000 Chinese women. This study was presented at the American Association Cancer Research Annual meeting in 2012 by researcher Sarah J.Nechuta. Sarah and her colleagues monitored the amount of cruciferous vegetables the breast cancer survivors consumed over a three year period and followed them up for over five years in total. They demonstrated that there was

a dose related response where additional benefits were derived by an increased intake of cruciferous vegetables.

The study found that Chinese women consuming the most cruciferous vegetables were the least likely to have a breast cancer recurrence.

Two other important findings were highlighted. Firstly, that the consumption of these vegetables are much higher in Chinese women compared to women in the USA and the type of cruciferous vegetables are different. Chinese women are more likely to eat cabbage, Bok Choi and turnip greens; whereas in the USA, women are more likely to eat broccoli, Brussel sprouts and salad leaves. The levels of antioxidants in these cruciferous vegetables may vary and how they are prepared will also contribute to the levels of antioxidants retained in them. For example, when broccoli is boiled most of its antioxidants are destroyed. This means that in order to get the maximum nutritional benefit from broccoli it is better to consume it in its raw state (for e.g. juicing), or lightly steamed or sautéed.

A further study published by the same author looked at some of the findings from a large scale project called the After Breast Cancer Pooling Project. A section of this study involved 11,390 USA and Chinese Breast cancer survivors who were asked to complete food questionnaires over a two year period, and then they were followed up for nine years. However this combined USA and Chinese data now concluded that cruciferous vegetable consumption was not associated with improved outcomes.

So we have conflicting results which can be very confusing. Such differences suggest that further research is needed to identify why the Chinese study shows a benefit and the pooled USA and Chinese data does not. Sometimes it is necessary to dig a bit deeper and further research could help to unravel the truth by including other relevant questions such as the types of cruciferous vegetables consumed and how they are prepared. These particular differences between the two countries vegetable consumption may help to get to the core of these contrasting results.

Researchers have also suggested that in addition to questionnaires a direct measurement of isothiocyanates in urine samples may be a more measurable and accurate way of assessing how much of the active antioxidants have actually been absorbed and also an indication of how much of the antioxidant content is destroyed by certain methods of food preparation. Another factor which is relevant is the food combinations present in a complete meal. For example, fat-soluble antioxidants such as beta-carotene that are also found in some cruciferous vegetables require the presence of fats in a meal in order to be absorbed.

By evaluating the available evidence I certainly believe the results show that it is worth increasing your intake of these vegetables. Juicing is an excellent way of preparing vegetables such as broccoli and kale, in this way the juice extracted contains the bioavailable antioxidants and they are not destroyed by heat. You can also add shredded uncooked cabbage to salads or prepare coleslaw with shredded red and white cabbage. To increase the health benefits further add some shredded carrots or raw beetroot to the coleslaw. As a flavoursome alternative to mayonnaise try some low fat organic dairy yoghurt and add a little Dijon mustard, a squeeze of lime, some seasoning and a sprinkling of herbs.

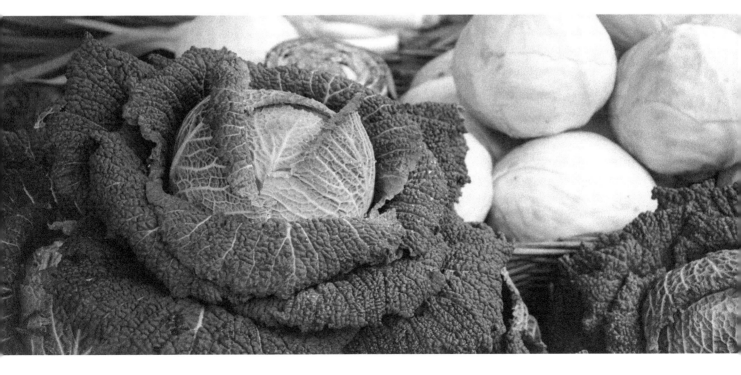

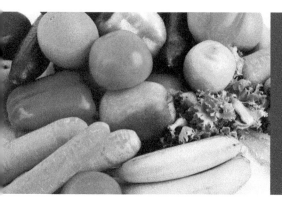

Yellow and Orange Fruits and Vegetables

Many studies have shown that diets containing good amounts of naturally occurring caretonoids have an inverse association with breast cancer rates (as the consumption goes up the incidence of breast cancer goes down).

Yellow and orange fruits and vegetables are particularly rich in carotenoids such as beta-carotene and xanthins. These nutrients are powerful antioxidants and their natural pigments are responsible for the food's vibrant colour. When these antioxidants are consumed they act as precursors to the antioxidant vitamin A. These plant based foods also contain good amounts of vitamin C which are seen especially in citrus fruits such as oranges and lemons. This group of foods also contain flavenoid and lycopene antioxidants.

The health benefits of caretonoids and vitamins A and C include improved eye health, healthy gums and mucous membranes, healthy skin and hair and a boost to the immune system. As well as this they act as antioxidants, scavenging free radicals and neutralising them.

Some of these studies have measured the levels of caretonoids circulating in the participant's bloodstreams as well as using food questionnaires; this quantifiable measure helps to support the evidence. Eight studies that all used blood tests to measure the levels of carotenoids were analysed together and published in the Journal of the National Cancer Institute by A.H.Eliassen and colleagues in 2012.

By pooling the results of these eight USA and Chinese studies they were able to provide comprehensive conclusions that women with higher circulating levels of carotenoids and lycopene were at a reduced risk of breast cancer. Several of these studies showed that the relationship was even stronger for more aggressive tumours.

A more recent review also led by A.H.Eliassen and published in the American Journal of Nutrition in 2015 supports these findings. This time a team of researchers completed a 20 year follow up of women from one of the eight pooled studies on circulating caretonoids and risk of breast cancer. This was called The Nurse's Health Study. In this study they obtained baseline blood tests (1990) measuring circulating carotenoid levels from 32,826 female nurses. In 2010, 20 years from the outset of the study, 2188 women had been diagnosed with breast cancer. They were able to confirm that those women with the highest concentrations of caretonoids in their bloodstreams had an 18-28% lower risk of getting breast cancer and this was especially so for more aggressive tumours.

Vegetables and Fruit Rich in Caretonoids

VEGETABLES	FRUITS
Orange and Yellow Peppers	Oranges
Sweet Potatoes	Lemons
Pumpkin	Nectarines, Satsumas, Clementines
Corn	Mango, Papaya, Peaches
Golden Beets	Pineapples
Butternut Squash	Bananas
Carrots	Honeydew, Cantaloupe Melons

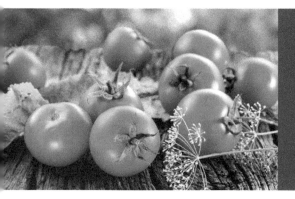

Tomatoes

The WHI study showed that carotenoids including lycopene were associated with a reduced risk of breast cancer and that in particular they reduced the incidence of hormone receptor positive breast cancers.

Tomatoes are particularly rich in a powerful carotenoid called lycopene which gives tomatoes and other fruit and vegetables their red colour. These include watermelon, mango, papaya, red peppers and red cabbage. There is increasing evidence that lycopene is associated with a reduced risk of breast cancer including evidence obtained from the Nurses' Health Study (as above). The Pooled Analysis also shows that lycopene was found to be one of the measurable and most potent carotenoids consumed by women who had a reduced risk of breast cancer. Many studies have also demonstrated a reduced risk of prostate cancer and longer survival after prostate cancer in men that regularly consume tomatoes.

Another group of researchers recruited almost 85,000 women into the Women's Health Initiative (WHI) Observational Study and evaluated the association between the dietary intakes of carotenoids, Vitamin C and E, and their risk of breast cancer. The women were followed up on average for 7-8 years.

The WHI study showed that carotenoids including lycopene were associated with a reduced risk of breast cancer and that in particular they reduced the incidence of hormone receptor positive breast cancers.

Importantly, unlike most fruits or vegetables that retain most of their nutritional benefits when eaten raw or slightly steamed, the amount of bioavailable lycopene from tomatoes is greatly increased by cooking them. Cooking tomatoes changes the lycopene into a form that is more easily absorbed by the body. Tomato purees, sauces, juice and ketchup are all particularly rich in lycopene. However, the benefits can be reduced if these products contain added sugars as seen in many tomato based condiments or processed sauces. On the other hand, if you make tomato based sauces yourself this means that you can reap the benefits and avoid the hidden sugars. Lycopene is a fat soluble antioxidant so it is also absorbed more effectively when cooked with a small amount of healthy fats such as extra virgin olive oil or in a meal containing some healthy fats such as avocados, oily fish, or lean meat.

An excellent way of consuming extra lycopene is to cook homemade tomato based sauces using fresh tomatoes, canned tomatoes, or passata. Tomatoes and tomato puree can also be added when making a curry. A puttanesca pasta sauce can be made very easily by gently sautéing fresh onions and garlic with olive oil, and then adding fresh or canned tomatoes and adding pitted olives, anchovies and a sprinkle of oregano and some seasoning.

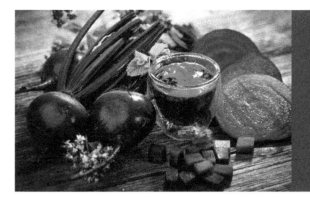

Beetroot

Beetroots have been used medicinally as far back as the Roman times and are well known for aiding the liver in its detoxification process.

Beetroots contain several powerful antioxidants including a unique source of antioxidants called betalains. In particular, a betalain called *betacyanin* gives beetroots there characteristically intense deep crimson-purple colour. Beetroots have been used medicinally as far back as the Roman times and are well known for aiding the liver in its detoxification process. Beetroots specifically stimulate the activity of the antioxidant enzyme glutathione peroxidise (see Chapter 20). Beetroots are also abundant in xanthin antioxidants and contain the antioxidant vitamin C, antioxidant manganese and also are a source of iron. Beetroots also contain nitrate which is very beneficial for blood flow and helps to dilate blood vessels; the effects include lowering blood pressure and improved stamina and so can help to boost energy levels. The many health benefits of beetroots include those listed opposite.

They induce enzymes that detoxify potential carcinogens

- Protect against oxidative stress
- Neutralise free radicals
- Anti-inflammatory
- Slow cancer cell growth

- Stabilise blood sugar
- Lower blood pressure
- Increase blood flow to the brain
- Improve stamina

Beetroots can heavily stain so it is worth wearing disposable gloves when preparing them. Since there are a lot of nutrients in the skin try to clean them by washing thoroughly then pat dry and remove any remaining dirt off the skin with a paper towel. If they are still soiled, scrub them gently with a soft nail brush. Another word of caution is that for about 10-15% of people that consume beetroots it turns their urine red or pink; this is called beeturia, it is harmless and will clear after 1-2 days. If you are prone to kidney stones it is advisable that you limit beetroot intake since they also contain a substance called oxalate which can trigger oxalate-containing kidney stones.

Beetroots are an excellent vegetable to add raw when juicing but can also be cooked. To avoid destroying the antioxidants cook them by steaming for about fifteen minutes and pierce with a skewer to check that they are done; otherwise roast them in the oven for up to an hour.

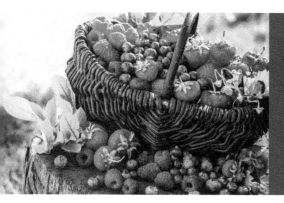

Berries

Ellagic acid is particularly effective in inhibiting the oxidative stress that can damage DNA. It can also scavenge free radicals and ROS and has antiviral, antibacterial, anti-inflammatory and anti-angiogenesis properties.

There are many different varieties of berry and they are all rich in a polyphenol antioxidant called Ellagic Acid. This antioxidant is particularly dominant in berry seeds such as seen in strawberries, blackberries and raspberries. Ellagic acid can also be found in grapes, black- currants, nuts and green tea. Cell and animal studies show that ellagic acid has a number of anti-cancer effects.

Ellagic acid is particularly effective in inhibiting the oxidative stress that can damage DNA. It can also scavenge free radicals and ROS and has antiviral, antibacterial, anti-inflammatory and anti-angiogenesis properties. Ellagic acid has also been shown to reduce the growth and proliferation of cancerous cells.

Berries are also rich in a number of other antioxidants including:

- Anthocyanins
- Beta-carotene
- Cryptoxanthins
- Vitamin C
- Flavonoids

This naturally existing combination of antioxidant nutrients cannot be surpassed by any pill. Ellagic acid is not destroyed by heat so muffins or other baked goods containing berries still contain good amounts; however some of the other nutrients may be destroyed.

Adding a handful of berries to some natural yoghurt or on top of porridge makes a nutritious breakfast. Berries also lend themselves to being made into a smoothie where their often sharp taste can be balanced with other fruits and yoghurt. I like to prepare a berry smoothie in a blender by combining 2 large handfuls of mixed berries, a banana and around 200ml of soya yogurt with about 100-200ml of rice or almond milk (adjusted to give the desired consistency). If you have time add a dessertspoon of chia seeds, and then put the smoothie into the fridge and allow the seeds to soak into the mixture for 30 minutes. This adds volume and satiety. The chia seeds also provide omega-3 fatty acids, antioxidants and fibre. Then on serving you can also add a heaped dessertspoon of milled linseed and stir thoroughly. I find that this is a real nutrient powerhouse and provides a delicious and energy boosting start to the day.

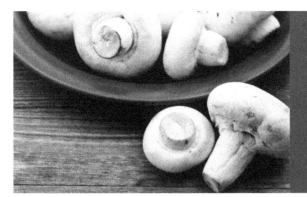

Mushrooms

Lab studies highlight that the glucans in mushrooms can inhibit aromatase enzyme and also inhibit breast cancer cell growth.

There are a large variety of mushrooms and they have all been shown to have a number of health benefits. In the UK most people consume button, chestnut or portobello mushrooms. In parts of Asia notably, China, Japan and Korea mushrooms form a regular part of their everyday diet and have been studied extensively in these populations. The mushrooms they tend to consume are shitake, mitake, enoki and oyster mushrooms which can also all be found easily in the UK, either in large supermarkets or in speciality grocers.

Mushrooms are a low calorie, high fibre wholefood that contain several important nutrients including good quantities of the antioxidant co-factor selenium, potassium, B Vitamins (riboflavin, niacin) and vitamin D. Mushrooms are classed as a fungus and are a unique plant food since they are the only plant food that naturally contain vitamin D. However their main anti-cancer properties are derived from substances called Glucans which stimulate the activity of cells in the immune system and an antioxidant called ergothioneine that can neutralise free radicals.

Cell studies have shown that these glucans can block tumour cell growth and they also have an anti-oestrogenic activity and so are particularly effective against breast cancer cells.

> *Lab studies highlight that the glucans in mushrooms can inhibit aromatase enzyme and also inhibit breast cancer cell growth.*

Mushrooms have been used for thousands of years in Eastern medicine to support the immune system. As a therapeutic food they are usually given as dried mushrooms or consumed as mushroom extract supplements. Interestingly, mushroom extracts are often used in Japan alongside adjuvant chemotherapy. Their use combined with chemotherapy is believed to improve the beneficial effects and also reduce some of the unpleasant side effects of chemotherapy. However, we need to exercise caution in interpreting some of these claims since many of the trials were not carried out using randomised or controlled research designs.

Many of the observational epidemiological studies have been carried out in those countries that consume the most mushrooms i.e. China, Japan and Korea. An analysis of these studies was published by Jiaoyuan Li and colleagues in the peer reviewed PLOS One Journal in 2014: with the title Dietary Mushroom Intake May Reduce the Risk of Breast Cancer: Evidence from a Meta-analysis of Observational Studies. The meta-analysis excluded any studies that scored low on the quality of study where quality was determined by factors such as the inclusion of information about the number of participants recruited and how the statistics were collated. After excluding unsatisfactory studies, ten good quality ones remained. They were able to conclude from these studies that as mushroom consumption increased the risk of breast cancer decreased in a straight line; indicating a dose response association as shown in the following graph.

This graph cited from the article shows how the Relative Risk (RR) of breast cancer reduces as mushroom consumption increases. A quarter of a cup of fresh sliced mushrooms is equivalent to twenty grams of mushrooms a day.

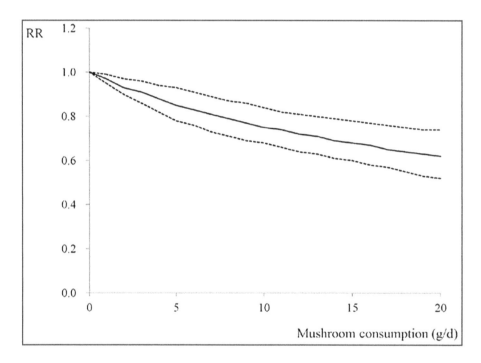

For further Information go to
http://www.ncbi.nlm.nih.gov/pmc/articles/PMC3972098/

The only reservations that the authors had was that the number of studies for the analysis was still relatively small and they indicated that they would like to see the findings updated and confirmed by further large-scale and well-designed prospective studies. Their view was that an increased number of women followed up over a longer period of time would help to provide more statistically significant evidence.

An Australian national science agency called CSIRO (Commonwealth Science and Industrial Research Organisation) has also recently compiled a report on mushrooms, Mushrooms and Health Report 2014. CSIRO are an internationally recognised organisation for quality research and their 73 page report discusses the many health benefits of mushrooms. Pages 26-29 specifically evaluate the available evidence on mushrooms and breast cancer including the results of the above meta-analysis.

(See http:// www.mushroomsandhealth.com /mushrooms-health-report/mushrooms-and-health-report-2014/). The available research shows benefits for both pre and post-menopausal women and particularly those that are oestrogen receptor positive.

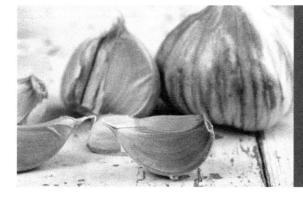

Allium Vegetables

Garlic in particular has been known for its beneficial health properties dating as far back as Ancient Egyptian times.

Vegetables from this group all contain allium sulphur compounds as discussed in chapter 20. The sulphur compounds give these vegetables their distinct and pungent aroma and flavour. Of this group, garlic in particular has been known for its beneficial health properties dating as far back as Ancient Egyptian times. It is even better known for its flavour and aroma, and therefore has a widespread use in cooking. Garlic's active compounds are only released once it is chopped, crushed and chewed and its absorption is improved if consumed with oil and luckily this reflects how it is used.

Allium compounds all have the following properties.

> Inhibit carcinogens

> Promote apoptosis

> Regulate blood sugar levels

> Reduce the growth of cancer cells

> Sulphur compounds support the antioxidant glutathione

The ability of this group to regulate blood sugar levels helps to achieve a reduction in the growth of cancer cells. By stabilising blood sugar levels it helps to reduce the stimulation of insulin secretion which is normally followed by the release of insulin-like growth factor (IGF). When IGF is produced in excess it can stimulate the growth of cancer cells. Many population studies show the benefits of allium vegetables especially for cancers of the oesophagus, stomach and bowel suggesting a localised effect within the digestive tract. However they achieve a more widespread effect too by boosting levels of the powerful antioxidant compound glutathione. Glutathione contains sulphur and so levels can be boosted by consuming sulphur containing foods such as those from the Allium group and cruciferous vegetables.

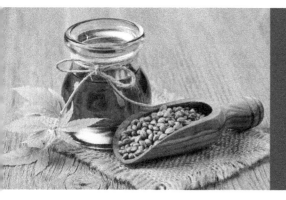

Linseed

These seeds are by far the richest dietary source of fat-soluble antioxidants called lignans. Lignan antioxidants can prevent the formation of free radicals as well as neutralising free radicals and ROS.

Linseed and flaxseed are one and the same but these two names are often used interchangeably, I will refer to them as linseeds. These seeds are by far the richest dietary source of fat-soluble antioxidants called lignans. Lignan antioxidants can prevent the formation of free radicals as well as neutralising free radicals and ROS. These lignans also behave in a way similar to soya and are also classed as phyto-oestrogens. Like soya they can block the effects of naturally produced, more powerful oestrogen on oestrogen sensitive cells such as breast, ovarian and uterine cells. Linseeds are also an excellent source of omega-3 fatty acids which are beneficial for cardiovascular health and also help to reduce cancer risk.

A study published in the Journal of National Cancer Institute, in 2007 by M.S. Touillaud and colleagues examined the association with dietary intakes of lignans and breast cancer incidence in a French population. The study was designed to look at a Western population since other studies had already showed that, Asian populations consuming relatively large amounts of soya phyto-oestrogens tended to have low rates of breast cancer. Countries which do not routinely consume soya get most of their phyto-oestrogens from plant lignans. The study involved 58 049 post-menopausal French women who formed a subgroup of the E3N-EPIC studies. They were followed up for over seven years. During that time 1469 women were diagnosed with breast cancer. Dietary questionnaires were used to calculate average daily intakes of different categories of food including lignans.

(See http://www.ncbi.nlm.nih.gov/pmc/articles/PMC2292813/)

> *The researchers were able to conclude that those women with the highest dietary intake of lignans had a statistically significant lower risk of post-menopausal breast cancers compared with women who had the lowest intake.*

This finding was mainly seen with hormone receptor positive breast cancer incidence rates. In a typical diet most lignans are obtained from cereals, whole grains, nuts, fruit and vegetables. However, adding one to two tablespoons of milled linseed a day to your diet acts as a much richer source of lignans along with the additional health benefits of omega-3s.

Linseed must be milled first of all into linseed powder in order for us to be able to absorb the lignans that they contain, this powdered form of linseed lends itself to be sprinkled over cereals and porridge or stirred into smoothies.

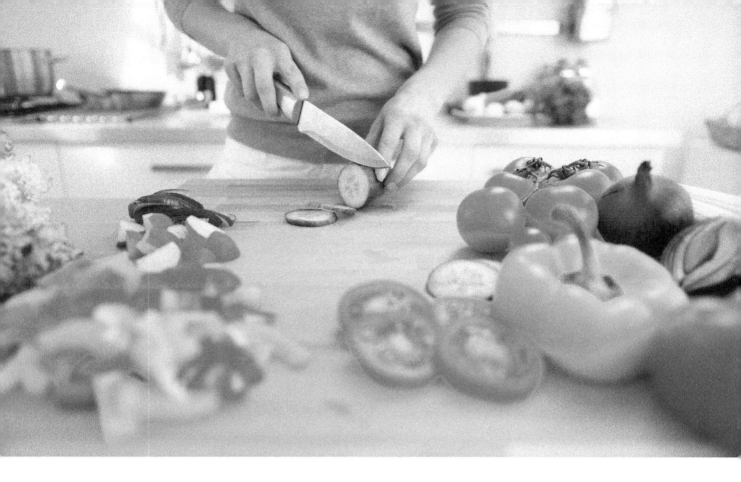

Eating for Health

Alongside other lifestyle factors involved in having a healthy mind, body and spirit there is now sufficient evidence that adding nutrient dense foods into your diet can reduce your risk of a breast cancer recurrence. Hence this chapter is very much about what you should actively try and add to your diet and should be used alongside the advice on healthy food swaps mentioned in the last few chapters. It is also going further than the '5 a Day' UK health campaign advising us to eat five pieces of fruit or portions of vegetables a day. The USA have changed their original 5 a day campaign to 'Fruit & Veggies-More Matters' and in Australia they have a '2 & 5' campaign which advises 2 pieces of fruit a day and 5 servings of vegetables a day.

I suggest you increase this figure to around eight to ten a day. If you are struggling to manage this quantity then juicing is an excellent way of extracting some extra antioxidants which can also be easily absorbed. Naturally occurring combinations of antioxidants found in plant foods have a synergy that is unbeatable. It is advisable to eat a variety of these foods so that you are not getting too much of one thing and not enough of the other, this will also keep you interested in this healthier way of eating. One approach is to consider consuming fruit and vegetables from every colour of the rainbow and you can then be certain that you are consuming a broad spectrum and excellent balance of antioxidants.

PART
6

Moving on ABC

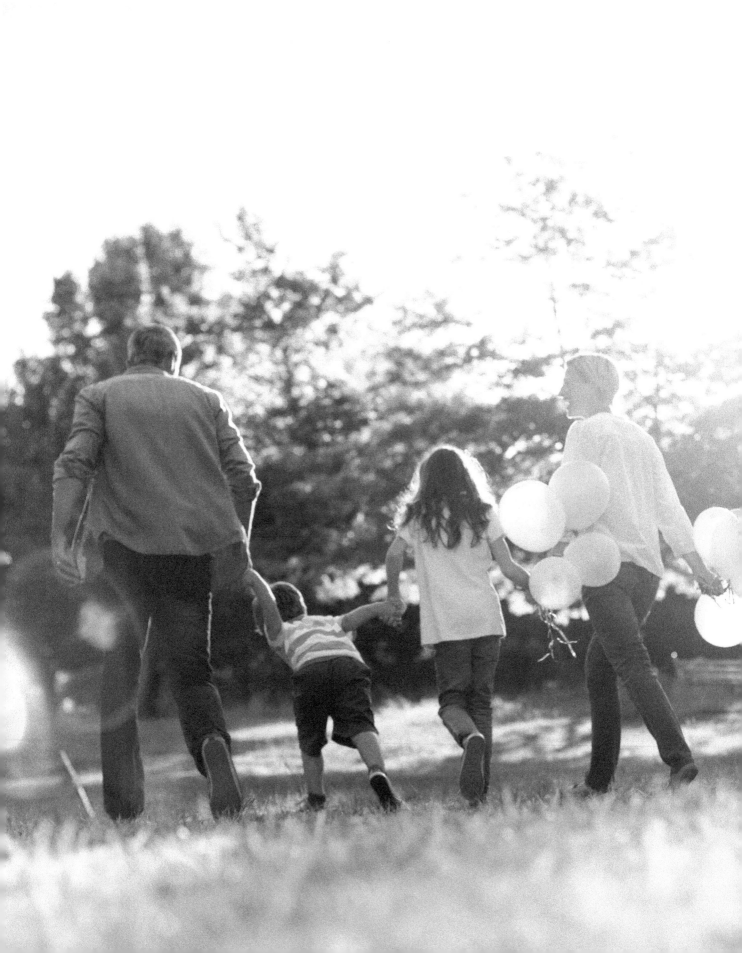

Moving on ABC

Over the last few years attention has begun to focus on living with and beyond cancer. There is an ever increasing population of cancer survivors, partly due to an increasing incidence of some cancers, and partly due to the rapidly improving treatments leading to higher survival rates.

Most cancer survivors share certain experiences. As I have found in my own journey, good aftercare is essential in order to aid the recovery and healing process. Sadly, it can be all too easy for cancer survivors to be held back by anxiety and fears, and to struggle to regain their confidence and self-esteem. Women often feel that they must continue to juggle their many roles in life and put pressure on themselves to do so. However if you are in emotional turmoil and suffering fatigue or other physical problems this is often much easier said than done.

Many health service providers are now starting to address the issues many cancer survivors face. In time this should lead to an improvement in the quality of cancer survivorship and more support being provided for survivors and their families. This would help us to deal more effectively with the difficulties we encounter after completing cancer treatment. Ideally, individualised after-care packages would provide a holistic management of problems ranging from physical symptoms or side effects of treatment, social and psychological support and general health education including advice on exercise, nutrition and relaxation. Any hardships could be anticipated and support made available to help survivors move forward in a more positive way. Although the complex needs of cancer survivors are starting to be recognised, services can often take some time to implement. Until this area of care is more formalised it may be helpful to try and find ways to help ourselves.

Writing this book has been extremely thought provoking and also therapeutic for me, albeit a much larger undertaking than I initially envisaged. Although somewhat difficult, I wanted to describe part of my journey in a little more detail in this final chapter to illustrate how important the help and encouragement of certain individuals was to me in helping me start life as a cancer survivor.

Since January 2014 when I first had the idea of writing this book I have had several major upheavals that have slowed things down. Just three months into the process I had my prophylactic mastectomy and re-construction. This left me sore and uncomfortable for several months and I was also still suffering with fatigue. I spent some of this time researching ideas and coming up with a rough plan for the book. By the summer I was feeling stronger and back on track with an outline for the book. I made good progress over the following six months which took me up to December 2014.

At this point my life was turned upside down again: my world was shattered when my mother passed away after an accidental home fire. It happened while she was on holiday in Pakistan, she was taken to hospital and then just a few days later she was air lifted by air ambulance back to the UK and admitted to the local burns unit. Although she had had a long journey and was covered in bandages she seemed to be bearing up well and was so relieved to see us, as we were her. However, initial tests showed that the burns had become infected with several 'superbugs' and were going to be difficult to treat. Despite the hospitals best efforts she developed septicaemia and was unable to fight it. My family and I just had a few days with her at the end and we were all together when she passed.

More than a year has now gone by since then and sometimes it just feels like she is on a long vacation and could walk through the door any minute. My mother inspired me and helped me in so many ways to become the person I am. She believed in me and pushed me so that I believed in myself and pursued my goals. She was a rock for me throughout my cancer journey; it was so upsetting for my mum to see me going through the chemotherapy but she took me each time to the hospital and stayed with me afterwards. When I got home all I wanted to do was just crawl into bed and my mum would get in next to me, just her being there was such a comfort for us both. Along with my younger sisters, she looked after my young boys and helped them enormously to deal with my illness. She cooked me healthy meals to stash in the fridge so I didn't have to worry about shopping and cooking. She even postponed her much needed knee replacement surgery so she could be there for me. I cannot really remember those first few months after she passed, I was just in a daze.

In a way, publishing this book has given me a way of thanking my mother for the fantastic role she has played in my life. We will all have individuals who we have been able to turn to in time of need. My mother was my star and she is the best example I can think of to illustrate the importance of having caring relatives and friends who can help us to have a good survival. Several months elapsed before I started to remember how much I wanted to write this book and how proud my mum was that I wanted to share my experiences in order

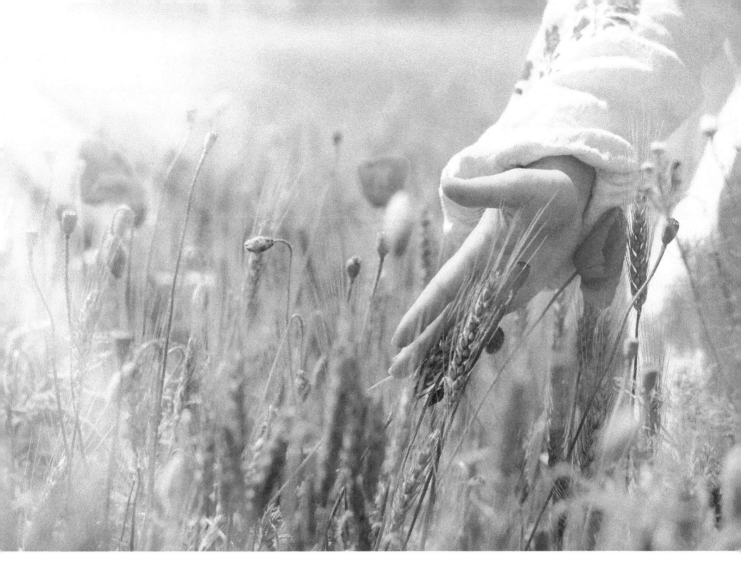

to help other people. I did eventually get to a turning point where I knew I must press on and that is what my mother would have wanted. Although some days were still difficult, I decided it was time to try and pick up where I left off.

Unabated, life's trials and tribulations continue and this book has taken me on a very personal journey. I sincerely hope that this book helps you to find the answers to many of the questions you may have or have had along the way and that the ideas that I have put forward will help you to make informed choices and get help when you need it. I believe that knowledge is power

and by sharing knowledge and supporting each other, breast cancer survivors can feel more empowered. Having cancer does not define us, however, I believe we can all become more in tune with ourselves and this may help us in the way we handle ourselves in the future. You can do this in whichever way that is right for you, either quietly, loudly , on your own, or in a crowd but do show yourself some self compassion. I hope that we are all on the way to a good life, and that this book has helped in the process. Keep well and look after yourself. xx

Photography Index

Images listed here are sourced through Shutterstock

Bibliography

CHAPTER 2

MK Singhal and V.Raina, Cure from breast cancer, not quite yet but getting there?
Ann Oncol (2009):1291-1292

http://annonc.oxfordjournals.org/content/20/8/1291.full

Breast Cancer Facts and Figures

http://www.cancer.org/acs/groups/content/@research/documents/document/acspc-042725.pdf

Oncotype Dx Test

http://www.breastcancer.org/symptoms/testing/types/oncotype_dx

NICE Diagnostic Guidance 10 (DG10)

https://www.nice.org.uk/Guidance/DG10

Fisher B et al, Twenty-year follow-up of a randomized trial comparing total mastectomy, lumpectomy, and lumpectomy plus irradiation for the treatment of invasive breast cancer.
N Engl J Med. 2002; 347:1233–1241

http://www.nejm.org/doi/full/10.1056/NEJMoa022152#t=article

Fisher B et al, Five-year results of a randomized clinical trial comparing total mastectomy and segmental mastectomy with or without radiation in the treatment of breast cancer.
N Engl J Med.1985 Mar 14;312(11):665-73

https://www.ncbi.nlm.nih.gov/pubmed/3883167?dopt=Abstract

CHAPTER 3

Office of National Statistics
Cancer Registration Statistics England 2014

http://www.ons.gov.uk/peoplepopulationandcommunity/healthandsocialcare/conditions anddiseases/bulletins/cancerregistrationstatisticsengland/2014

Improved Survival rates

http://webarchive.nationalarchives.gov.uk/20160105160709/http://www.ons.gov.uk/ons/rel/vsob1/cancer-statistics-registrations--england--series-mb1-/no--42--2011/sty-breast-cancer-survival.html

Cancer Research UK Accessed June 2016
Breast Cancer Incidence UK

http://www.cancerresearchuk.org/health-professional/cancer-statistics/statistics-by-cancer-type/breast-cancer#heading-Zero

Increased Breast Cancer Rates in under 50s

http://www.cancerresearchuk.org/about-us/cancer-news/press-release/2013-05-03-breast-cancer-in-women-under-50-tops-10000-cases-for-first-time

Female and Male common cancers compared

http://www.cancerresearchuk.org/health-professional/cancer-statistics/incidence/common-cancers-compared#heading-Two

http://www.cancerresearchuk.org/health-professional/cancer-statistics/incidence/common-cancers-compared#heading-One

Lung Cancer Incidence Statistics

http://www.cancerresearchuk.org/health-professional/cancer-statistics/statistics-by-cancer-type/lung-cancer/incidence#heading-Two

IARC World Cancer Report 2014

World Health Organisation 2015,

GLOBOCAN Cancer Fact Sheets, World Breast Cancer rates.

http://globocan.iarc.fr/old/FactSheets/cancers/breast-new.asp

http://globocan.iarc.fr/Pages/glossary.aspx

EUCAN Cancer Fact Sheets

http://eu-cancer.iarc.fr/EUCAN/CancerOne.aspx?Cancer=46&Gender=2

The World Factbook, Birth Rates across Europe

https://www.cia.gov/library/publications/the-world-factbook/fields/2054.html#13

Melanie Nichols, Nick Townsend1, Peter Scarborough, and Mike Rayner, Cardiovascular Disease in Europe: epidemiological update. European Heart Journal doi:10.1093/eurheartj/ehu299

http://www.oxfordjournals.org/our_journals/eurheartj/press_releases/freepdf/prpaper.pdf

2012 European Cardiovascular Disease Statistics

http://www.escardio.org/The-ESC/Initiatives/EuroHeart/2012-European-Cardiovascular-Disease-Statistics

Professor David Whiteman, Australian Melanoma Rates Approved. Australian Cancer Research Foundation

https://acrf.com.au/2016/australian-melanoma-rates-improve/

Ann M.Bode, Ya Cao, and Zigang Dong, Update on Cancer Prevention Research in the United States and China:The 2009 China-U.S. Forum on Frontiers OF Cancer Research. Cancer Prevention Research: 3 (12) December 2010 American Association for Cancer Research.

http://cancerpreventionresearch.aacrjournals.org/content/3/12/1630.full.pdf

Christopher I. Li Kathleen E. Malone, and Janet R. Daling, Differences in Breast Cancer Hormone Receptor Status and Histology by Race and Ethnicity among Women 50 Years of Age and Older.

Cancer Epidemiology Biomarkers and Prevention 11 (7)

http://cebp.aacrjournals.org/content/11/7/601.full.pdf+html

Mary A. Gerend and Manacy Pai, Social Determinants of Black-White Disparities in Breast Cancer Mortality: A Review Cancer Epidemiology Biomarkers and Prevention November 2008 17; 2913

http://cebp.aacrjournals.org/content/17/11/2913.full.pdf+html?sid=a760b0f4-8847-4440-a421-25c03642c611

Joseph et al. Outcome analysis of breast cancer patients who declined evidence-based treatment, World Journal of Surgical Oncology 2012, 10:118

http://www.wjso.com/content/10/1/118

CHAPTER 4

Ruddy KJ,Winer EP, Male Breast Cancer: risk factors, biology, diagnosis, treatment, and survivorship. Ann Oncol, Jun2013:24(6):1434-43

http://annonc.oxfordjournals.org/content/24/6/1434.full.pdf+html

NICE Clinical Guidance 164 Published 2013, Updated Aug 2015

https://www.nice.org.uk/guidance/CG164/chapter/1-Recommendations

Karrin B Michels, Contralateral Mastectomy for women with hereditary breast cancer. BMJ 2014;348:g1379.

http://www.bmj.com/content/348/bmj.g1379

Kelly Metcalfe et al, Contralateral mastectomy and survival after breast cancer in carriers of BRCA1 and BRCA2 mutations: retrospective analysis. BMJ 2014;348:g226

http://www.bmj.com/content/348/bmj.g226?trendmd-shared=0

National Cancer Institute

BRCA1 and BRCA2: Cancer Risk and Genetic Testing

http://www.cancer.gov/about-cancer/causes-prevention/genetics/brca-fact-sheet

Allen N.E. et al, Moderate alcohol intake and cancer incidence in women. J Natl Cancer Inst, 2009, 101 (5): p 296-305

http://www.ncbi.nlm.nih.gov/pubmed/19244173

Romieu et al, Alcohol intake and breast cancer in the European prospective investigation into cancer and nutrition. Int J Cancer 2015 Oct 15;137(8):1921-30

http://www.ncbi.nlm.nih.gov/pubmed/25677034?&report=abstract

Change for Life, Alcohol units and guidelines.

http://www.nhs.uk/Change4Life/Pages/alcohol-lower-risk-guidelines-units.aspx

Unit and Calorie Calculator

https://www.drinkaware.co.uk/understand-your-drinking/unit-calculator

CHAPTER 5

Jonathan Koffel, Understanding Research Design Studies

https://hsl.lib.umn.edu/biomed/help/understanding-research-study-designs.

International Agency for Research on Cancer. IARC

Overview of Study Designs

http://www.iarc.fr/en/publications/pdfs-online/epi/cancerepi/CancerEpi-5.pdf

The Cochrane Collaboration

http://www.cochrane.org/about-us

The EPIC Study

http://epic.iarc.fr/

NICE Guidance

https://www.nice.org.uk/

CHAPTER 6

Salma Fahridin and Helena Britt, Cancer Screening in general practice. Australian Family Physician Vol 38. No 4, April 2009

A.Van Steen, R. Van Tiggelen, Short History of Mammography. JBR-BTR, 90: 151-153

http://www.mojamammografia.pl/dl,Historia.pdf

Professor V Beral (Chairman)et al, Advisory Committee on Breast Cancer Screening. Screening for Breast Cancer in England: Past and Future. NHSBSP Feb 2006

http://salute.regione.emilia-romagna.it/screening/tumori-femminili/documentazione/report-linee-guida-manuali-operativi/screening-for-breast-cancer-in-england-past-and-future/screen_report_bc2006.pdf

Peter C. Gotzsche et al, Screening for breast cancer with mammography. Nordic Cochrane Centre 2012

http://nordic.cochrane.org/screening-breast-cancer-mammography.

Peter C. Gotzsche, KJ Jorgensen, Screening for breast cancer with mammography. Cochrane Database Systematic Review.

http://onlinelibrary.wiley.com/doi/10.1002/14651858.CD001877.pub5/full

Professor Sir Michael G Marmot et al. The UK Panel on Breast Cancer Screening. The Benefits and Harms of Breast Cancer Screening: an independent review. Report jointly commissioned by Cancer Research UK and Department of Health (England).

http://www.cancerresearchuk.org/prod_consump/groups/cr_common/@nre/@pol/documents/generalcontent/breast-screening-report.pdf

Harald Weedon-Fekjaer, Pal R Romnundstad, Lars J Vatten, Modern mammography screening and breast cancer mortality: population study . BMJ 2014; 348:g3701

http://www.ncbi.nlm.nih.gov/pubmed/24951459

Joann G Elmore, Russel P Harris, The harms and benefits of modern screening mammography. BMJ 2014;338:g3824

http://www.bmj.com/content/348/bmj.g3824

CHAPTER 7

National Cancer Institute, Lymphedema (PDQ) Patient Version

http://www.cancer.gov/about-cancer/treatment/side-effects/lymphedema/lymphedema-pdq

Useful websites

http://www.lymphoedema.org/
http://www.lymphnet.org/
https://www.lymphoedema.org.au/

CHAPTER 8

Hormonal therapies for the adjuvant treatment of early oestrogen-receptor-positive breast cancer.

https://www.nice.org.uk/guidance/ta112
https://www.nice.org.uk/guidance/ta112/resources/hormonal-therapies-for-the-adjuvant-treatment-of-early-oestrogenreceptorpositive-breast-cancer-82598069519557

Estrogen and Progesterone Receptor Testing for Breast Cancer.

http://www.cancer.net/research-and-advocacy/asco-care-and-treatment-recommendations-patients/estrogen-and-progesterone-receptor-testing-breast-cancer

M. Elizabeth H Hammond et al, American Society of Clinical Oncology/College of American Pathologists Guideline Recommendations for Immunohistochemical Testing of Estrogen and Progesterone Receptors in Breast Cancer. Journal of Clinical Oncology June 1, 2010 vol. 28 no. 16 2784-2795

http://jco.ascopubs.org/content/28/16/2784.full

EBCTCG Relevance of breast cancer hormone receptors and other factors to the efficacy of adjuvant tamoxifen: patient-level meta-analysis of randomised trials. Lancet. 2011 Aug 27; 378(9793): 771–784.

http://www.ncbi.nlm.nih.gov/pmc/articles/PMC3163848/

Hormone therapy for breast cancer. National Cancer Institute: Accessed June 2016.

http://www.cancer.gov/types/breast/breast-hormone-therapy-fact-sheet

Long term data from 20 trials confirm tamoxifen's long-lasting benefit. National Cancer Institute.

http://www.cancer.gov/types/breast/research/tamoxifen-long-lasting-benefit

EBCTCG, Effects of adjuvant tamoxifen and of cytotoxic therapy on mortality in early breast cancer.
N Engl J Med 1988;319:1681-1692

http://www.nejm.org/doi/full/10.1056/NEJM198812293192601

Gail MH et al, Weighing the benefits and risks of tamoxifen for preventing breast cancer.
JNCI J Natl Cancer Inst (1999) 91(21): 1829-1846.

http://jnci.oxfordjournals.org/content/91/21/1829.long

Fisher B et al, Tamoxifen for the Prevention of Breast Cancer: Current Status of the National Surgical Adjuvant Breast and Bowel Project P-1 Study (NSABP P-1). J Natl Cancer Inst (16 November 2005) 97 (22): 1652-1662.

http://jnci.oxfordjournals.org/content/97/22/1652.full.pdf+html

McCowan C et al, The value of high adherence to tamoxifen in women with breast cancer: a community based cohort study. Br J of Cancer; 2013 Sep 3; 109(5): 1172–1180

http://www.ncbi.nlm.nih.gov/pmc/articles/PMC3778308/

King MC et al, Tamoxifen and Breast Cancer Incidence among Women with Inherited Mutations in BRCA1 and BRCA2 National Surgical Adjuvant Breast and Bowel Project (NSABP-P1) Breast Cancer Prevention Trial. JAMA. 2001;286(18):2251-2256

http://jama.jamanetwork.com/article.aspx?articleid=1108388

Antidepressants and Tamoxifen, Harvard Health Publications , June 2010.

http://www.health.harvard.edu/newsletter_article/antidepressants-and-tamoxifen

Source for table Desmarais JE et al, Journal of Clinical Psychiatry (Dec 2009): Vol. 70, No 12, pp1688-97.

Kelly CM: Selective serotonin reuptake inhibitors and breast cancer mortality in women receiving tamoxifen: a population based cohort study. BMJ. 2010. 340:c693.

http://www.bmj.com/content/340/bmj.c693

Population pharmokinetic modelling to assess the impact of CYP2D6 and CYP3A metabolic phenotypes on the pharmokinetics of tamoxifen and endoxifen. B J Clin Phamacol 2014 Sep; 78(3): 572–586.

http://www.ncbi.nlm.nih.gov/pmc/articles/PMC4243908/

Monroe KR et al, Prospective study of grapefruit intake and risk of breast cancer in postmenopausal women: the Multiethnic Cohort Study. Br J of Cancer (2007) 97, 440–445

http://www.nature.com/bjc/journal/v97/n3/abs/6603880a.html

Lilja JJ, Kivosto KT, Neuvonen PJ, Duration of effect of grapefruit juice on the pharmacokinetics of the CYP3A4 substrate simvastatin. Clin. Pharmacol Ther. 2000 Oct;68(4):384-90.

http://www.ncbi.nlm.nih.gov/pubmed/11061578

CHAPTER 9

Women's Health Programme, Monash University, Testosterone and androgens in women. Oct 2010

http://med.monash.edu.au/sphpm/womenshealth/docs/testosterone-and-androgens-in-women.pdf

Dowsett M, Cuzick J , Ingle J, et al. Metanalysis of breast cancer outcomes in adjuvant trials of aromatase inhibitors versus tamoxifen. J Clin Oncol. 2010, 509-18,28 (3):

http://jco.ascopubs.org/content/28/3/509.long

Alan S Coates et al, Five years of letrozole compared with tamoxifen as initial adjuvant therapy for postmenopausal women with endocrine-responsive early breast cancer: Update of Study BIG 1-98. J Clin Oncol February 10, 2007 vol. 25 no. 5 486-492

http://jco.ascopubs.org/content/25/5/486.full

Cuzick J, Sestak I, Baum M, et al.for the ATAC/LATTE Investigators. Effects of anastrozole and tamoxifen as adjuvant treatment for early stage breast cancer: 10 year analysis of the ATAC trial. Lancet Oncol. 2010 .11(12): 1135-41

http://www.thelancet.com/journals/lanonc/article/PIIS1470-2045(10)70257-6/fulltext

The Arimidex, Tamoxifen, Alone or in Combination (ATAC) Trialists' Group. Effect of anastrozole and tamoxifen as adjuvant treatment for early-stage breast cancer: 100-month analysis of the ATAC trial.

Lancet Oncol. 2008. 9(1): 45-53

http://www.thelancet.com/journals/lanonc/article/PIIS1470-2045(07)70385-6/abstract

Boccardo Fet al. Switching to anastrozole versus continued tamoxifen treatment of Early Breast Cancer: Preliminary Results of the Italian Tamoxifen Anastrozole Trial. J Clin Oncol. Sept 2005; 23(22):5138-47 ·

https://www.researchgate.net/publication/7734570_Switching_to_Anastrozole_Versus_Continued_Tamoxifen_Treatment_of_Early_Breast_Cancer_Preliminary_Results_of_the_Italian_Tamoxifen_Anastrozole_Trial

Hormonal therapy side effects linked to a lower risk of recurrence. BreastCancer.org

http://www.breastcancer.org/research-news/20081029b

P. Niravath, Aromatase inhibitor induced arthralgia: a review. Ann Oncol March 2013.

http://annonc.oxfordjournals.org/content/early/2013/03/06/annonc.mdt037.full.pdf+html

Effect of aromatase inhibitors on the lipid profile of post menopausal breast cancer patients.

Clinical Lipidology; April 2010 ,Vol. 5, No. 2, Pages 245-254

http://www.futuremedicine.com/doi/abs/10.2217/clp.10.4?journalCode=clp

IBIS-11 Prevention. International Breast Cancer Prevention.

http://www.ibis-trials.org/thetrials/ibistrials/ibis-2-prevention

Hormonal therapies for the adjuvant treatment of early oestrogen-receptor-positive breast cancer.

https://www.nice.org.uk/guidance/ta112

https://www.nice.org.uk/guidance/ta112/resources/hormonal-therapies-for-the-adjuvant-treatment-of-early-oestrogenreceptorpositive-breast-cancer-82598069519557

McMillan Cancer Support, HER2 positive breast cancer.

http://www.macmillan.org.uk/cancerinformation/cancertypes/breast/aboutbreastcancer/typesandrelatedconditions/her2%20positive.aspx

NICE Guideline TA107 (Aug 2006), Trastuzumab for the adjuvant treatment of early-stage HER2-positive breast cancer.

https://www.nice.org.uk/guidance/ta107/chapter/1-guidance

Nice Guideline TA34 (March 2002),Trastuzumab for the adjuvant treatment of advanced stage HER2-positive breast cancer.

https://www.nice.org.uk/guidance/TA34

Goldhirsch A et al, 2 Year versus 1 Year of adjuvant trastuzumab for HER2 positive breast cancer

(HERA): an open label randomised control trial.Lancet. 2013 Sep 21;382(9897)

http://www.ncbi.nlm.nih.gov/pubmed/23871490

Baselga J et al, Adjuvant trastuzumab: a milestone in the treatment of HER-2 positive early breast cancer. Oncologist. 2006; 11 Suppl 1:4-12

http://theoncologist.alphamedpress.org/content/11/suppl_1/4.long

Ismael G et al, Subcutaneous versus intravenous administration of (neo) adjuvant trastuzumab in patients with HER2-positive, clinical stage I-III breast cancer (HannaH study): a phase 3, open-label, multicentre, randomised trial. Lancet Oncol. 2012 Sep;13(9): 869-78

http://www.ncbi.nlm.nih.gov/pubmed/22884505

Hall PS et al, Updated cost-effectiveness analysis of trastuzumab for early breast cancer: a UK perspective considering duration of benefit, long-term toxicity and pattern of recurrence. Pharmacoeconomics. 2011May; 29(5):415-32

http://www.ncbi.nlm.nih.gov/pubmed/21504241

Triple-Negative Breast Cancer, Living Beyond Breast Cancer, Reviewed by Edith P. Mtichell et al, Updated Aug 2015.

http://www.lbbc.org/learn/types-breast-cancer/triple-negative-breast-cancer

Calcium in the Vegan diet- The Vegetarian Resource Group

http://www.vrg.org/nutrition/calcium.php

CHAPTER 10

Collaborative Group on Hormonal Factors in Breast Cancer. Breast cancer and hormone replacement therapy: collaborative reanalysis of data from 51 epidemiological studies of 52,705 women with breast cancer and 108,411 women without breast cancer. Lancet 2001 Oct 27 :358 (9291): 1389-99

http://www.thelancet.com/journals/lancet/article/PIIS0140-6736(01)06524-2/abstract

Beral. Vet al. Million Women Study. Breast cancer and hormone replacement therapy in the Million Women Study. Lancet 2003, 362 (9382)):p 419-27

http://www.ncbi.nlm.nih.gov/pubmed/12927427

Writing Group for the Women's Health Initiative Investigators, Risks and Benefits of Estrogen Plus Progestin in Healthy Postmenopausal Women Principal Results From the Women's Health Initiative Randomized Controlled Trial . JAMA. 2002;288(3):321-333

http://jama.jamanetwork.com/article.aspx?articleid=195120

Women's Health Concerns. Article reviewed by British Menopause Society. HRT: What you should know about the benefits and risks . Accessed June 2015

https://www.womens-health-concern.org/help-and-advice/factsheets/hrt-know-benefits-risks/

Jacqueline McGlade, Executive Director European Environment Agency EEA, Increase in cancers and fertility problems may be caused by household chemicals and pharmaceuticals.

http://www.eea.europa.eu/media/newsreleases/increase-in-cancers-and-fertility

International Programme of Chemical Safety IPCS (2002). Global assessment of the state of the science of endocrine disruptors. Geneva, Switzerland, World Health Organization,

http://www.who.int/ipcs/publications/en/ch1.pdf?ua=1

Kortenkamp A et al, Ten Years of Mixing Cocktails: A Review of Combination Effects of Endocrine-Disrupting Chemicals. Environ Health Perspect. 2007 Dec; 115(Suppl 1): 98–105.

http://www.ncbi.nlm.nih.gov/pmc/articles/PMC2174407/

REACH Registration Evaluation Authorisation and restriction of Chemicals.

http://www.hse.gov.uk/reach/

Chemsec , the International Chemical Secretariat, is a non-profit organisation dedicated to working towards a toxic free environment.

http://chemsec.org/hazardous-chemicals/

Breast Cancer UK works to save lives and reduce breast cancer rates by tackling the environmental and chemical causes of the disease. Information about Endocrine Disrupting Chemicals.

http://www.breastcanceruk.org.uk/science-and-research/endocrine-disrupting-chemicals/

Breast Cancer Fund The Breast Cancer Fund works to prevent breast cancer by eliminating our exposure to toxic chemicals and radiation linked to the disease.

http://www.breastcancerfund.org/clear-science/biology-of-breast-cancer/endocrine-disrupting-compounds/?referrer=https://www.google.co.uk/

CHAPTER 11

Darbre PD, et al., Concentrations of parabens in human breast tumors. Journal of Applied

Toxicology, vol. 24, pp 5-13, 2004.

http://www.dr-baumann.ca/science/
Concentrations%20of%20Parabens%20in%20
Human%20Breast.pdf

Barr L., et al., Measurement of paraben
concentrations in human breast tissue at
serial locations across the breast from axilla
to sternum. J Appl Toxicol, vol. 32, no. 3, pp
219–232, 2012.

http://www.ncbi.nlm.nih.gov/pubmed/22237600

Calafat, Antonia M., et al. Urinary
concentrations of four parabens in
the US population: NHANES 2005-
2006. Environmental health perspectives 118.5
(2010): 679.

http://www.ncbi.nlm.nih.gov/pmc/articles/
PMC2866685/

Environment and Human Health Inc.

http://www.ehhi.org/reports/plastics/phthalates_
intro.shtml

Danish Environmental Protection Agency

http://eng.mst.dk/topics/chemicals/legislation-
on-chemicals/fact-sheets/fact-sheet-pvc-and-
phthalates/

Brophy JT et al, Breast cancer risk in relation to
occupations with exposure to carcinogens and
endocrine disruptors: a Canadian case-control
study. Environ Health. 2012 Nov 19; 11:87

http://www.ncbi.nlm.nih.gov/pubmed/23164221

National Institute of Environmental Health
Sciences, Bisphenol A

http://www.niehs.nih.gov/health/topics/agents/
sya-bpa/

Lita M. Proctor, The Human Microbiome: A
True Story about You and Trillions of Your
Closest (Microscopic) Friends. Sept 2013 on
action bioscience website.

http://www.actionbioscience.org/genomics/
the_human_microbiome.html

Maura Meade-Callahan, Microbes: What they
do and how antibiotics change them. Jan 2001

http://www.actionbioscience.org/evolution/
meade_callahan.html

Public Health England, General Information on
PFOS and PFOA. Toxicology Dept 2009.

https://www.gov.uk/government/uploads/system/
uploads/attachment_data/file/338258/PFOS___
PFOA_General_Information_phe_v1.pdf

National Institute of Environmental Health
Sciences, Perfluorinated Chemicals. Sept 2012

https://www.niehs.nih.gov/health/materials/
perflourinated_chemicals_508.pdf

National Cancer Institute, Antiperspirant
Fact sheet.

http://www.cancer.gov/about-cancer/causes-
prevention/risk/myths/antiperspirants-fact-sheet

Mirick DK, Davis S, Thomas DB, Antiperspirant
use and the risk of breast cancer. J Natnl
Cancer Instit. 2002 Oct 16; 94(20):1578-80.

http://jnci.oxfordjournals.org/content/94/20/1578.
long

Darbre PD, Bakir A, Iskakova E, Effect of
aluminium on migratory and invasive properties
of MCF-7 human breast cancer cells in culture.
J Inorg Biochem. 2013 Nov; 128:245-9.

http://www.ncbi.nlm.nih.gov/pubmed/23896199

CHAPTER 12

Safe Cosmetics

http://www.safecosmetics.org/

Environmental Working Group

http://www.ewg.org/

CLean Make Up, Colby College Environmental
Studies Program

http://web.colby.edu/cleanmakeup/

Cosmetics Toiletry and Perfumery Association

http:/www.ctpa.org.uk/

Personal Care Products Council

http://www.personalcarecouncil.org/

Jo Lewin- Nutritional Therapist, What to eat for
Healthy Hair.

http://www.bbcgoodfood.com/howto/guide/
what-eat-healthy-hair

Rele AS, Mohile RB, Effect of mineral oil,
sunflower oil, and coconut oil on prevention of
hair damage. J Cosmet Sci. 2003 Mar-April;54
(2):175-92

http://journal.scconline.org/pdf/cc2003/
cc054n02/p00175-p00192.pdf

Daisy Whitbread and Paul House, Useful Top
Ten Lists.

Nutrition information on this website is sourced from the U.S. Agricultural Research Service Nutrition Data Releases 20,21,25,26,27

https://www.healthaliciousness.com

CHAPTER 13

Fatigue- Patient Version, National Cancer Institute.

http://www.cancer.gov/about-cancer/treatment/side-effects/fatigue/fatigue-pdq

Cramp F, Byron-Daniel J. Exercise for the management of cancer-related fatigue in adults.

Cochrane Database Syst. Rev, 2012 Nov 14:11

http://onlinelibrary.wiley.com/doi/10.1002/14651858.CD006145.pub3/full

Sheryl M. Ness Cancer Related Fatigue: Create a personal exercise plan.

http://www.mayoclinic.org/diseases-conditions/cancer/expert-blog/exercise-for-cancer-related-fatigue/bgp-20090995

Fatigue, National Comprehensive Cancer Network

https://www.nccn.org/patients/resources/life_with_cancer/managing_symptoms/fatigue.aspx

Yeo TP, Cannady S. Cancer-related fatigue: impact on patient quality of life and management approaches.

https://www.dovepress.com/cancer-related-fatigue-impact-on-patient-quality-of-life-and-managemen-peer-reviewed-fulltext-article-NRR

Mokkinhoff.E.M et al, Physical activity and breast cancer: a systematic review. Epidemiology 2007, 18 (1): p 137-57

http://www.ncbi.nlm.nih.gov/pubmed/17130685

Bower JE et al, Yoga for persistent fatigue in breast cancer survivors: A randomised control trial. Cancer 2012 Aug 1;118(15):3766-75

http://www.ncbi.nlm.nih.gov/pubmed/22180393/

Molassiotis A et al, Acupuncture for cancer-related fatigue in patients with breast cancer: a pragmatic randomized controlled trial. J Clin Oncol 2012 Dec 20;30(36):4470-6

http://www.ncbi.nlm.nih.gov/pubmed/23109700

CHAPTER 14

David A. Padgett and Ronald Glaser. How stress influences the immune response. Trends in Immunology Aug 2003: vol 24 (8)444-448.

http://www.direct-ms.org/sites/default/files/Stress%20and%20immunity.pdf

Surteees PG et al, No evidence that social stress is associated with breast cancer incidence.

Breast Cancer Res Treat. 2010 Feb; 120(1):169-74

http://www.ncbi.nlm.nih.gov/pubmed/19572196

Imai K et al, Natural cytotoxic activity of peripheral-blood lymphocytes and cancer incidence: an 11-year follow-up study of a general population. Lancet 2000 Nov 25; 356(9244):1795-9.

http://www.ncbi.nlm.nih.gov/pubmed/11117911

Basse PH et al, Cancer immunotherapy with Interleukin-2-activated natural killer cells. Mol Biotechnol 2002 jun; 21(2):161-70.

http://www.ncbi.nlm.nih.gov/pubmed/12059115

Heberman RB, Cancer Immunotherapy with natural killer cells. Semin Oncol 2002 Jun;29(3 Suppl 7):27-30.

http://www.ncbi.nlm.nih.gov/pubmed/12068385

CHAPTER 15

Mary Jane Massie, Prevalence of Depression in Patients With Cancer. J Natl Cancer Inst Monogr (2004)2004 (32): 57-71.

http://jncimono.oxfordjournals.org/content/2004/32/57.full

Shadiya Mohamed Saleh Baqutayan, The Effect of Anxiety on Breast Cancer Patients. Indian J Psychol Med. 2012 Apr-Jun; 34(2): 119–123.

http://www.ncbi.nlm.nih.gov/pmc/articles/PMC3498772/

Thomas A. Richards, Ph.D., Psychologist, What is the Difference between Panic Disorder and Social Anxiety Disorder?

http://anxietynetwork.com/content/differences-between-panic-and-social-anxiety

Anxiety and Panic Disorders Health Centre

http://www.webmd.com/anxiety-panic/default.htm

Judith Potts, Under stress, our own bodies turn against us. Telegraph,Health and Lifestyle , June 20th 2014.

Jennifer McDowall. Oestrogen Receptors, InterPro Protein Archive

https://www.ebi.ac.uk/interpro/potm/2003_4/Page_1.htm

Steindorf K et al, Physical activity and breast cancer risk: the European Prospective Investigation into Cancer and Nutrition. Int J of Cancer 2013 Apr 1;132(7):1667-78

http://www.ncbi.nlm.nih.gov/pubmed/22903273

A Fournier et al, Recent Recreational Physical Activity and Breast Cancer Risk in Postmenopausal Women in the E3N Cohort.

http://cebp.aacrjournals.org/content/early/2014/07/31/1055-9965.EPI-14-0150.full.pdf

https://www.sciencedaily.com/releases/2014/08/140811124814.htm

Michelle D Holmes et al, Physical activity and survival after breast cancer diagnosis. JAMA May 2005, Vol 293, no. 20

http://jama.jamanetwork.com/article.aspx?articleid=200955

Yoga for Health, National Centre for Complementary and Alternative Medicine, Accessed June 2016

https://nccih.nih.gov/health/yoga

Kiecolt-Glaser J et al, Yoga's impact on inflammation, mood, and fatigue in breast cancer survivors: a randomized controlled trial. J Clin Oncol. 2014 Apr 1;32(10):1040-9

http://www.ncbi.nlm.nih.gov/pubmed/24470004

Buffart LM et al, Physical and psychosocial benefits of yoga in cancer patients and survivors, a systematic review and meta-analysis of randomized controlled trials. BMC Cancer 2012 Nov 27: 12:559

http://bmccancer.biomedcentral.com/articles/10.1186/1471-2407-12-559

Support Groups;ASCO's patient information website,Cancer.Net (www.cancer.net) -- brings the expertise and resources of American Society of Clinical Oncology (ASCO) to people living with cancer and those who care for and care about them.

http://www.cancer.net/coping-with-cancer/finding-support-and-information/support-groups

Rosyln Guy, A Qusetion of Proof,The Age Newspaper, Australia March 29 2004.

http://www.theage.com.au/news/science/a-question-of-proof/2004/03/28/1080412236273.html

CHAPTER 16

Madeleine Bunting, Why we will come to see mindfulness as mandatory. Guardian Tues 6th May 2014

http://www.theguardian.com/commentisfree/2014/may/06/mindfulness-hospitals-schools

Carlson LE et al, Randomised control trial of Mindfulness-based recovery versus supportive expressive group therapy for distressed survivors of breast cancer. J Clin Oncol. September 1, 2013 vol. 31no. 25 3119-3126

http://jco.ascopubs.org/content/31/25/3119.long

Wurtzen H et al, Mindfulness significantly reduces self-reported levels of anxiety and depression: results of a randomised control trial among 336 Danish women treated for stage 1-111 breast cancer. Eur J Cancer 2013 Apr;49(6):1365-73.

http://www.ncbi.nlm.nih.gov/pubmed/23265707

Kenne Sarenmalm E et al , Mindfulness based stress reduction study design of a longitudinal randomised controlled complementary intervention in women with breast cancer. BMC Complementary and Alternative Medicine Oct 2nd 2013 13:248

http://bmccomplementalternmed.biomedcentral.com/articles/10.1186/1472-6882-13-248

H. Cramer et al, Mindfulness-based stress reduction for breast cancer-a systematic review and meta-analysis. Curr Oncol. 2012 Oct; 19(5):e343-e352

http://www.ncbi.nlm.nih.gov/pmc/articles/PMC3457885/

Ruby Wax Ted Talk, What's so funny about mental illness

https://www.ted.com/talks/ruby_wax_what_s_so_funny_about_mental_illness?language=en

Useful Websites

www.franticworld.com

www.breathworks-mindfulness.org.uk

www.headspace.com

CHAPTER 17

Sugar and Cancer, Oncology Nutrition; Academy of Nutrition and Dietetics.

https://www.oncologynutrition.org/erfc/healthy-nutrition-now/sugar-and-cancer/

Klement RJ, Kämmerer U, Is there a role for carbohydrate restriction in the treatment and prevention of cancer? Nutr Metab (Lond). 2011; 8: 75.

http://www.ncbi.nlm.nih.gov/pmc/articles/PMC3267662/

Buckland G et al, Adherence to the Mediterranean diet and risk of breast cancer in the European prospective investigation into cancer and nutrition cohort study. Inter. Journal of Cancer; 2013; 132(12): 2918-2927

http://www.ncbi.nlm.nih.gov/pubmed/23180513/

Cottet V et al, Postmenopausal breast cancer risk and dietary patterns in the E3N-EPIC prospective cohort study. Am J Epidemiol. 2009 Nov 15;170(10):1257-67

https://www.researchgate.net/publication/38010988_Postmenopausal_Breast_Cancer_Risk_and_Dietary_Patterns_in_the_E3N-EPIC_Prospective_Cohort_Study

Glcemic Index and Glycemic load for a 100+ foods

http://www.health.harvard.edu/diseases-and-conditions/glycemic_index_and_glycemic_load_for_100_foods

Romieu et al, Dietary glycemic index and glycemic load and breast cancer risk in the European Prospective Investigation into Cancer and Nutrition (EPIC). Am J Clinical Nutrition 2012; 96(2): 345-355.

http://www.ncbi.nlm.nih.gov/pubmed/22760570

Nicole M Avena, Pedro Rada, Bartley G Hoebel. Evidence for sugar addiction: Behavioural and neurochemical effects of intermittent, excessive sugar intake.

http://www.ncbi.nlm.nih.gov/pmc/articles/PMC2235907/

Melanie Greenberg, Why Our Brains Love Sugar - And Why Our Bodies Don't. How sugar affects our brain chemistry making us want more and more. Psychology Today, Feb 5th 2013.

https://www.psychologytoday.com/blog/the-mindful-self-express/201302/why-our-brains-love-sugar-and-why-our-bodies-dont

Useful Websites

http://www.actiononsugar.org/

https://www.gov.uk/government/uploads/system/uploads/attachment_data/file/470179/Sugar_reduction_The_evidence_for_action.pdf

https://news.liverpool.ac.uk/2014/01/09/sugar-is-the-new-tobacco-says-expert/

World Cancer Research Fund

http://www.wcrf.org/

http://www.wcrf.org/sites/default/files/Curbing-Global-Sugar-Consumption.pdf

CHAPTER 18

Aseem Malhotra,Saturated fat is not the major issue. BMJ 2013;347:f6340

http://www.bmj.com/content/347/bmj.f6340?sso=

The Mayo Clinic: Dietary Fats which type to choose.

http://www.mayoclinic.org/healthy-lifestyle/nutrition-and-healthy-eating/in-depth/fat/art-20045550?pg=1

Sieri s et al, Dietary fat and breast cancer risk in the European Prospective Investigation into Cancer and Nutrition. AM J of Clinical Nutrition 2008; 88(5): 1304-1312

http://www.ncbi.nlm.nih.gov/pubmed/18996867

S Rinaldi et al, IGF-I, IGFBP-3 and breast cancer risk in women: The European Prospective Investigation into Cancer and Nutrition (EPIC). Endocrine-Related Cancer; 2006; 13(2): 593-605

http://erc.endocrinology-journals.org/content/13/2/593.full

NF Boyd et al, Dietary fat and breast cancer risk revisited: a meta-analysis of the published literature. Br J Cancer. 2003 Nov 3; 89(9): 1672–1685.

http://www.ncbi.nlm.nih.gov/pmc/articles/PMC2394401/

EF Taylor et al, Meat Consumption and risk of breast cancer in the Uk Women's Cohort Study. Br J Of Cancer April 10. 2007; 96(7):1139-1146.

http://www.ncbi.nlm.nih.gov/pmc/articles/PMC2360120/

Binukumar and Mathew; licensee BioMed Central Ltd. Dietary fat and risk of breast cancer. 2005World Journal of Surgical Oncology 20053:45.

http://wjso.biomedcentral.com/articles/10.1186/1477-7819-3-45

RJ de Souza et al, Intake of saturated and trans unsaturated fatty acids and risk of all cause mortality, cardiovascular disease, and type 2 diabetes: systematic review and meta-analysis of observational studies. BMJ 2015;351:h3978

http://www.bmj.com/content/351/bmj.h3978

James N Kiage et al, Intake of trans fat and all-cause mortality in the Reasons for Geographical and Racial Differences in Stroke (REGARDS) cohort. Am J Clin Nutr. 2013 May; 97(5): 1121–1128.

http://www.ncbi.nlm.nih.gov/pmc/articles/PMC3628378/

V Chajés et al, Association between serum trans-monounsaturated fatty acids and breast cancer risk in the E3N-EPIC Study. Am J of Epidemiol June 2008;167(11):1312-1320

http://www.ncbi.nlm.nih.gov/pmc/articles/PMC2679982/

Kohlmeier L et al, Adipose tissue trans-fatty acids and breast cancer in the in the European Community Multicenter Study on Antioxidants, Myocardial Infarction, and Breast Cancer. Cancer Epidemiol Biomarkers Prev.1997 Sep;6(9):705-10.

http://cebp.aacrjournals.org/content/6/9/705.long

Compassion in World Farming, Know Your Labels.

http://www.ciwf.org.uk/your-food/know-your-labels/

CHAPTER 19

Marji McCullough The Bottom Line on Soy and Breast Cancer Risk. American Cancer Society, Expert Opinions. August 2nd 2012.

http://blogs.cancer.org/expertvoices/2012/08/02/the-bottom-line-on-soy-and-breast-cancer-risk/

Soy Foods, Diet and tamoxifen. Oncology Nutrition; Academy of Nutrition and Dietetics.

https://www.oncologynutrition.org/erfc/hot-topics/soy-foods-diet-and-tamoxifen/

Shu XO et al, Soy food intake and breast cancer survival. JAMA. 2009;302(22):2437-43

http://www.ncbi.nlm.nih.gov/pmc/articles/PMC2874068/

Guha N et al, Soy isoflavones and risk of cancer recurrence in a cohort of breast cancer survivors: the Life After Cancer Epidemiology study. Breast Cancer Res Treat. 2009 Nov; 118 (2): 395-405.

http://www.ncbi.nlm.nih.gov/pmc/articles/PMC3470874/

Coral A Lamartiniere, Protection against breast cancer with genestein: a component of soy. Am J Clin Nutr 2000 Jun;71(6 Suppl):1705S-7S

http://ajcn.nutrition.org/content/71/6/1705s.full

Professor Carlo Leifert,M Baranski et al, Higher antioxidant and lower cadmium and lower incidence of pesticide residues in organically grown crops: a systematic literature review and meta-analyses. Br J Nutr 2014 Sep 14; 112(5): 794–811.

http://www.ncbi.nlm.nih.gov/pmc/articles/PMC4141693/

http://www.ncl.ac.uk/press/news/2015/10/organicvsnon-organicfood/

Benbrook CM at al, Organic production enhances milk nutritional qualityby shifting fatty acid composition: a United States-wide, 18-month study. PloS One 2013 Dec 9;8(12):e82429

http://journals.plos.org/plosone/article?id=10.1371/journal.pone.0082429

G Butler et al, Fat composition of organic and conventional retail milk in northeast England, Journal of Dairy Science, Jan 2011, Vol. 94(1): 24-36

http://www.journalofdairyscience.org/article/S0022-0302(10)00670-3/abstract

CHAPTER 20

Khalid Rahman, Studies on free radicals, antioxidants and co-factors. Clin Interv Aging. 2007 Jun; 2(2): 219–236.

http://www.ncbi.nlm.nih.gov/pmc/articles/PMC2684512/

Dr Stephen Sinatras Heart MD institute, Antioxidants and Free radicals. Published 24th Sept 2009

https://heartmdinstitute.com/diet-nutrition/antioxidants-and-free-radicals/

An introduction to Reactive Oxygen Species-Measurement of ROS in cells. BioTek Website, Published 26th Jan 2014

http://www.biotek.com/resources/articles/reactive-oxygen-species.html

LH Kushi etal, Lifestyle Factors and Survival in Women with Breast Cancer. J. Nutr. January 2007 ; 137 (1) 236S-242S

http://jn.nutrition.org/content/137/1/236S.full

Robert Thomas, Elizabeth Butler, Fabio Macchi and Madeine Williams, Phytochemicals in cancer prevention and management? BJMP 2015;8(2):a815

http://bjmp.org/files/2015-8-2/bjmp-2015-8-2-a815.pdf

C Manach et al, Polyphenols: Food sources and bioavailability. Am J of Clin Nutr. May 2004; 79(5): 727-747

http://ajcn.nutrition.org/content/79/5/727.full

Yan Cui et al, Selected antioxidants and risk of hormone redeptor-defined invasive breast cancers among postmenopausal women in the Women's Health Initiative Observational Study. AM J CLin Nutr. 2008 April; 87(4): 1009-1018.

http://www.ncbi.nlm.nih.gov/pmc/articles/PMC2753414/

Cai-Xia Zhang ,Suzanne C Ho et al, Greater vegetable and fruit intake is associated with a lower risk of breast cancer among Chinese women. Int. J. Cancer: 125, 181–188 (2009)

http://onlinelibrary.wiley.com/doi/10.1002/ijc.24358/pdf

Emaus MJ et al. Vegetable and fruit consumption and the risk of hormone receptor-defined breast cancer in the EPIC cohort. Am J Clin Nutr 2016 Jan;103(1):168-77

http://www.ncbi.nlm.nih.gov/pubmed/26607934

Sabina Sieri et al, Dietary Patterns and Risk of Breast Cancer in the ORDET Cohort, Cancer Epidemiol Biomarkers Prev April 2004 13; 567

http://cebp.aacrjournals.org/content/13/4/567.full.pdf+html

Hayes DJ et al The cancer chemopreventive actions of phytochemicals derived from glucosinolates.Eur J Nutr, 2008 May;47 Suppl 2:73-88

http://www.ncbi.nlm.nih.gov/pubmed/18458837

Xiang Wu, Qing-hua Zhou, KE Xu, Are isothiocyanates potential anti-cancer drugs? Acta PharmacologicaSinica 2009, 30:501-512.

http://www.ncbi.nlm.nih.gov/pmc/articles/PMC4002831/

H. Fritz et al, Soy, Red Clover and Isoflavones and Breast Cancer: A systematic review. PloS One. 2013; 8(11):e81968

http://www.ncbi.nlm.nih.gov/pmc/articles/PMC3842968/

Patisaul HB, Jefferson W. The pros and cons of phytooestrogens, Front Neuroendocrinology 2010: 31(4):400-419

http://www.ncbi.nlm.nih.gov/pmc/articles/PMC3074428/

CHAPTER 21

Min-Jing L et al, Green tea compounds in breast cancer prevention and treatment. World J Clin Oncol. 2014 Aug 10; 5(3): 520–528

http://www.ncbi.nlm.nih.gov/pmc/articles/PMC4127621/

Qi Dai et al , Is Green Tea Drinking Associated With a Later Onset of Breast Cancer?Ann Epidemiol 2010 Jan; 20(11): 74-81

http://www.ncbi.nlm.nih.gov/pmc/articles/PMC2848451/

Bansall SS, Gupta, RC, Curcumin Implants, not Curcumin Diet Inhibits Estrogen-Induced Mammary Carcinogenesis in ACI Rats, Cancer Prev Research.2014 April;7(4):456-465.

http://www.ncbi.nlm.nih.gov/pmc/articles/PMC3992985/

Nechuta S, Caan BJ, Chen WY, et al. Post-diagnosis Cruciferous Vegetable Consumption and Breast Cancer Outcomes: a Report from the After Breast Cancer Pooling Project. Cancer epidemiology, biomarkers & prevention: a publication of the American Association for Cancer Research, cosponsored by the American Society of Preventive Oncology. 2013;22(8):1451-1456.

http://www.ncbi.nlm.nih.gov/pmc/articles/PMC3732536/

Jane V. Higdon et al, Cruciferous Vegetables and Human Cancer Risk: Epidemiologic Evidence and Mechanistic Basis. Pharmacol Res. 2007 Mar

http://www.ncbi.nlm.nih.gov/pmc/articles/PMC2737735/

Sarah J. Nechuta, Cruciferous vegetable consumption linked to improved breast cancer survival rates.

American Association for Cancer research, published April 2012.

http://www.eurekalert.org/pub_releases/2012-04/aafc-cvc032812.php

Eliassen AH et al, Plasma Carotenoids and risk of breast cancer over 20 year of follow up, Am J of Nutr 2015 Jun;101(6):1197-205

http://www.ncbi.nlm.nih.gov/pmc/articles/PMC4441811/

Eliassen AH et al. Circulating caretenoids and risk of breast cancer: Pooled analysis of eight prospective studies. J Natl Cancer Inst 2012; 104(24):1905-1916.

http://jnci.oxfordjournals.org/content/104/24/1905.long

HM Zhang, L Zhao et al, Research progress on the anticarcinogenic actions and mechanisms of ellagic acid. Cancer Biol Med. 2014 Jun; 1192):92-100

http://www.cancerbiomed.org/index.php/cocr/article/view/641/679

J Li et al, Dietary Mushroom Intake may reduce the risk of breast cancer: Evidence from a meta-analysis of observational studies. PloS OneApril 2014, 1;9(4):e93437

http://journals.plos.org/plosone/article?id=10.1371/journal.pone.0093437

Hong SA et al, A case control study on the dietary intake of mushrooms and breast cancer risk in Korean women. Int J Cancer Feb 2008; 122(4):919-23

http://onlinelibrary.wiley.com/doi/10.1002/ijc.23134/full

Shin A et al, Dietary mushroom intake and the risk of breast cancer based on hormone receptor status. Nutr Cancer 201; 62(4):476-83.

http://www.ncbi.nlm.nih.gov/pubmed/20432168

Mushrooms and Health CSIRO Report 2014

http://www.mushroomsandhealth.com/files/Files/FINAL%20Mushrooms%20and%20Health%20Report%202014%2003062014%20(1).pdf

MS Touilland et al, Dietary lignan intake and postmenopausal breast cancer risk by estrogen and progesterone receptor status, J Natl Cancer Inst 2007 Mar, 99(6):475-486

http://www.ncbi.nlm.nih.gov/pmc/articles/PMC2292813/

Breast Health and Lignans

www.lignans.net/breast-cancer-prevention.html

Top high lignan foods that lower breast cancer

http://www.integrativecanceranswers.com/top-high-lignan-foods-that-lower-breast-cancer-risk/

Meta-analyses of lignans and enterolignans in relation to breast cancer risk. Am J Cl Nutr.uly 2010.92(1): 141-153

http://ajcn.nutrition.org/content/92/1/141.long

Useful Books

Mindfulness: A Practical Guide to Finding Peace in a Frantic World ,Professor Mark Williams and Dr Danny Penman. (Published 2011)

Mindfulness Based Cognitive Therapy for Cancer: Gently Turning Towards by Trish Bartley. (published 2012)

Sane New World:Taming the Mind by Ruby Wax ,published 2014).

Sleep Better Naturally, Lisa Helmenis, Published 2006.

Anticancer: A New Way of Life, David Servan-Schreiber, published 2007.

Foods to Fight Cancer, Professor Richard Béliveau and Dr Denis Gingras, published 2007.

Eat for Health, Joel Fuhrman, published 2008.

Eat to Boost Your Immunity, Kirsten Hartvig, published 2002.

The Juicemaster: Turbo charge your life in 14 days, Jason Vale, published 2005.

Farmageddon, Philip Lymbery and Isabel Oakeshott, published 2014

Not on the Label: What Really Goes Into the Food on Your Plate, Felicity Lawrence, published 2004.

The China Study: Startling Implications for Diet, Weight loss and Long-Term Health, T.Colin Campbell and Thomas M Campbell, published 2006.